D1518710

Respiratory Medicine

Series Editor:
Sharon I.S. Rounds

For further volumes:
http://www.springer.com/series/7665

Atul C. Mehta • Prasoon Jain
Editors

Interventional Bronchoscopy

A Clinical Guide

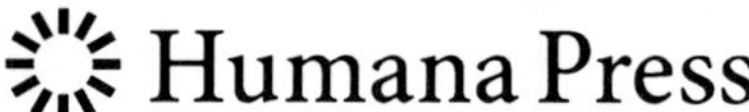

Editors
Atul C. Mehta, MBBS, FACP, FCCP
Respiratory Institute
Lerner College of Medicine
Cleveland Clinic, Cleveland, OH, USA

Prasoon Jain, MBBS, MD, FCCP
Pulmonary and Critical Care
Louis A Johnson VA Medical Center
Clarksburg, WV, USA

ISBN 978-1-62703-394-7 ISBN 978-1-62703-395-4 (eBook)
DOI 10.1007/978-1-62703-395-4
Springer New York Heidelberg Dordrecht London

Library of Congress Control Number: 2013934706

Printed on acid-free paper

Humana Press is a brand of Springer
Springer is part of Springer Science+Business Media (www.springer.com)

"..to today's students and tomorrows bronchoscopists."

Atul C. Mehta

"..to my mother and father."

Prasoon Jain

Preface

A revolution is taking place in the field of bronchoscopy. The strides made over the past decade in this field have exponentially improved the diagnostic as well as therapeutic capability of flexible bronchoscopy. It is now possible to see beyond the bronchial wall using endobronchial ultrasound and navigate to small peripheral lesions using virtual bronchoscopy and electromagnetic navigational bronchoscopy. The therapeutic role of bronchoscope is no longer limited to palliate symptoms of advanced lung cancer. There are exciting developments in the potential role of bronchoscopy in the treatment of bronchial asthma, chronic obstructive pulmonary disease (COPD), and bronchopleural fistula.

The advances in bronchoscopic techniques and refinement of knowledge in this field could not have come at a better time. We are in the midst of a worldwide lung cancer epidemic. With lung cancer screening we are expected to encounter increasing numbers of patients with lung nodules that are too small to reach with conventional bronchoscopic methods. Bronchial asthma and COPD continue to threaten the well-being of a significant proportion of the population around the globe. It is our belief that advanced bronchoscopy techniques have an important current and future role in diagnosis and management of many these patients.

In this book, we invited some of the world's leading experts to critically review the important diagnostic and therapeutic bronchoscopic techniques that have emerged over the past decade. The book is written for pulmonologists, pulmonary fellows in training, and for all those who perform diagnostic and therapeutic bronchoscopy. We provide a balanced view of the current status, limitation, and the future of the new bronchoscopic techniques that have been adopted in mainstream practice over the past few years.

Rapid growth in any medical field raises many pertinent questions. Bronchoscopy is no exception. One must ask whether the new techniques are more effective in providing diagnosis or in improving outcome than the existing techniques. The safety issues as well as limitations of the new procedure must be understood. As most of the new bronchoscopic techniques are expensive, the cost issues must be addressed. Presently, the economic implication of adopting any expensive technique cannot be overlooked. Society and third-party payers alike are increasingly demanding economic justification for choosing a more expensive technique over an existing less expensive technique. In the global arena, many of the emerging techniques are simply out of reach of resource-poor societies. Throughout the book the authors have addressed some of these issues to guide the reader to make informed and judicious decisions in adopting new techniques and make sound decisions regarding allocation of health care resources.

We strongly and unapologetically feel that the emergence of new techniques in bronchoscopy does not imply that existing and conventional bronchoscopic techniques such as transbronchial lung biopsy and conventional transbronchial needle aspiration have become obsolete and should be abandoned. In fact, the emergence of new techniques provides a unique opportunity to refine and redefine the clinical role of the existing techniques. We firmly believe that the intelligent and effective use of time-tested conventional bronchoscopic methods still has and will continue to have an important role in routine bronchoscopy practice. It is essential for every bronchoscopist to have a sound understanding of the fundamental principles of the conventional procedures before embarking upon more advanced techniques. Due to this reason, considerable sections have been devoted to the conventional bronchoscopic techniques in this book.

We sincerely thank all the contributing authors who share their expertise in this book. With their assistance, we have done our best to provide a balanced and state-of-the art review of this rapidly expanding field. We hope the readers will find the information thought provoking, practical, and readily applicable in their clinical practice. We are excited about the advances in the field of bronchoscopy, but we truly believe that it is only the beginning. The best is yet to come.

Cleveland, OH, USA — Atul C. Mehta
Clarksburg, WV, USA — Prasoon Jain

Contents

Contributors

Fumihiro Asano, M.D., F.C.C.P. Department of Pulmonary Medicine, Gifu Prefectural General Medical Center, Gifu, Japan

John F. Beamis Jr., M.D. Department of Pulmonology, Hawaii Permanente Medical Center, Honolulu, HI, USA

Prashant N. Chhajed, M.D., D.N.B., D.E.T.R.D., F.C.C.P. Lung Care and Sleep Centre, Fortis Hiranandani Hospital, Navi Mumbai, Maharashtra, India

Cliff K. C. Choong, M.B.B.S., F.R.C.S., F.R.A.C.S. Department of Surgery (MMC), The Valley Hospital, Monash University, Melbourne, VIC, Australia

Joseph Cicenia, M.D. Respiratory Institute - Department of Advanced Diagnostic Bronchoscopy, Cleveland Clinic, Cleveland, OH, USA

Yaser Abu El-Sameed, M.B.B.S. Respirology Division, Medicine Institute, Sheikh Khalifa Medical City, Abu Dhabi, UAE

Erik Folch, M.D., M.Sc. Division of Thoracic Surgery and Interventional Pulmonology, Beth Israel Deaconess Medical Center, Harvard Medical School, Boston, MA, USA

Thomas R. Gildea, M.D., M.S. Bronchoscopy, Cleveland Clinic, Respiratory Institute, Cleveland, OH, USA

Sarah Hadique, M.D. Pulmonary and Critical Care Medicine, West Virginia University, Morgantown, WV, USA

Edward F. Haponik, M.D. Pulmonary and Critical Care Medicine, Wake-Forest School of Medicine, Winston-Salem, NC, USA

Cheng He, M.B.B.S., B.Med.Sc., P.G.Dip.Surg.Anat. Department of Surgery (MMC), Monash Medical Center, Monash University, Clayton, VIC, Australia

Prasoon Jain, M.B.B.S., M.D., F.C.C.P. Pulmonary and Critical Care, Louis A Johnson VA Medical Center, Clarksburg, WV, USA

Arvind H. Kate, M.D., F.C.C.P. Lung care and sleep centre, Fortis Hiranandani Hospital, Navi Mumbai, Maharashtra, India

Sumita B. Khatri, M.D., M.S. Asthma Center, Cleveland Clinic, Respiratory Institute, Cleveland, OH, USA

Noriaki Kurimoto, M.D., F.C.C.P. Department of Chest Surgery, St. Marianna University, Kawasaki, Kanagawa, Japan

Pyng Lee, M.D. Yong Loo Lin School of Medicine, National University of Singapore, Singapore

Division of Respiratory and Critical Care Medicine, National University Hospital, Singapore, Singapore

A. Lukas Loschner, M.D. Section of Pulmonary, Critical Care, Environmental and Sleep Medicine, Carilion Clinic, Virginia Tech Carilion School of Medicine, Roanoke, VA, USA

Adnan Majid, M.D., F.C.C.P. Division of Thoracic Surgery and Interventional Pulmonology, Beth Israel Deaconess Medical Center, Harvard Medical School, Boston, MA, USA

Praveen M. Mathur, M.B.B.S. Pulmonary/CCM Department, Indiana University Hospital, Indianapolis, IN, USA

Atul C. Mehta, M.B.B.S. Respiratory Institute, Lerner College of Medicine, Cleveland Clinic, Cleveland, OH, USA

Sonali Sethi, M.D. Respiratory Institute - Department of Interventional Pulmonary, Cleveland Clinic, Cleveland, OH, USA

Santhakumar Subramanian, M.D., F.C.C.P., I.D.C.C. KG Hospital, Arts College Road, Coimbatore, Tamilnadu, India

Part I

Introduction

Interventional Pulmonology: Current Status and Future Direction

1

John F. Beamis Jr. and Praveen M. Mathur

Abstract

This chapter outlines the development of interventional pulmonology over the last three decades beginning with the introduction of the Nd:YAG laser for use in therapeutic bronchoscopy. Mention will be made of early pioneers who set the stage for modern interventional pulmonology. The chapter reviews the current scope of practice of interventional pulmonology with emphasis on newer bronchoscopy techniques for diagnosis and staging of thoracic malignancy. The current status of training in interventional pulmonology will be discussed along with issues regarding credentialing and the need for a formal 1-year interventional pulmonology fellowship.

Keywords

Interventional pulmonology • Flexible bronchoscopy • Rigid bronchoscopy • Pleuroscopy (medical thoracoscopy) • Endobronchial ultrasound • Autofluorescence bronchoscopy • Lung cancer • Navigational bronchoscopy • Electrocautery • Cryotherapy • Stents (airway)

Introduction

Interventional pulmonology (IP) has evolved over the last three decades into a multifaceted subspecialty of thoracic medicine and surgery that involves diagnostic and therapeutic bronchoscopy, pleuroscopy, and several other procedures outlined in Table 1.1. Advances in technology and the epidemic of lung cancer in the later half of the last century were major stimuli in the development of IP. In addition, emergence of lung transplantation as a therapeutic option in advanced and end-stage lung diseases over the past two decades also became an engine to stimulate the research and development in the field of IP. Lung transplant recipients need to undergo multiple bronchoscopies for diagnosis and surveillance for rejection and management of airway complications. It can be argued that the success of lung transplantation would not

J.F. Beamis Jr., M.D. (✉)
Department of Pulmonology, Hawaii Permanente Medical Center, 3288 Moanalua Rd., Honolulu, HI 96819, USA
e-mail: jbeamisc@gmail.com

P.M. Mathur, M.B.B.S.
Pulmonary/CCM Department, Inidana University Hospital, Indianapolis, IN, USA

A.C. Mehta and P. Jain (eds.), *Interventional Bronchoscopy: A Clinical Guide*, Respiratory Medicine 10, DOI 10.1007/978-1-62703-395-4_1, © Springer Science+Business Media New York 2013

Table 1.1 The scope of interventional pulmonology components

Advanced diagnostic bronchoscopy
Autofluorescence bronchoscopy[a]; narrow-band imaging[a]; radial EBUS[a]; linear EBUS-TBNA[a], OCT[b]; navigational bronchoscopy[a]
Therapeutic bronchoscopy
Rigid bronchoscopy[a]; laser[a]; electrocautery[a]; argon plasma coagulation[a]; cryotherapy[a]; brachytherapy[a]; photodynamic therapy[a]; balloon bronchoplasty[a]; stents[a]—silicone, SEMS (covered, uncovered); foreign body removal[a]; bronchial thermoplasty[a]; bronchoscopic lung volume reduction methods[b]; airway valves for bronchopleural fistula[a]; whole lung lavage[a]
Pleural procedures
Pleuroscopy[a]; indwelling pleural catheter[a]
Critical care procedures
Percutaneous dilatational tracheotomy[a]

EBUS endobronchial ultrasound, *TBNA* transbronchial needle aspiration, *OCT* optical coherence tomography
[a]Clinically available
[b]Investigational only

have been possible without the aid of expert bronchoscopy services.

IP is more than performance of procedures. It often involves total care of patients with advanced malignancies, critical central airway obstruction, and respiratory compromise from pleural effusions. IP requires more training and experience than is available in most pulmonary fellowships or thoracic surgery residencies. While the number of IP practitioners has increased both in the USA and many other countries their distribution remains spotty. Many patients in need remain without access to the benefits of IP.

In this chapter we review the current status of IP practice and training as the specialty has developed over the last three decades along with historical perspective and comment on the future of the specialty.

Definition of Interventional Pulmonology

IP was first defined in a monograph in 1995 [1] and again in the European Respiratory Society/American Thoracic Society guidelines [2]. Interventional pulmonology can be defined as "the art and science of medicine as related to the performance of diagnostic and invasive therapeutic procedures that require additional training and expertise beyond that required in a standard pulmonary medicine training program." Although this definition is over 20 years old it remains cogent despite the fact that the number of IP procedures has surged. In addition to therapeutic procedures for malignancies there has been more emphasis on diagnosis and increasing interest in treating benign disorders such as asthma and emphysema using IP techniques.

The Development of Interventional Pulmonology

The Pioneers

Dr. Gustave Killian, a German otolaryngologist, was the first to provide translaryngeal access to the tracheobronchial tree when in 1897 he performed the first rigid bronchoscopy to remove a bone from the main bronchus of a patient. Killian's procedure gained worldwide attention. Among his disciples was Chevalier Jackson, a Pittsburgh otolaryngologist who was to be known as the "Father of American Bronchoesophagology" [3–5]. Jackson moved to Philadelphia where he eventually became Professor of Otolaryngology at all five of the local medical schools. Jackson designed rigid bronchoscopes and accessories that have been the standard for over 100 years. His techniques of foreign body removal and dilation of airway strictures have also stood the test of time. Possibly his greatest contributions were his development of strict safety standards and the instructional courses he organized which are a model for modern-day IP courses.

A major factor in the growth of pulmonary medicine as a subspecialty was the invention of the flexible fiber-optic bronchoscope by Dr. Shigeto Ikeda, a thoracic surgeon at Tokyo's National Cancer Institute [6]. Originally designed as a diagnostic tool, the flexible bronchoscope has proven to be invaluable in therapeutic bronchoscopy [7].

In the last century a number of technologies were developed that had potential for treatment of airway disorders via bronchoscopy. In the 1920s Yankauer reported on the implantation of radium into an endobronchial tumor using a bronchoscope. The radium was placed in capsules attached to a string that exited through the mouth. Although effective, this technique exposed the treatment team to radiation [8]. Neel and Sanderson from Mayo Clinic used cryotherapy through rigid bronchoscopes or bronchotomy to treat airway tumors [9, 10]. Hooper and Jackson described early experience with endobronchial electrocautery [11, 12]. Laforet et al. [13] described the use of the carbon dioxide laser to treat an obstructing mucoepidermoid tumor of the trachea. All of these methods of treating endobronchial pathology showed promise in expert hands but were never widely embraced.

Just as therapeutic bronchoscopy has over 100 years of history, medical thoracoscopy, an important procedure within IP, has also been performed for over 100 years. Hans-Christian Jacobeus, a Swedish pulmonologist, is said to have performed the first thoracoscopy in 1910. His technique became widely accepted as a method to lyse pleural adhesions in the pre-antibiotic era of tuberculosis therapy [14, 15]. There is now evidence that an Irish physician might have preceded Jacobeus in exploring the pleural space by 50 years [16]. Once systemic therapy for tuberculosis was introduced thoracoscopy procedures waned dramatically. However, aided by improved video technology and stimulated by the interest in minimally invasive surgery, a number of groups expanded the indications for thoracoscopy to other conditions such as treatment of empyema and malignant pleural effusions and diagnosis of pleural diseases [17, 18].

Interventional Pulmonology Through the Decades

1980s

Many would date the dawn of IP to two reports from France in the early 1980s describing the utility of the neodymium:yttrium–aluminum–garnet laser (Nd:YAG) laser for treating airway obstruction from lung cancer. Toty and associates performed laser therapy on 164 patients with benign and malignant airway stenosis. Excellent results in treating central airway tumors (benign and malignant) and iatrogenic stenosis using the laser through a rigid bronchoscope were reported. The authors felt that the main indication for laser therapy was "... in the treatment of asphyxiating and intractable forms of cancers, previously operated on and irradiated" [19]. Dumon et al. [20] from Marseilles described their experience treating 111 patients with a variety of benign and malignant airway disorders. The results were excellent and authors stated "serious complications have yet to occur." Because of Dumon's clinical skills, and his willingness to share his experience with others through speaking engagements, hands-on courses, and in print, Marseilles quickly became the main attraction for those interested in therapeutic bronchoscopy. Other European physicians, many disciples of Dumon, quickly developed large series of laser-treated patients [21]. Within a short time laser bronchoscopy crossed the Atlantic to centers in the USA [22–25].

Throughout the 1980s, stimulated by the continuing epidemic of lung cancer and improvements in technology, multiple centers of laser bronchoscopy were established throughout Europe and North America. Safety standards were developed by Dumon [26] and others. Despite the renewed interest in rigid bronchoscopy for debulking airway tumors [27] many US bronchoscopists preferred to use the laser through the flexible bronchoscope [28, 29].

1990s

After 10 years of worldwide experience with laser bronchoscopy it became evident that other endobronchial therapies were needed to fight the epidemic of lung cancer in its attack on the central airway. Coagulating a central tumor with the Nd:YAG laser and resecting it with rigid or flexible bronchoscopy techniques resulted in immediate but often short-term airway patency. Patients with external compression or loss of cartilage support could not be treated with laser. Other methods to maintain or open the central airway obstruction were needed. A renewed interest in endobronchial brachytherapy surfaced. Compared to crude placement of radiation sources in prior decades, newer afterloading techniques using Iridium-192 were developed [30]. Ever the innovator, Dumon developed a silicone stent that was deliverable via the rigid bronchoscope and proved valuable for long-term treatment of benign and malignant stenosis [31, 32]. A number of self-expandable metal stents became available. Wallstents® and Palmaz® stents [33, 34] proved relatively easy to insert using flexible bronchoscopy but were soon replaced by Ultraflex® stents made of nitinol (Boston Scientific, Natick, MA, USA) [35].

Stimulated by the success of laser some older technologies were updated and proved successful in treating endobronchial disease. Electrocautery using probes or snares, often with flexible bronchoscopy, proved to be as effective as laser in experienced hands and more cost effective [36–38]. Homasson and others in Europe used new cryotherapy probes with rigid bronchoscopy to treat airway tumors [39, 40]. Mathur et al. introduced flexible cryoprobes that could be passed through the working channel of a flexible bronchoscope [41]. The argon plasma coagulator proved to be another tool to coagulate and ablate endobronchial tumors [42, 43]. All of these methods offered alternatives to laser therapy in that start-up costs were less, applications through flexible bronchoscopy were available, and in most cases effectiveness was similar, although no true comparison studies were reported.

In the 1990s there was renewed interest among North American pulmonologists in performing medical thoracoscopy (now called pleuroscopy) [44]. Advances in minimally invasive surgical technology along with techniques developed by European masters including Boutin [45] and Loddenkemper [46] facilitated this interest. Although the procedure was commonplace in Europe, the idea of internists performing surgery in the chest generated considerable controversy in the USA [47, 48]. The controversy was eventually resolved as differences between video-assisted thoracic surgery (VATS) and medical thoracoscopy were appreciated and most pulmonologists limited their scope of practice to performing parietal pleural biopsy and talc pleurodesis.

Also in this decade, bronchoscopists, knowing the difficulties of treating airways obstructed with advanced cancers, began to look for early, possibly curable endobronchial cancers. Exciting work by Lam et al. showed that areas of severe dysplasia and cancer in situ could be detected with autofluorescence bronchoscopy using the lung imaging fluorescence endoscope (LIFE) [49, 50]. Dysplastic lesions could be followed and might resolve with smoking cessation; more invasive lesions could be treated with a variety of methods including photodynamic therapy, electrocautery, or brachytherapy.

The introduction of endobronchial ultrasonography in the early 1990s would, by the next decade, prove to be a major advance in IP and bronchology in general. Hürter and Hanrath passed balloon-tipped ultrasound catheters through the working channel of flexible bronchoscopes to image airway walls to detect invasion, to study peripheral lesions, and to guide stent placement [51]. Shannon et al. [52] demonstrated that this method of endobronchial ultrasound (now called radial EBUS) could image mediastinal structures including vessels and lymph nodes and facilitate transbronchial lymph node aspiration (TNBA) described earlier by Wang [53].

2000s

The new century brought rapid advancements in the application of radial EBUS. Herth et al. [54] outlined the advantages of using EBUS in therapeutic bronchoscopy. Miyazu et al. used radial EBUS to assess the depth of airway wall invasion by early lung cancer to determine treatment with local photodynamic therapy versus surgical resection or radiation [55]. Herth's group also showed that EBUS could be used to localize peripheral pulmonary nodules and lesions with results similar to those using fluoroscopy [56]. Kurimoto et al. passed the EBUS probe through a guided sheath to improve sampling of peripheral pulmonary lesions [57]. In a systematic review and meta-analysis of the use of radial EBUS for diagnosing peripheral lesions Steinfort et al. noted an overall specificity of 100 % and a sensitivity of 73 %. These authors concluded that, although the diagnostic yield was less than that using computed tomography-guided percutaneous biopsy, the favorable safety record of EBUS-transbronchial lung biopsy (TBLB) was "... supporting initial investigation of patients with peripheral pulmonary lesions using EBUS-TBLB" [58].

Possibly more important than radial EBUS in the management of thoracic malignancy was the introduction by Olympus Ltd. (Tokyo, Japan) of the linear EBUS bronchoscope which allowed real-time ultrasound guidance for TBNA of mediastinal and hilar lymph nodes. This procedure was originally reported by Krasnik et al. [59] in a small group of patients. Subsequently Yasufuku [60, 61] in Japan and the Heidelberg/Boston collaboration of Herth and Ernst [62–64] have validated linear EBUS-TBNA in large series of lung cancer patients. The linear EBUS-TBNA procedure has changed the way lung cancer is staged and has also been shown to be effective in diagnosing other conditions that present with mediastinal and hilar adenopathy such as lymphoma [65], extra-thoracic malignancy [66], sarcoidosis [67], and tuberculosis [68]. In a meta-analysis by Adams et al. linear EBUS-TBNA was shown to have a specificity of 100 % and an overall sensitivity of 88 % when used to sample mediastinal lymph nodes in patients with known or suspected lung cancer [69]. In another systematic review Varela-Lema et al. noted similar results and suggested that EBUS-TBNA could replace mediastinoscopy for lung cancer staging in many cases [70].

In recent years the clinical presentation of lung cancer has shifted from central lesions to more peripheral lesions. This has stimulated bronchoscopists to develop methods to diagnose peripheral pulmonary nodules and masses that have improved diagnostic yields, improved compared to classic techniques using fluoroscopy and transbronchial biopsies. In addition to radial EBUS new techniques of navigational bronchoscopy and ultrathin bronchoscopy were developed in this decade. Schwarz et al. [71] described the superDimension bronchus system (superDimension, Inc, Mineapolis, MN) which used virtual bronchoscopy and electromagnetic navigation to approach targeted peripheral lesions for sampling. The Cleveland Clinic group used this system to sample peripheral lesions with a mean size of 22.8 mm ± 12.6 mm in 60 patients and noted a yield of 74% [72]. Asano described a virtual bronchoscopy navigation system (VBN System, Olympus Medical Systems, Tokyo, Japan) that gave similar yields [73]. Using an ultrathin bronchoscope guided by the LungPoint navigation system (Bronchus Technologies Inc., Mountain View, CA) Eberhardt et al. had a diagnostic yield of 80 % in 25 patients with peripheral lesions with a mean size of 28 mm [74].

Benign airway tumors and benign tracheal stenosis can be treated with methods similar to those used to treat cancer. A major development in this decade was the attempt to treat emphysema and asthma with interventional bronchoscopy techniques. However, treating asthma and emphysema required novel techniques. Bronchial thermoplasty, which utilizes radiofrequency energy delivered to the subsegmental and segmental airways by a catheter passed through the working channel of a standard flexible bronchoscope resulting in ablation of airway smooth muscle, has been shown in a multicenter, randomized double-blind sham-controlled study to reduce severe exacerbations and healthcare utilization in moderate and severe asthmatics [75, 76]. This technology has now been approved by the Federal Drug Administration (FDA) and is marketed as the Alair Bronchial Thermoplasty System (Boston Scientific, Natick, MA).

Attempts at using bronchoscopy to treat severe emphysema have not been successful. Stimulated by the results of National Emphysema Treatment Trial [77] several bronchoscopic lung volume reduction techniques have been studied including airway occlusion using valves, collapsing segments with biodegradable gels, and creating extra anatomic tracts between the bronchial tree and hyperinflated parenchyma. None of these techniques have demonstrated sufficient efficacy or safety profiles to warrant FDA approval [78].

Training in Interventional Pulmonology

When laser bronchoscopy was introduced in the early 1980s many US bronchoscopists traveled to Europe, particularly to Marseilles, to learn the technique. Dumon and his early disciples soon organized courses to share their experience with the pulmonology community. The first US course was at Lahey Clinic in 1983. Soon multiple courses were available throughout the USA. All these courses offered didactic review of laser principle indications, technique and complications of the procedure, and hands-on experience using inanimate and animal models [79]. Kvale [80] outlined a typical laser bronchoscopy course and expressed concern regarding training and credentialing for this new procedure. Over the last three decades IP courses have expanded their scope dramatically. Courses now cover multiple endobronchial therapies: laser, electrocautery, cryotherapy, stents, and balloon dilation and advanced diagnostic procedures: linear and radial EBUS, and autofluorescence. Simulation is often utilized. Some courses also cover pleuroscopy and percutaneous tracheotomy. But does a 2–5-day course provide enough experience for a pulmonologist to return home and perform a new procedure on a patient?

In questionnaire surveys of program directors of the US pulmonary/critical care medicine fellowships and affiliate members of the American College of Chest Physicians (ACCP) Pastis et al. [81, 82] reported that the US pulmonary fellows were generally pleased with their training experience in routine flexible bronchoscopy but did not have enough experience in "interventional" procedures to meet competency standards proposed in the ACCP guidelines [83]. Unlike their European colleagues who often have exposure to rigid bronchoscopy and pleuroscopy during fellowship, most American pulmonary and critical care medicine fellows will require further training to gain competence in IP procedures. This has prompted the development of interventional pulmonology fellowships. The first formal US IP fellowship was organized at Lahey Clinic in 1996. Currently there are 19 active IP fellowships in North America (Table 1.2). Gildea [84] has argued that in a high-IP-volume institution such as Cleveland Clinic every fellow has an opportunity for involvement in IP procedures and a specific IP fellowship is not required. In contrast Feller-Kopman [85] has outlined the benefits of a formal 1-year IP fellowship which includes exposure to a greater variety and number of procedures, better research opportunities, networking, and a process similar to training in other interventional specialties such as cardiology and gastroenterology. The authors favor a formal year of IP fellowship.

Table 1.2 Current North American interventional pulmonology fellowships

- Beth Israel Deaconess Medical Center, Boston, MA
- Cancer Treatment Centers of America, Philadelphia, PA
- Centre Hospitalier de l'University of Montreal, Montreal, QB, CA
- Chicago Chest Center, Elk Grove, IL
- Cleveland Clinic Foundation Respiratory Institute, Cleveland, OH
- Duke University Medical Center, Durham, NC
- Emory University School of Medicine, Atlanta, GA
- Henry Ford Hospital, Detroit, MI
- Johns Hopkins Hospital, Baltimore, MD
- Lahey Clinic, Burlington, MA
- McGill University Royal Victoria Hospital, Montreal, QB, CA
- National Jewish Health, Denver, CO
- Ohio State University, Columbus, OH
- University of Calgary, Calgary, AB, CA
- University of Texas MD Anderson Cancer Center, Houston, TX
- University of Arkansas for the Medical Sciences, Little Rock, AK
- University of Pennsylvania Medical Center, Philadelphia, PA
- Virginia Commonwealth University, Richmond, VA
- Washington University School of Medicine, St Louis, MO

[Based on data from Fellowships. American Association for Bronchology and Interventional Pulmonology; 2007. http://aabronchology.org/fellowships.php. Last accessed 18 Sept 2012]

Lamb et al. [86] recently outlined principles and objectives of training in IP. The authors emphasized that, in addition to acquiring procedural skills, IP fellows must develop a broad knowledge base in areas such as thoracic malignancy, complex airway disorders, and pleural diseases along with a working understanding of the various technologies employed in IP and how they interact with benign and malignant tissue. 2011 was a landmark year for IP fellowships as it was the first year that fellows were chosen through the National Resident Matching Program (http://www.nrmp.org/fellow/match_name/msmp/about.html). The goal is for IP fellowships to be eventually accredited by the American Council for Graduate Medical Education. In the more distant future a formal board examination may be developed which might facilitate IP recognition by the American Board of Medical Specialties.

Current Status of Interventional Pulmonology

The following chapters will address the current practice of many IP bronchoscopic procedures in detail. Here, we summarize our impression of the status of IP in the second decade of the twenty-first century. Guidelines from the ERS/ATS [2] and the ACCP [83] were based on expert consensus and are now a decade old but remain valid and continue to reflect much of the current practice.

- Although laser and other endobronchial therapies revitalized rigid bronchoscopy, the use of this versatile instrument, except in Europe, remains limited. Standard pulmonary critical care medicine fellowships and cardiothoracic surgery residencies in the USA offer limited or no exposure to this procedure. The flexible bronchoscope has become the main therapeutic bronchoscopy tool in many institutions. At Lahey Clinic where both rigid and flexible bronchoscopies are performed there has been a shift to more flexible bronchoscopy procedures (Fig. 1.1) [87]. Recent British Thoracic Society Guidelines have reviewed the current practice for therapeutic and advanced diagnostic procedures using the flexible bronchoscope [88].
- There are many options for ablative endobronchial therapy: laser, electrocautery, brachytherapy, cryotherapy, and argon plasma coagulation. Laser remains the most powerful. As original Nd:YAG lasers wear out many groups have shifted to the new neodymium: yttrium–aluminum–perovskite (Nd:YAP) laser which is more portable and less expensive than the Nd:YAG laser and provides similar if not better coagulation of endobronchial tumors [89].
- The Dumon-type silicone stent has stood the test of time for the treatment of external airway compression or loss of cartilage support but still requires rigid bronchoscope insertion. The Ultraflex® stent was the most widely used self-expanding metal stent (SEMS) for a number of years but recently is becoming supplanted by the AERO® stent, a totally covered nitinol SEMS (Merit Medical Systems, Inc., South Jordon, UT). Both can be inserted with the flexible bronchoscope [90].
- Pleuroscopy by internists in the USA remains an uncommon, underutilized procedure despite excellent experience in a relatively few US centers and throughout Europe. With the development of the semirigid thoracoscope [91, 92] that has an appearance similar to that of a common video flexible bronchoscope and has been shown to be just as effective as rigid instruments in managing pleural diseases [93], it is hoped that more pulmonologists will incorporate this safe and highly sensitive and specific procedure into their practice. Janssen has stated, "any pulmonologist who deals with pleural disease nowadays should be able to perform thoracoscopy" [94]. We echo his statement. Despite the potential for local roadblocks, the procedure, as described by Michaud with an accompanying video [95], should be part of any IP program, at least at Level I practice as outlined in the British Thoracic Society Guideline of 2010 [96].
- Autofluorescence bronchoscopy (AFB) is another procedure that has been introduced to clinical practice but remains underutilized.

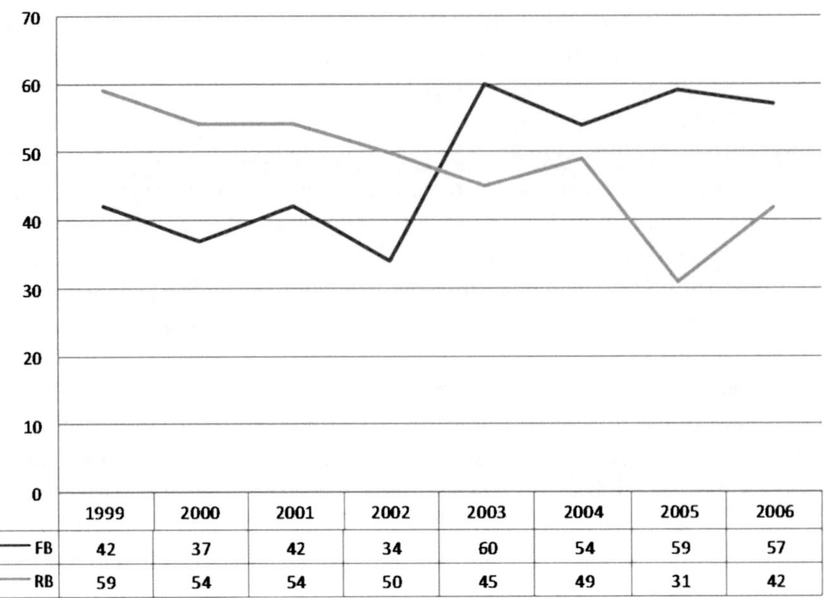

	1999	2000	2001	2002	2003	2004	2005	2006
FB	42	37	42	34	60	54	59	57
RB	59	54	54	50	45	49	31	42

Fig. 1.1 Number of interventional bronchoscopies performed during study period demonstrating a shift toward flexible bronchoscopy. *FB* flexible bronchoscopy, *RB* rigid bronchoscopy [reprinted from Zias N, Chroneou A, Gonzalez AV, Gray AW, Lamb CR, Riker DR, Beamis JF. Changing patterns in interventional bronchoscopy. Respirology 2009;14:595–600. With permission from John Wiley and Sons]

AFB has been shown to be highly sensitive but not particularly specific in detecting preneoplastic airway lesions [97, 98]. Only one system, the D-Light system, has been approved for use in the USA (Karl Storz Endoscopy America, Inc., El Segundo, CA). Other systems are available for use in Europe and Japan. Newer technologies, such as narrow-band imaging and optical coherence tomography, have been developed to improve the specificity of AFB. The recent evidence that CT screening for lung cancer improves mortality [99] may spark the development of formal lung cancer screening programs that probably should incorporate AFB to screen for early airway lesions.

- Linear EBUS is quickly becoming the standard of care for mediastinal staging of patients with lung cancer and for sampling mediastinal lymph nodes. Although this procedure can and should be performed by most bronchoscopists, the IP pulmonologist seems to be taking the lead in incorporating EBUS into day-to-day practice. In addition to its role as a staging instrument linear EBUS-TBNA is being used to obtain more tissue in advanced or recurrent lung cancer cases to guide targeted lung cancer therapy in the new era of personalized cancer therapy [100].
- As the clinical presentation of lung cancer has shifted from central squamous cancers to predominantly peripheral adenocarcinomas there has been an increasing use of IP techniques to diagnose peripheral lesions. Electromagnetic navigation, radial EBUS-TBNA, and ultrathin bronchoscopes are all being used to obtain tissue from peripheral lesions. The preferred technique varies among institutions and often these techniques are used together. They are in competition with transthoracic needle aspiration performed by interventional radiologists.

The Future of Interventional Pulmonology

The future if IP seems very bright. The lung cancer epidemic continues, only slightly abated in developed countries and on the rise in developing countries. For the foreseeable future, patients will continue to present with cancerous central airway lesions that require ablative therapy or stenting. EBUS is here to stay, both for staging and diagnosis, and is rapidly being brought from the academic centers to the community. IP instrumentation is expensive but setting up an IP program at a local hospital or a cancer center can be accomplished as recently outlined by Colt [101]. A major concern is what to do in developing countries where cancer, particularly lung cancer, is being diagnosed more frequently. Volunteerism on the part of IP trained personnel and generosity on the part of industry will have to remain the only means of transporting IP to developing countries for the foreseeable future.

Although it was relatively easy to define IP in 1995, it remains difficult to define who is an interventional pulmonologist. Is it someone who has completed an IP fellowship? Is it someone who has taken a several day course and now feels able to perform EBUS and place an SEMS? Is it a recent pulmonary/CCM graduate who has enthusiastically followed the local IP doctor and now feels comfortable setting up a program in his/her new job? Is it someone in an academic center of excellence or someone in a community hospital? Is it a member of the American Association for Bronchology and Interventional Pulmonology? This is an important question that needs to be defined in the future. Possibly a board exam will help answer the question but that seems many years away and may not be appropriate for those already in practice.

In the future IP practice must become more evidence based. Most of the medical literature in IP (and most of the articles quoted in this chapter) is from single-institution case series. IP research is shifting to randomized, controlled multicenter studies, often with sham controls [75, 102]. This type of research can best serve patients and can only lead to improved stature of IP within the medical world.

We have been fortunate to be involved with the IP community since the beginning and have seen the specialty blossom and new generations of interventional pulmonologists join the ranks. Over the last three decades we have collaborated with and become friends with IP practitioners from many countries. IP is an international specialty. The diseases that IP confronts are global and in the future we must make sure that the care that IP offers is also global.

References

1. Mathur PN, Beamis J. Preface. In: Mathur PN, Beamis J, editors. Interventional pulmonology. Chest Clinics of North America. London: Saunders; 1995. p. ix–xii.
2. Bolliger CT, Mathur PN, Beamis JF, Becker HD, Cavaliere S, Colt H, et al. ERS/ATS statement on interventional pulmonology. European Respiratory Society/American Thoracic Society. Eur Respir J. 2002;19:356–73.
3. Tyson EB. The development of the bronchoscope. J Med Soc N J. 1957;54:26–30.
4. Jackson C. Bronchoscopy: past, present and future. N Engl J Med. 1928;199:759–63.
5. Zolliner F. Gustav Killian: father of bronchoscopy. Arch Otolaryngol. 1965;82:656–9.
6. Ikeda S. Flexible bronchofiberscope. Ann Otol Rhinol Laryngol. 1970;79:916–23.
7. Rand IA, Barber PV, Goldring J, et al. British Thoracic Society guidelines for advanced diagnostic and therapeutic flexible bronchoscopy in adults. Thorax. 2011;66 Suppl 3:iii1–21.
8. Yankauer S. Two cases of lung tumor treated bronchoscopically. N Y Med J. 1922;1922:741–2.
9. Gorenstein A, Neel HB, Sanderson DR. Transbronchoscopic cryosurgery of respiratory strictures. Experimental and clinical studies. Ann Otol Rhinol Laryngol. 1976;85:670–8.
10. Carpenter RJ, Neel HB, Sanderson DR. Cryosurgery of bronchopulmonary structures. An approach to lesions inaccessible to the rigid bronchoscope. Chest. 1977;72:279–84.
11. Hooper RG, Jackson FN. Endobronchial electrocautery. Chest. 1985;87:712–4.
12. Hooper RG, Jackson FN. Endobronchial electrocautery. Chest. 1988;94:595–8.
13. Laforet EG, Berger RL, Vaughan CW. Carcinoma obstructing the trachea: treatment by laser resection. N Engl J Med. 1976;294:941.
14. Jacobaeus HC. U¨ ber die Mo¨glichkeit, die Zystoskopie bei Untersuchung sero¨ser Ho¨hlungen anzuwenden.Mu¨nch med Wschr 1910;57:2090–92.
15. Seijo LM, Sterman DH. Interventional pulmonology. N Engl J Med. 2001;344:740–9.
16. Hoksch B, Birken-Bertsch H, Muller JM. Thoracoscopy before Jacobaeus. Ann Thorac Surg. 2002;74:1288–90.
17. Swierenga J, Wagenaar JPM, Bergstein PGM. The value of thoracoscopy in the diagnosis and treatment

of diseases affecting the pleura and lung. Pneumonologie. 1974;151:11–8.
18. Mathur PN, Boutin C, Loddenkemper R. Medical thoracoscopy: techniques and indications in pulmonary medicine. J Bronchol Intervent Pulmonol. 1994;1:228–38.
19. Toty L, Persone C, Colchen A, Vourc'h G. Bronchoscopic management of tracheal lesions using the neodynium yttrium aluminium garnet laser. Thorax. 1981;36:175–8.
20. Dumon JF, Reboud E, Garbe L, et al. Treatment of tracheobronchial lesions by laser photoresection. Chest. 1982;81:278–84.
21. Cavaliere S, Foccoli P, Farina PL. Nd:YAG laser bronchoscopy: a five year experience with 1,396 applications in 1000 patients. Chest. 1988;94: 15–21.
22. McDougall JC, Cortese DA. Neodynium YAG laser therapy of malignant airway obstruction: a preliminary report. Mayo Clin Proc. 1983;58:35–9.
23. Gelb AF, Epistein JD. Laser treatment of lung cancer. Chest. 1984;86:662–6.
24. Kvale PA, Eichenhorn MS, Radke JA, Mika V. YAG laser photoresection of lesions obstructing the central airways. Chest. 1985;87:283–8.
25. Beamis JF, Vergos KV, Rebeiz EE, Shapshay SM. Endoscopic laser therapy for obstructing tracheobronchial lesions. Annals Otol Rhinol Laryngol. 1991;100:413–9.
26. Dumon JF, Shapshay S, Bourcereau J, et al. Principles for safety in application of neodymium-YAG laser in bronchology. Chest. 1984;86:163–8.
27. Cortese DA. Rigid versus flexible bronchoscopy in laser bronchoscopy: Pro rigid bronchoscopic laser application. J Bronchol. 1994;1:72–5.
28. Joyner LR, Maran AG, Sarama R, Yakaboski A. Neodymium-YAG laser treatment of intrabronchial lesions: a new mapping technique via the flexible fiberoptic bronchoscope. Chest. 1985;87:418427.
29. Unger M. Rigid versus flexible bronchoscopy in laser bronchoscopy: pro flexible bronchoscopic laser application. J Bronchol. 1994;1:69–71.
30. Lo TCM, Girschovich L, Lealey GA, Beamis JF, Webb-Johnson DC, Villanueva AG, et al. Low dose rate vs. high dose rate intraluminal brachytherapy for malignant endobronchial tumors. Radiother Oncol. 1995;35:193–7.
31. Dumon JF. A dedicated tracheobronchial stent. Chest. 1990;97:328–32.
32. Diaz-Jimenez JP, Munoz EF, Ballarin JIM, et al. Silicone stents in the management of obstructive tracheobronchial lesions: 2-year experience. J Bronchol. 1994;1:15–8.
33. Dasgupta A, Dolmatch BL, AbipSaleh WJ, et al. Self-expandable metallic airway stent insertion employing flexible bronchoscopy: preliminary results. Chest. 1998;114:106–9.
34. Susanto I, Peters JI, Levine SM, et al. Use of balloon-expandable metallic stents in the management of bronchial stenosis and bronchomalasia after lung transplantation. Chest. 1998;114:1330–5.
35. Miyazawa T, Yamakido M, Ikeda S, et al. Implantation of ultraflex nitinol stents in malignant tracheobronchial stenosis. Chest. 2000;118:958–65.
36. Gerasin VA, Shafirovsky BB. Endobronchial electrocautery. Chest. 1988;93:270–4.
37. Van Boxem T, Muller M, Venmans B, et al. Nd:YAG laser vs. bronchoscopic electrocautery for palliation of symptomatic airway obstruction: a cost effective study. Chest. 1999;116:1108–12.
38. Coulter, Mehta AC. The heat is on: impact of endobronchial electrosurgery on the need for Nd:YAG laser photoresection. Chest. 2000; 118:516–21.
39. Homasson JF, Renault P, Angebault M, et al. Bronchoscopic cryotherapy for airway strictures caused by tumors. Chest. 1988;90:159–64.
40. Vergnon JM, Schmitt T, Alamartine E, et al. Initial combined cryotherapy and irradiation for unresectable non-small cell lung cancer: preliminary results. Chest. 1992;102:1436–40.
41. Mathur PN, Wolf KM, Busk MF, et al. Fiberoptic bronchoscopic cryotherapy in the management of tracheobronchial obstruction. Chest. 1996;110: 718–23.
42. Crosta C, Spaggiari L, DeStefano A, Fiori G, Ravizza D, Pastorino U. Endoscopic argon plasma coagulation for palliative treatment of malignant airway obstructions: early results in 47 cases. Lung Cancer. 2001;33:75–80.
43. Morice RC, Ece T, Ece F, Keus L. Endobronchial argon plasma coagulation for treatment of hemoptysis and neoplastic airway obstruction. Chest. 2001; 119:781–7.
44. Menzies R, Charbonneau M. Thoracoscopy for the diagnosis of pleural disease. Ann Intern Med. 1991;114:271–6.
45. Boutin C, Viallat JR, Aelony Y. Practical thoracoscopy. Berlin; Heidelberg; New York: Springer; 1991.
46. Brandt HJ, Loddenkemper R, Mai J. Atlas of diagnostic thoracoscopy indications—Technique. New York: Thieme; 1985.
47. Lewis JW. Thoracoscopy: a surgeon's or pulmonologist's domain: pro-pulmonologist. J Bronchol. 1994; 1:152–4.
48. Faber LP. Thoracoscopy: a surgeon's or pulmonologist's domain: pro-surgeon. J Bronchol. 1994;1: 155–9.
49. Palcic B, Lam S, Hung J, MacAulay C. Detection and localization of early lung cancer by imaging techniques. Chest. 1991;99:742–3.
50. Lam S, Kennedy T, Unger M, Miller YE, Gelmont D, Rusch V, et al. Localizarion of bronchial intraepithelial neoplastic lesions by fluorescence bronchoscopy. Chest. 1998;113:696–702.
51. Hürter T, Hanrath P. Endobronchial sonography: feasibility and preliminary results. Thorax. 1992;47: 565–7.

52. Shannon JJ, Bude RO, Orens JB, Becker FS, Whyte RI, Rubin JM, et al. Endobronchial ultrasound-guided needle aspiration of mediastinal adenopathy. Am J Respir Crit Care Med. 1996;153:1424–30.
53. Wang K, Brower R, Haponik E, Siegelman S. Flexible transbronchial needle aspiration for staging of bronchogenic carcinoma. Chest. 1983;84:571–6.
54. Herth F, Becker HD, LoCicero J, Ernst A. Endobronchial ultrasound in therapeutic bronchoscopy. Eur Respir J. 2002;20:118–21.
55. Miyazu Y, Miyazawa T, Kurimoto N, Iwamoto Y, Kanoh K, Hohno N. Endobronchial ultrasounography in the assessment of centrally located early-stage lung cancer before photodynamic therapy. Am J Respir Crit Care Med. 2002;165:832–7.
56. Herth FJF, Ernst A, Becker HD. Endobronchial ultrasound-guided transbronchial lung biopsy in solitary pulmonary nodules and peripheral lesions. Eur Respir J. 2002;20:972–4.
57. Kurimoto N, Miyazawa T, Okimasa S, Maeda A, Oiwa H, Miyazu Y, et al. Endobronchial ultrasonography using a guide sheath increases the ability to diagnose peripheral pulmonary lesions endoscopically. Chest. 2004;126:959–65.
58. Steinfort DP, Khor YN, Manser RL, Irving LB. Radial probe endobronchial ultrasound for the diagnosis of peripheral lung cancer: systematic review and meta-analysis. Eur Respir J. 2011;37:902–10.
59. Krasnik M, Vilmann P, Larsen SS, Jacobsen GK. Preliminary experience with a new method of endoscopic transbronchial real time ultrasound guided biopsy for diagnosis of mediastinal and hilar lesions. Thorax. 2003;58:1083–6.
60. Yasufuku K, Chiyo M, Sekine Y, Chhajed PN, Shibuya K, Iizasa T, et al. Real-time endobronchial ultrasound-guided transbronchial needle aspiration of mediastinal and hilar lymph nodes. Chest. 2004;126:122–8.
61. Yasufuku K, Nakajima T, Chiyo M, Sekine Y, Shibuya K, Fujisawa T. Endobronchial ultrasonography: current status and future directions. J Thorac Oncol. 2007;2:970–9.
62. Herth FJF, Krasnik M, Yasufuku K, Rintoul R, Ernst A. Endobronchial ultrasound-guided transbronchial needle aspiration: how I do it. J Bronchol. 2006;13: 84–91.
63. Ernst A, Anantham D, Eberhardt R, Krasnik M, Herth FJF. Diagnosis of mediastinal adenopathy—real-time endobronchial ultrasound guided needle aspiration versus mediastinoscopy. J Thorac Oncol. 2008;3:577–82.
64. Ernst A, Eberhardt R, Krasnik M, Herth FJF. Efficacy of endobronchial ultrasound-guided transbronchial needle aspiration of hilar lymph nodes for diagnosing and staging cancer. J Thorac Oncol. 2009;4: 947–50.
65. Steinfort DP, Conron M, Tsui A, Pasricha SR, Renwick WEP, Antippa P, et al. Endobronchial ultrasound-guided transbronchial needle aspiration for the evaluation of suspected lymphoma. J Thorac Oncol. 2010;5:804–9.
66. Navani N, Nankivell M, Woolhouse I, Harrison RN, Munavvar M, Oltmanns U, et al. Endobronchial ultrasound-guided transbronchial needle aspiration for the diagnosis of intrathoracic lymphadenopathy in patients with extrathoracic malignancy: a multicenter study. J Thorac Oncol. 2011;6: 1505–9.
67. Tremblay A, Stather DR, MacEachern P, Khalil M, Field SK. A randomized controlled trial of standard vs. endobronchial ultrasonography-guided transbronchial needle aspiration in patients with suspected sarcoidosis. Chest. 2009;136:340–6.
68. Navani N, Molyneaux PL, Breen RA, Connell DW, Jepson A, Nankivell M, et al. Utility of endobronchial ultrasound-guided transbronchial needle aspiration in patients with tuberculous intrathoracic lymphadenopathy. Thorax. 2011;66:889–93.
69. Adams K, Shah PL, Lim E. Test performance of endobronchial ultrasound and transbronchial needle aspiration biopsy for mediastinal staging in patients with lung cancer: systematic review and meta-analysis. Thorax. 2009;64:757–62.
70. Varela-Lema L, Fernandez-Villar A, Ruano-Ravina A. Effectiveness and safety of endobronchial ultrasound-transbronchial needle aspiration: a systematic review. Eur Respir J. 2009;33:1156–64.
71. Schwarz Y, Greif J, Becker HD, Ernst A, Mehta A. Real-time electromagnetic navigation bronchoscopy to peripheral lung lesions using overlaid CT images: the first human study. Chest. 2006;129:988–94.
72. Guildea TR, Mazzone PJ, Karnak D, Meziane M, Mehta AC. Electromagnetic navigation diagnostic bronchoscopy: a prospective study. Am J Respir Crit Care Med. 2006;174:982–9.
73. Asano F. Virtual bronchoscopic navigation. Clin Chest Med. 2010;31:75–85.
74. Eberhardt R, Kahn N, Gompelmann D, Schumann M, Heusel CP, Herth FJF. LungPoint—a new approach to peripheral lesions. J Thorac Oncol. 2010;5:1559–63.
75. Castro M, Rubin AS, Laviolette M, Fiterman J, DeAndrade LM, Shah PL, et al. Effectiveness and safety of bronchial thermoplasty in the treatment of severe asthma: a multicenter, randomized, double-blind, sham-controlled clinical trial. Am J Respir Crit Care Med. 2010;181:116–24.
76. Wahidi MM, Kraft M. Bronchial thermoplasty for severe asthma. Am J Respir Crit Care Med. 2012; 185:709–14.
77. National Emphysema Treatment Trial Research Group. A randomized trial comparing lung-volume-reduction surgery with medical therapy for severe emphysema. N Engl J Med. 2003;348: 2059–73.
78. Berger RL, DeCamp MM, Criner GJ, Celli BR. Lung volume reduction therapies for advanced emphysema: an update. Chest. 2010;138:407–17.

79. Beamis JF, Shapshay SM, Setzer S, Dumon JF. Teaching models for Nd:YAG laser bronchoscopy. Chest. 1989;95:1316–8.
80. Kvale PA. Training in laser bronchoscopy and proposals for credentialing. Chest. 1990;97:983–9.
81. Pastis NJ, Nietert PJ, Silvestri GA. Variation in training for interventional pulmonary procedures among US pulmonary/critical care fellowships: a survey of fellowship diretors. Chest. 2005;127:1614–21.
82. Pastis NJ, Nierert PJ, Silvestri GA. Fellows' perspective of their training in interventional pulmonary procedures. J Bronchol. 2005;12:88–95.
83. Ernst A, Silvestri GA, Johnstone D. Interventional pulmonary procedures: guidelines from the American College of Chest Physicians. Chest. 2003;123: 1693–717.
84. Gildea TR. Is a dedicated 12-month training program required in interventional pulmonology? Con: dedicated training. J Bronchol. 2004;11:65–6.
85. Feller-Kopmn D. Is a dedicated 12-month training program required in interventional pulmonology? Pro: dedicated training. J Bronchol. 2004;11:62–4.
86. Lamb CR, Feller-Kopman D, Ernst A, Simoff MJ, Sterman DH, Wahidi MM, et al. An approach to interventional pulmonary fellowship training. Chest. 2010;137:195–9.
87. Zias N, Chroneou A, Gonzalez AV, Gray AW, Lamb CR, Riker DR, et al. Changing patterns in interventional bronchoscopy. Respirology. 2009;14: 595–600.
88. DuRand IA, Barber PV, Goldring J, Lewis RA, Mandal S, Munavvar M, et al. British Thoracic Society guideline for advanced diagnostic and therapeutic flexible bronchoscopy. Thorax. 2011;66: iii1–21.
89. Lee HJ, Malhotra R, Grossman C, Shepherd RW. Initial report of neodymium:yttrium-aluminum-perovskite (Nd:YAP) laser use during bronchoscopy. J Bronchol Intervent Pulmonol. 2011;18:229–32.
90. Gildea TR, Downie G, Eapen G, Herth F, Jantz M, Freitag L. A prospective multicenter trial of a self-expanding hybrid stent in malignant airway obstruction. J Bronchol. 2008;15:221–4.
91. Ernst A, Hersh CP, Herth FJF, Thurer R, LoCicero J, Beamis J, et al. A novel Instrument for the evaluation of the pleural space: an experience in 34 patients. Chest. 2002;122:1530–4.
92. Mohan A, Chandra S, Agarwal D, Naik S, Munavvar M. Utility of semirigid thoracoscopy in the diagnosis of pleural effusions: a systematic review. J Bronchol Intervent Pulmonol. 2010;17:195–201.
93. Khan MAI, Ambalavanan S, Thomson D, Miles J, Munavvar M. A comparison of the diagnostic yield of rigid and semirigid thoracoscopes. J Bronchol Intervent Pulmonol. 2012;19:98–101.
94. Janssen JP. Why do you or do not need thoracoscopy. Eur Respir Rev. 2010;19(117):213–6.
95. Michaud G, Berkowitz DM, Ernst A. Pleuroscopy for diagnosis and therapy for pleural effusions. Chest. 2010;138:1242–6.
96. Rahman NM, Ali NJ, Brown G, Chapman SJ, Davies RJ, Downer NJ, et al. Local anesthetic thoracoscopy: British Thoracic Society pleural disease guideline 2010. Thorax. 2010;65 Suppl 2:ii54–60.
97. Islam S, Beamis JF. Autofluorescence bronchoscopy. Minerva Pneumol. 2005;44:1–16.
98. Sutedja TG, Venmans BJ, Smit EF, Postmus PE. Fluorescence bronchoscopy for early detection of lung cancer: a clinical perspective. Lung Cancer. 2001;34:157–68.
99. National Lung Cancer Screening Trial Research Team. Reduced lung-cancer mortality with low-dose computed tomographic screening. N Engl J Med. 2011;365:395–409.
100. Bulman W, Saqi A, Powell CA. Acquisition and processing of endobronchial ultrasound-guided transbronchial needle aspiration specimens in the era of targeted lung cancer chemotherapy. Am J Respir Crit Care Med. 2012;185:606–11.
101. Colt HG. Development and organization of an interventional department. Respirology. 2010;15:887–9.
102. Shah PL, Slebos DJ, Cardoso PF, et al. Bronchoscopic lung-volume reduction with exhale airway stents for emphysema (EASE trial): randomised, sham-controlled, multicentre trial. Lancet. 2011;378(9795): 997–1005.

Transbronchial Lung Biopsy

2

Prasoon Jain, Sarah Hadique, and Atul C. Mehta

Abstract

Transbronchial Lung biopsy (TBBx) also known as "Bronchoscopic Lung Biopsy" is one of the most important sampling procedures performed during flexible bronchoscopy. In majority of cases, TBBx is performed under conscious sedation in an outpatient setting. TBBx is performed for obtaining tissue specimen from peripheral lung masses and focal or diffuse lung infiltrates. The technique is useful in patients with suspected lung cancer, fungal and mycobacterial lung infections, unexplained infiltrates in immunocompromised hosts and in patients with suspected pulmonary sarcoidosis, lymphangitic carcinomatosis, and in selected cases of pulmonary Langerhan's cell histiocytosis, lymphangioleiomyomatosis, and cryptogenic organizing pneumonia. TBBx also plays important role in assessment of rejection and infectious complications following lung transplantation.

TBBx is not useful for histological diagnosis of idiopathic pulmonary fibrosis or for distinguishing histological subtypes of idiopathic interstitial pneumonia. The diagnostic yield is also suboptimal in lung nodules smaller than 2 cm in diameter. Several recent techniques such as radial probe endobronchial ultrasound with guide sheath, electromagnetic navigation bronchoscopy, and virtual bronchoscopy navigation have been devised to improve the diagnostic yield of TBBx for solitary lung nodule. Hemoptysis and pneumothorax are the two leading complications of TBBx, occurring in less than 2 % of cases. Every bronchoscopists must be able to perform TBBx.

P. Jain, M.B.B.S., M.D., F.C.C.P. (✉)
Pulmonary and Critical Care, Louis A Johnson
VA Medical Center, Clarksburg, WV 26301, USA
e-mail: prasoonjain.md@gmail.com

S. Hadique, M.D.
Pulmonary and Critical Care Medicine,
West Virginia University, Morgantown, WV, USA

A.C. Mehta, M.B.B.S.
Respiratory Institute, Lerner College of Medicine,
Cleveland Clinic, Cleveland, OH 44195, USA

A.C. Mehta and P. Jain (eds.), *Interventional Bronchoscopy: A Clinical Guide*, Respiratory Medicine 10,
DOI 10.1007/978-1-62703-395-4_2, © Springer Science+Business Media New York 2013

Keywords
Transbronchial biopsy • Lung cancer • Solitary lung nodule • Tumor–bronchus relationship

Introduction

Transbronchial Lung Biopsy (TBBx) also known as Bronchoscopic Lung Biopsy (BLBx) is one of the most important applications of flexible bronchoscopy. A diagnostic TBBx may obviate the need for an open lung biopsy. Even though the procedure is generally safe, serious and sometimes life-threatening complications may occur during TBBx. Therefore, decision to proceed with TBBx should be taken only after a careful risk–benefit analysis. In this chapter, we discuss the technique, clinical applications, limitations, and complications of transbronchial biopsy.

Technique

Performing TBBx is an essential skill for every bronchoscopist. Apart from mastering the technique, all bronchoscopists must have a thorough understanding of indications, clinical uses, and the limitations of the procedure. Also, one must be ready to manage its immediate complications, such as bleeding and pneumothorax. Several studies have established the safety of TBBx in an outpatient setting under moderate sedation [1, 2].

Patient Evaluation

A detailed history, physical examination, and chest roentgenograms (Chest X-Ray and Computed Tomography of Chest) are essential before TBBx. The purpose, risks, and the limitations of TBBx should be thoroughly discussed with the patient before the procedure. The patients must understand that underlying diagnosis cannot be confirmed in all instances with this technique. Routine complete blood counts, coagulation profile, blood chemistry, arterial blood gas analysis, pulmonary function tests, and electrocardiogram are not required prior to the procedure. The decision to perform these tests should be based on individual clinical evaluation. For instance, evaluation of clotting mechanism is indicated for patients with bleeding diathesis, those receiving anticoagulation therapy and for those who are at a high risk of bleeding due to liver disease or renal insufficiency.

General contraindications to TBBx are listed in Table 2.1. Patients with low platelet count should receive platelet transfusion immediately before the procedure to increase platelet count to at least 50,000/mm^3. We have also encountered excessive bleeding in presence of platelet count more than 1 million/mm^3. Correction of clotting mechanism may need administration of vitamin K and fresh frozen plasma. There is no need to stop aspirin [3], but a very high incidence of bleeding after TBBx has been reported in patients receiving clopidogrel [4], which must be held for at least 5–7 days prior to TBBx. A practical approach to identification and correction of coagulopathy prior to TBBx is summarized in Table 2.2.

Because of the higher risk of bleeding in uremic patients after transbronchial biopsy, serum creatinine should be measured when renal insufficiency is suspected. According to a survey,

Table 2.1 Contraindications for transbronchial biopsy

• Refractory hypoxemia
• Uncorrected coagulopathy (see Table 2.2)
• Uncontrolled cardiac arrhythmia
• Active myocardial ischemia
• Severe pulmonary hypertension
• Uncontrolled bronchospasm
• Uncooperative patient
• Inability to control cough
• Lack of adequate facilities for patient resuscitation
• Abnormal platelet counts (<50 K or >1 million)

Table 2.2 General guidelines for detection and correction of coagulopathy before transbronchial biopsy

History and physical examination
• Known bleeding or clotting disorder
• Prior history of epistaxis, petechial hemorrhage, GI bleed, hematuria, menorrahagia
• Excessive bleeding during prior surgeries
• Transfusion of blood products
• Renal insufficiency
• Liver disease
• Hematological malignancy
• Immunocompromised state
• Medications: aspirin, nonsteroidal anti-inflammatory drugs (NSAIDs), clopidogrel (Plavix), ticlopidine (Ticlid), prasugrel (Effient), dabigatran (Pradaxa), rivaroxaban (Xarelto) Coumadin, unfractionated heparin, low-molecular-weight heparin
Laboratory tests (based on clinical assessment)
• Platelet counts
• Prothrombin time (PT-INR)
• Activated partial thromboplastin time (aPTT)
• Renal functions
• Liver function tests
Specific recommendations[a]
• Proceed with TBBx only when: PT-INR < 1.5, aPTT < 50 s, platelet counts > 50 K
• No need to stop aspirin or NSAIDs
• Stop clopidorel, ticlodipine, and prasugrel for 5–7 days
• Hold Coumadin for 3 days; check PT-INR before the procedure
• Hold unfractionated heparin for 6 h and check aPTT before the procedure
• Hold low-molecular-weight heparin for at least 12 h
• Hold dabigatran and rivaroxaban for 2 days (hold for a longer period in presence of renal insufficiency)
• Transfuse platelets if counts are <50 K and check counts immediately prior to TBBx
• Reconsider decision to perform TBBx in patients with uremia. For BUN >30 mg/dl and creatinine >3.0 mg/dl, administer DDAVP: 0.3 μg/kg IV in 50 ml of saline and administer over 30 min; start infusion 60 min prior to procedure, or 3 μg/kg intranasal spray 30 min prior to TBBx

[a]Consult prescribing physician (e.g., cardiologist) before holding anti-platelet agents or anticoagulants. Consider bridge therapy in selected patients using standard clinical guidelines. Discuss the risk of holding anticoagulation with the patient

about one-half of bronchoscopists consider uremia a contraindication to transbronchial biopsies [5]. Specifically, BUN level of >30 mg/dl and creatinine level of >3.0 mg/dl (both together) are thought to increase the risk of bleeding after TBBx due to associated platelet dysfunction. For example, in a study reported in 1977, significant bleeding was encountered in 45 % of immunocompromised uremic patients undergoing bronchoscopic lung biopsy [6]. Somewhat more reassuring are results from a small retrospective study in which only 1 of 25 patients (4 %) with end stage renal disease had major and 1 (4 %) had minor bleeding after transbronchial biopsies [7]. Similarly, no association was found between the risk of bleeding and elevated serum creatinine in 45 immunocompromised patient who underwent transbronchial biopsies for evaluation of lung infiltrates [8]. The risk of bleeding in uremic patients may be reduced by intravenous infusion of 0.3 μg/kg desamino-8-D-arginine (DDAVP) over 30 min, starting 1 h before the TBBx. The same medication can also be administered in form of a nasal spray at a dose of 3 μg/kg about 30 min prior to the procedure (Table 2.2).

A vast majority of bronchoscopists consider pulmonary hypertension an absolute or relative contraindication to TBBx [5]. However, there is little evidence of excessive risk of bleeding after TBBx in these patients. For example, in a prospective, blinded study, the presence of pulmonary hypertension on echocardiography did not increase the risk of bleeding after TBBx [9]. However, patients with clinically evident pulmonary hypertension or cor-pulmonale were excluded from the study. Similarly, in a retrospective study, there was no significant increase in bleeding complications with TBBx in 24 patients with variable severity of pulmonary hypertension, as compared to 32 control subjects [10]. Since there were only a handful of patients with severe pulmonary hypertension in this study, the authors concluded that TBBx is safe in patients with mild to moderate pulmonary hypertension.

Radiologic Investigations

Chest radiograph is essential in all patients prior to transbronchial biopsies. Routine chest Computed Tomography (CT) scan is also useful in patients with localized lung infiltrates and in patients suspected to have lung cancer. In these cases, CT shows the location of lung infiltrate or mass and its relation with the bronchopulmonary segment, which is a useful information to have during TBBx [11] One study reported higher diagnostic yield from TBBx when the site of biopsy was chosen on the basis of chest CT scan in human immunodeficiency virus (HIV)-infected patients with localized lung infiltrates [12].

Biopsy Forceps

More alveolar tissue is obtained when the TBBx is performed with a large as compared to the small biopsy forceps [13]. The difference in the size of the biopsy specimen does not always translate into higher overall diagnostic yield or complications [14]. One problem with large biopsy forceps is difficulty in opening its cusps in the small peripheral airways, thus reducing the likelihood of obtaining desired alveolar specimen of lung parenchyma [15]. Alligator forceps tend to provide larger lung tissue specimen than cup forceps of comparable size. Cusps of the alligator forceps tear the tissue while that of the cup forceps cut the tissue; latter limiting the volume of the biopsy specimen. Our preference is to use alligator biopsy forceps for TBBx in most cases.

Fluoroscopic Guidance

Some investigators have performed TBBx without fluoroscopic guidance [16]. However, we recommend performing the biopsy under fluoroscopic guidance. The use of fluoroscopy during TBBx clearly improves the diagnostic yield of TBBx for focal lung infiltrates and lung masses [17]. The diagnostic yield of TBBx is similar with or without fluoroscopic guidance for diffuse lung infiltrates. Nevertheless, even in diffuse lung disease, fluoroscopy helps the bronchoscopist to select different areas for biopsy and allows the operator to obtain biopsy from the periphery of lung near the pleural surface. Moreover, fluoroscopy reduces the risk of pneumothorax during TBBx. The main drawback of using fluoroscopy for TBBx is its availability in resource-limited settings and radiation exposure to the patient and the staff [18]. There is no evidence that radiation exposure during diagnostic bronchoscopy has any long-term ill-effects on the patients or the bronchoscopy staff. The fluoroscopy time can be reduced with proper training and instructions [19]. Future health risks can be minimized with sound radiation hygiene practices [20]. Nevertheless, TBBx can be successful performed without fluoroscopic guidance. This is a common practice when the procedure is performed on intensive care unit patients with diffuse parenchymal disease.

Biopsy Technique

The technical aspects of TBBx have been reviewed elsewhere [21, 22]. A thorough airway examination should precede the TBBx because bleeding after lung biopsy may preclude adequate airway examination. Adequate control of cough with topical application of lidocaine and systemic administration of opiates is essential for optimal biopsy procedure and to reduce the risk of pneumothorax.

The choice of biopsy site depends on radiological and fluoroscopic findings. Under no circumstance should TBBx be attempted from both lungs during the same bronchoscopic procedure on the same date due to delayed risk of bilateral pneumothorax. Selection of the site for the TBBx is simple while dealing with focal disease. However, in cases of diffuse, five lobe disease selection of the site for the TBBx requires some consideration. In the latter event, we prefer to perform the biopsy from the dependent parts of the lungs; right and left lower lobes. In an event of bleeding, the blood is at least contained in this area before spilling into the other lobes. Also we prefer left over the right lower lobe as the longer length of the left main bronchus allow more volume for blood to accumulate before it spills into the contralateral side. This also allows more time to recognize and react to the complication. On the contrary we try to avoid performing the biopsy from the right upper lobe segments. Bleeding from this particular site soils both lungs and limits the reactionary time.

Once the biopsy site is chosen, the distal end of the bronchoscope is wedged into the specific segmental bronchus. Subsequent procedure is performed under fluoroscopic guidance when available. The assistant is asked to introduce and advance the forceps through the biopsy port into the working channel. Mild resistance is usually felt when the biopsy forceps reaches the distal end of flexible bronchoscope, especially during TBBx from the upper lobes and from the superior segment of lower lobes. This is because the distal bending section needs to be flexed at a sharp angle to reach these segments. In this situation, one should not apply excessive force to push the biopsy forceps out of the scope as it can damage the inner channel of the instrument. Instead, the operator should reduce the degree of flexion of the bending section by easing off from angulation control lever and gently advance the biopsy forceps through the distal end. Although this simple maneuver is usually successful, it can compromise the wedged position of bronchoscope. If this maneuver is unsuccessful, the best course is to pull the bronchoscope back into the lobar or main stem bronchus, and push the biopsy forceps a few centimeters beyond the distal end of the bronchoscope and push the biopsy forceps into the desired sub-segmental bronchus. The bronchoscope can then be advanced onto the wedged position using the biopsy forceps as a guide wire. This maneuver allows the biopsy forceps to be introduced into the difficult-to-reach bronchopulmonary segments while minimizing the risk of damage to the bronchoscope.

To obtain the specimen from a diffuse lung infiltrate under fluoroscopic guidance, the biopsy forceps is advanced into the lung parenchyma towards the pleura till resistance is met. The forceps is then pulled proximally by approximately 1.5–2 cm and the patient is instructed to take a deep breath and hold breath at maximum inspiration. This maneuver dilates the peripheral airway allowing cusps of the forceps open wide. While patient is holding breath, the assistant is instructed to open the biopsy forceps. The patient is then asked to breathe out and during expiration, the biopsy is gently advanced into the area of interest under fluoroscopic guidance, making sure that the forceps tip does not cross the pleural margins. While patient is breathing, resistance to advancing biopsy forceps is met. This is due to the fact that the open cusps are anchored at the bifurcation of the respiratory or the terminal bronchioles. At this stage the assistant is asked to close the biopsy cusps and the forceps is gently retracted. Usually a "tug" is felt when the lung tissue is sheared off. This sensation, however, does not guarantee that a good biopsy specimen has been retrieved. One should carefully look for actual movement of the lung infiltrate on fluoroscopy screen as the biopsy forceps is pulled back. In our experience, this movement of the infiltrate during TBBx strongly predicts the successful sampling of the diseased lung parenchyma. Lung tissue is obtained by actually tearing off the respiratory/terminal bronchioles. There is no need to make forceful and jerky movements while withdrawing the biopsy forceps.

To obtain the biopsy from a focal lesion, such as a lung cancer, the forceps is advanced till the margin of the mass is reached (Fig. 2.1). At this time, resistance is felt and it is not possible to push the forceps any further. At this time, "C" arm of the fluoroscopy unit is rotated to look at the movement of biopsy forceps and the lung mass relative to each other on the fluoroscopy screen. If the forceps is seen to move away from the lung mass with this maneuver, the forceps need to be repositioned. The forceps is in good position for biopsy if lung mass and the forceps move together as fluoroscope is rotated. After confirming the proximity of biopsy forceps and lung mass, the biopsy forceps is pulled back 0.5–1 cm and the assistant is asked to open the forceps cusps. The cusps of open biopsy forceps are pushed firmly into the mass and the contact between the forceps and the mass is verified on fluoroscopic screen. The forceps is closed and is gently retracted. Respiratory maneuvers are usually unnecessary for the biopsy of lung masses. Again, as the biopsy forceps is retracted, the movement of lung mass on fluoroscopy predicts the successful sampling from the lung mass.

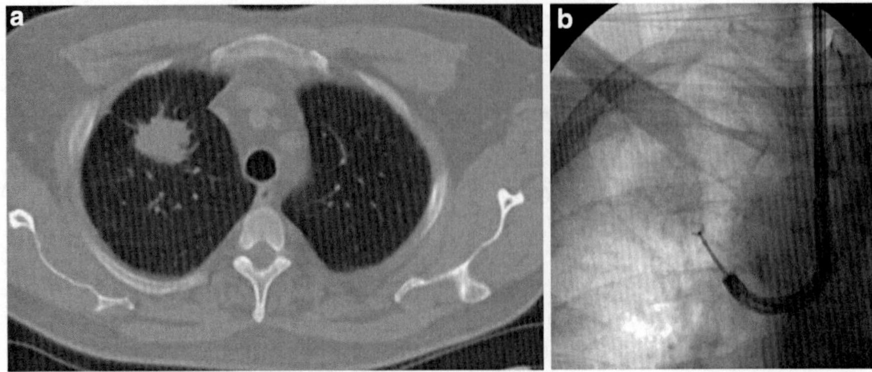

Fig. 2.1 (**a**) Chest CT showing right upper lobe lung nodule. (**b**) Biopsy forceps is advanced to the lesion under fluoroscopic guidance to obtain biopsy

Further biopsies should be obtained from the area of interest while maintaining the wedged position as much as possible. The purpose of wedging the bronchoscope is to create a tight seal around the distal part of the bronchoscope to tamponade the bleeding source and to prevent blood from spilling into more proximal airways. It is prudent to keep the bronchoscope wedged for at least 4 min (normal bleeding time) after all biopsies are taken from a lung segment. No suction should be performed at this time.

Number of Biopsy Specimens

There is limited information on the optimal number of transbronchial biopsies. In general, four to six biopsy specimens are adequate in majority of patients with diffuse lung disease [24]. In one study, 53 % of diagnoses were provided with the first specimen, and 33 % of diagnoses were provided with the second specimen [25]. In patients with stage II and III sarcoidosis 4–6 TBBx specimens provide optimal diagnostic yield [26]. However, for stage I sarcoidosis up to ten biopsy specimens may be needed for maximum diagnostic yield [27]. For localized peripheral lung mass and lung infection, a minimum of 6 and if feasible, up to 10 biopsy specimens should be obtained [28]. In a large study, the diagnostic yield from localized lesions increased from 23 % with 1–3 specimens to 73 % with 6–10 specimens [24].

Post-biopsy Fluoroscopy

A fluoroscopic examination should be performed at the conclusion of the procedure to rule out pneumothorax. The patient should be observed in the recovery room for at least 1½ h. A routine chest radiograph has a low diagnostic yield for pneumothorax after uncomplicated TBBx procedure in clinically stable patients [23], but is indicated for chest discomfort, dyspnea, excessive hemoptysis, or unexplained hypoxemia after the transbronchial biopsies.

Specimen Handling

The lung biopsy specimens are collected by opening the cusps and gently shaking the forceps in sterile saline. A toothpick may be used to retrieve the specimen from the biopsy forceps. Due to infection control concerns, using a needle to remove biopsy specimens should be avoided. After all biopsies are obtained, the specimens can be transferred to a container with 10 % formalin for routine pathological examination. Undue delay in immersion of biopsy specimens in the fixative solution should be avoided as much as possible. When infectious disease is likely, one or more tissue specimen may be submitted to the microbiology laboratory in sterile Ringer's lactate. Biopsy specimens for special studies such as electron microscopy, immunostaining and flowcytometry should be collected and transported in consultation with the receiving pathology laboratory.

Quality of Biopsy Specimen

The quality and adequacy of transbronchial biopsies are difficult to assess during the procedure. The usual size of tissue fragment from TBBx varies from 1 to 3 mm. Due to their small size, TBBx are inherently limited for assessment of disease processes such as interstitial pulmonary fibrosis in which pathological diagnosis requires identification of typical architectural changes in the lung parenchyma.

Sometimes, the biopsy material contains predominantly bronchial mucosa with very little or no alveolar tissue. This happens when TBBx is obtained from proximal area of the lung. Of course, biopsies with little or no alveolar tissues are not expected to provide meaningful information about the pathological process involving lung parenchyma. It is proposed that lung biopsy specimens with alveolar tissue are more likely to float when placed in 10 % formalin and show representative pathological changes than biopsy specimen with no alveolar tissue. For example, in one study, the TBBx specimens with alveolar tissue were more likely to float on 10 % formalin than specimens without alveolar tissue, and in patients with sarcoidosis, specimens containing non-caseating granuloma were more likely to float than specimens without non-caseating granuloma [29]. However, the practical value of float sign remains unproven because another study that had more heterogeneous patient population could not reproduce these results [25]. Besides more proximal biopsy may cause more bleeding while too distal biopsy increases the risk for pneumothorax.

Most pathologists accept a kidney biopsy specimen containing 5 or more glomeruli as an adequate specimen. No such consensus exists for TBBx. One group has proposed that TBBx specimen containing 20 or more alveoli should be considered adequate as it is more likely to detect a pulmonary infection than a specimen with fewer alveoli [30]. However, this concept has not been validated for other diagnoses such as pulmonary malignancies and most experts continue to believe that diagnostic yield from TBBx is more closely related to the number of the specimens obtained rather than actual number of alveoli in each biopsy specimen.

Clinical Applications of TBB

Lung biopsy is required for appropriate diagnosis and management of a variety of pulmonary diseases. Samples of lung tissue for diagnostic purpose may be obtained through the TBBx, CT-guided fine needle aspiration (CT-FNA), and video-assisted thoracoscopic or surgical lung biopsy. With few exceptions, surgical lung biopsy is the gold standard for obtaining lung tissue for patients with interstitial lung diseases but it is invasive, costly, requires general anesthesia and hospital admission. The application of CT-FNA is largely limited to peripheral pulmonary nodules or masses. The specimen from CT-FNA is generally insufficient for tissue diagnosis of benign disease processes. Pneumothorax develops in up to a quarter and chest tube is required in about 10 % of patients after CT-FNA [31]. In contrast, TBBx has wider clinical applications, the complication rate is low and the procedure can safely be performed in an outpatient bronchoscopy suite under conscious sedation. Serial lung biopsies are also best obtained with the transbronchial approach.

Several large case series have addressed the diagnostic yield of TBBx in heterogeneous groups of patients with a variety of underlying disease processes [24, 32–36]. Even though TBBx provided adequate lung specimen in 70–90 % of cases, a specific diagnosis could not be rendered in a significant proportion of the patients. The overall diagnostic yield for specific diagnosis varies widely, depending on the size, location and extent of lung infiltrates, and the nature of underlying lung disease. The results of TBBx also depend on the experience and technical skills of the bronchoscopist. Caution is warranted in interpreting the literature on diagnostic

Table 2.3 Pulmonary diseases in which transbronchial biopsies are useful

Malignancy
• Lung cancer
• Metastasis
Infections
• Tuberculosis
• Non-tubercular mycobacterial infections
• Fungal infection
• Pneumocystis pneumonia
• Viral infections such as CMV pneumonitis
Acute lung transplant rejection
Undiagnosed infiltrates in mechanically ventilated patients
Diffuse lung diseases
• Sarcoidosis
• Lymphangitic carcinomatosis
• Pulmonary alveolar proteinosis
• Pulmonary Langerhan's histiocytosis
• Alveolar microlithiasis
• Amyloidosis
• Lymphangioleiomyomatosis
• Bronchiolitis obliterans with organizing pneumonia

yield of TBBx because most authors have included nonspecific fibrosis or organizing pneumonia in the diagnostic yield and only a few have applied more stringent criteria for pathologic interpretation of TBBx specimens. Nonspecific findings on TBBx are often unhelpful and can lead to erroneous clinical decisions. Pulmonary disorders in which a confident diagnosis is possible with TBBx are listed in Table 2.3. In case of diffuse lung diseases, TBBx is more likely to establish the diagnosis of diseases such as sarcoidosis and lymphangitic carcinomatosis than in pulmonary vasculitis and diffuse lung diseases such as idiopathic pulmonary fibrosis for which low-magnification architectural overview is essential for diagnosis. In pulmonary Langerhans' cell histiocytosis (PLCH), and lymphangioleiomyomatosis (LAM), the TBBx are reliable but have a low diagnostic yield due to sampling error. Therefore, the presence of typical histological findings in these conditions is sufficient for diagnosis, but their absence does not exclude the diagnosis. The diagnostic role of TBBx in selected conditions is discussed below.

Lung Cancer

Flexible bronchoscopy is the most widely used technique for diagnosis of peripheral lung cancer. Usually, a combination of sampling procedures such as bronchial washing, brush, TBBx and peripheral TBNA are performed in these patients to maximize the diagnostic yield. According to an evidence-based review, FB provided diagnostic specimen in 36–88 %, with an average of 78 % in 16 studies of patients with peripheral lung cancers [37]. TBBx is the most useful sampling method for the diagnosis of peripheral lung cancer. The average diagnostic yield from TBBx is 57 % with a range of 17–77 % in patients with peripheral lung cancers. When performed in conjunction with bronchial washing and brushing, TBBx provides exclusive diagnosis in up to 19 % of the patients [38]. TBBx provides exclusive diagnosis in 7 % of patients if peripheral-transbronchial needle aspiration (P-TBNA) is also performed in addition to other sampling methods.

Although CT-guided fine needle aspiration (CT-FNA) is the diagnostic procedure of choice, flexible bronchoscopy with TBBx will provide diagnosis in 30–40 % of patients with superior sulcus tumor [39, 40]. Bronchoscopy with TBBx has a high diagnostic yield in patients with lymphangitic carcinomatosis [41, 42]. There is a limited data on usefulness of TBBx in metastatic pulmonary tumors but in one study the biospy provided diagnostic tissue in only 2 of 12 (17 %) of such patients [43].

The diagnostic yield of TBBx for lung cancer increases with the number of biopsy specimens. In one study, the diagnostic yield was 21 % when 1–3 TBBx specimens were obtained and 78 % when 6–10 specimens were obtained [24]. In another study, the diagnostic yield increased from 45 % with the first specimen to 70 % with multiple TBBx specimens [28]. Based on these studies, 6–10 TBBx should be obtained in these patients for an optimal diagnostic yield.

The size of the lesion is the single most factors affecting the sensitivity of bronchoscopy for diagnosis of peripheral lung cancers. Pooled data from ten studies shows a diagnostic yield of 34 %

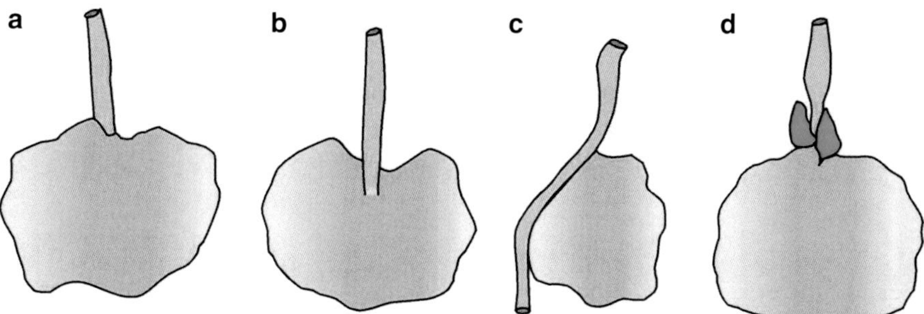

Fig. 2.2 Tumor–bronchus relationship: (**a**) Type I: bronchus is patent up to the tumor, (**b**) Type II: the bronchus is contained within the tumor mass, (**c**) Type III: the bronchus is compressed, narrowed and displaced by the tumor mass, but the bronchial mucosa is intact (**d**) Type IV in which the proximal bronchus is narrowed by the submucosal and peribronchial spread of the tumor, fibrosis, or enlarged lymph nodes

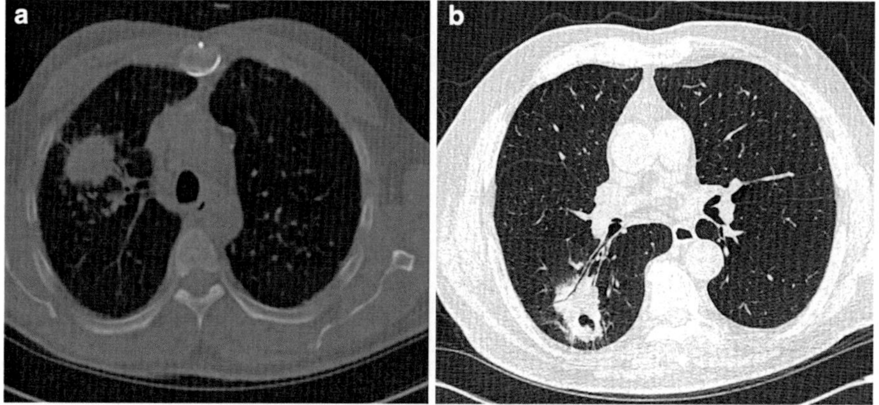

Fig. 2.3 Chest CT showing (**a**) Type I tumor–bronchus relationship, (**b**) Type II tumor–bronchus relationship

for lesions <2 cm and 63 % for lesions ≥2 cm in diameter [37]. Due to a very low yield was reported for lesions ≤2 cm in diameter located in outer one-third of the lung, some authors suggest an alternative approach such as CT-FNA for obtaining tissue diagnosis [44].

Tumor–bronchus relationship also affects the diagnostic yield of TBBx in peripheral lung cancers. Tsuboi and associates examined surgically resected specimens in 47 patients and identified four types of tumor–bronchus relationship: type I, in which the bronchus is patent up to the tumor, type II, in which, the bronchus is contained within the tumor mass, type III, in which the bronchus is compressed, narrowed and displaced by the tumor mass, but the bronchial mucosa is intact, and type IV in which the proximal bronchus is narrowed by the submucosal and peribronchial spread of the tumor, fibrosis, or enlarged lymph nodes [45] (Fig. 2.2). The authors also noted that more than 60 % of tumors that were <3 cm in diameter had only one bronchus involved, whereas three or more bronchi could be identified approaching 60 % of tumors that were >3 cm in diameter [45]. High-resolution chest computed tomography demonstrates different types of tumor–bronchus relationship with a high degree of accuracy [46] (Fig 2.3).

Bronchus sign on CT refers to the finding of a bronchus leading directly to or contained within the peripheral lung mass [47]. The diagnostic yield of bronchoscopy for peripheral lesions is 0–44 % when the bronchus sign is absent, as compared with 60–82 % when it is

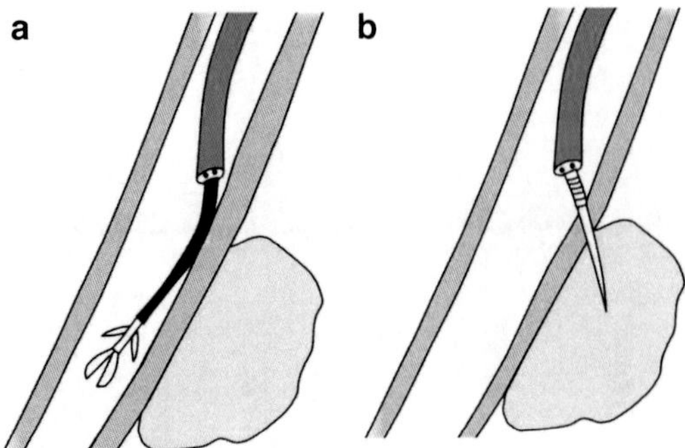

Fig. 2.4 (**a**) Biopsy forceps is displaced away from the lesion with type III tumor–bronchus relationship. (**b**) Transbronchial needle is seen to pierce the bronchial wall and obtain sample from the tumor

present [46–50]. Peripheral-TBNA procedure has a higher success rate in obtaining tissue diagnosis from peripheral masses with type III or IV tumor–bronchus relationship than with conventional sampling procedure including TBBx [51]. In one study, P-TBNA provided diagnostic tissue from 20 of 26 (77 %) lesions, whereas TBBx provided diagnosis in 5 of 26 (19 %) of lesions with type III or IV tumor–bronchus relationship [48]. The higher success of P-TBNA in lesions with type III or IV tumor–bronchus relationship may be related to the ability of TBNA needle to pierce the displaced bronchial wall or traverse the narrowed and stenotic segment of the bronchus to reach the core of the tumor, which may not possible with standard TBBx forceps (Fig 2.4).

Lung Infections

Non-resolving Pneumonia

Flexible bronchoscopy is frequently performed for further evaluation of non-resolving pneumonia [52]. TBBx provides useful information in these cases. For example, in one study, TBBx provided diagnosis in 57 % of patients with community-acquired pneumonia who failed antimicrobial therapy [53]. TBBx specimens can demonstrate mycobacterial or fungal infection, and may provide tissue diagnosis of other conditions that can mimic pneumonia such as bronchioloalveolar cancer (Adenocarcinoma in situ), cryptogenic organizing pneumonia, and hypersensitivity pneumonitis. In cavitary lesions, obtaining biopsies from the wall of the cavity increases the chances of detecting underlying lung pathology (Fig 2.5).

Tuberculosis

Flexible bronchoscopy is frequently performed for patients with smear negative pulmonary tuberculosis. In most cases, a combination of bronchial washing, bronchoalveolar lavage and TBBx is performed to maximize the diagnostic yield. TBBx provides rapid diagnosis in 17–60 % of cases with confirmed active tuberculosis [54–57] and is the exclusive source of diagnostic specimen in 10–20 % of these patients [58–60]. TBBx also provides rapid diagnosis in miliary tuberculosis. Furthermore, in a significant proportion of patients, TBBx uncovers other disease processes such as lung cancer and fungal infection that can mimic tuberculosis. Therefore, it is appropriate to perform TBBx whenever flexible bronchoscopy is performed in patients suspected to have sputum negative tuberculosis.

Non-tubercular Mycobacteria

The diagnosis of non-tubercular mycobacterial infection is difficult to establish because the NTM are shed intermittently in the sputum. Further, the presence of NTM in the sputum often raises the possibility of contamination or colonization rather than true infection [61].

Flexible bronchoscopy with TBBx is frequently needed to confirm the diagnosis in these cases. According to the current American Thoracic Society/Infectious Disease Society guidelines, in the presence of appropriate clinical setting, the diagnosis of NTM requires one of the following microbiological criteria: (1) positive culture results from at least two separate sputum samples, or (2) positive culture results from at least one bronchial wash or lavage, or (3) transbronchial biopsies showing granulomatous inflammation, stainable acid-fast bacilli and positive NTM cultures or mycobacterial histological features and one or more sputum or bronchial wash culture positive for NTM [62].

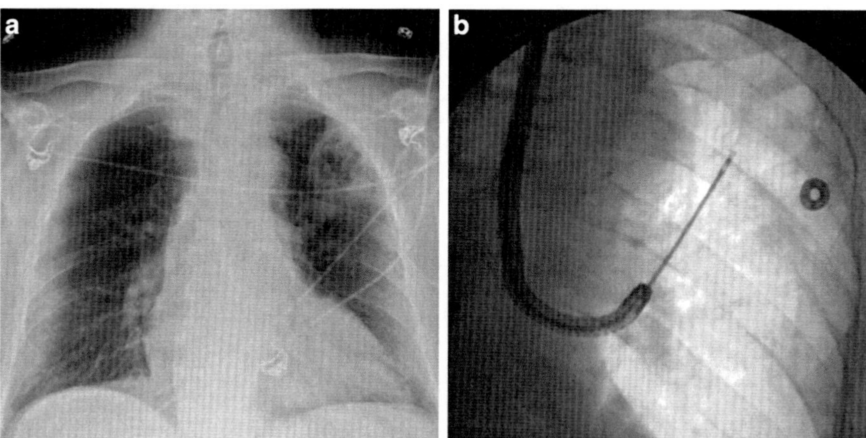

Fig. 2.5 (**a**) Chest radiograph showing a left upper lobe cavitary lesion in an immunocompromised patient. (**b**) Transbronchial biopsy is obtained from the wall of cavitary lesion

Accordingly, TBBx should be performed whenever bronchoscopy is needed in patients suspected to have NTM infection.

Fungal Infections

Bronchial washing and bronchoalveolar lavage are the most valuable bronchoscopic procedures for the diagnosis of pulmonary fungal infections [63–66]. A modest improvement in diagnostic yield is achieved with addition of TBBx in these patients [67–69]. We routinely perform TBBx whenever FB is required for patients with suspected fungal infection of the lung.

Infections in Immunocompromised Hosts (Non-HIV)

Immunocompromised hosts are subject to a wide spectrum of serious and life-threatening opportunistic pulmonary infections. FB with BAL provides diagnostic information in up to two-third of these patients with minimum procedure-related complications. While the diagnostic value of BAL is well established, the role of TBBx in altering management and improving outcome in these patients is a matter of some controversy. TBBx provides diagnostic information in 15–68 % of immunosuppressed patients with pulmonary infiltrates [8, 70–80]. Unfortunately, potential for serious procedure-related complications with TBBx limits its utility in these patients.

In a prospective study, Stover and associates performed bronchoscopy in 97 immunocompromised patients with lung infiltrates [70]. Bronchoalveolar lavage was diagnostic in 61 of 92 (66 %) diseases, whereas TBBx were diagnostic in 36 of 57 (63 %) diseases, for a combined yield of 83 %. We performed bronchoscopy in 104 immunocompromised patients with lung infiltrates [8]. TBBx was performed in 45 of these patients. The overall diagnostic yield of bronchoscopy was 56 %. TBBx provided specific diagnosis in 38 % of patients. The combined yield of BAL and TBBx (70 %) was better than diagnostic yield from BAL (38 %) alone. In this study, TBBx was exclusively diagnostic in 13 % of procedures and was more likely to detect noninfectious causes of lung infiltrates in the immunocompromised hosts than BAL. The procedure-related complications were encountered in 31 % of patients who underwent TBBx, but there were no procedure-related deaths. In a large retrospective study, Cazzadori and associated reviewed their experience with TBBx in 142 immunocompromised patients with lung infiltrates [72]. Overall, the diagnostic yields of TBBx and BAL were 68 % and 36 %, respectively. The only complications were pneumothorax in 3 patients and bleeding in 1 patient.

Notwithstanding, the limitations of TBBx in these patients must be noted. First, not all studies have found TBBx to be useful in immunocompromised with lung infiltrates. For example, in a retrospective study, White and associates reviewed the results of bronchoscopy in 52 bone marrow transplant (BMT) patients with lung infiltrates. A total of 68 bronchoscopies were performed [81]. TBBx was performed in addition to BAL in 42 procedures. Only 1 additional diagnosis was made with TBBx in this study. Complications were encountered in 15 % of patients. In another study, TBBx was performed in 71 patients with hemopoietic stem cell transplantation [82]. The pathologic findings were nonspecific in 82 % of patients. Specific diagnoses were obtained in less than 10 % of patients undergoing the procedure. Complications were encountered in 8 % of patients. These data cast some doubt on the value of routine TBBx in BMT patients with lung infiltrates.

Second, most immunocompromised patients who require bronchoscopy are critically ill and have associated comorbid conditions that place them at a high risk for procedure-related complications [8]. In many instances, TBBx cannot be performed in these patients due to safety considerations. Studies have consistently shown higher complications rate with TBBx, than with bronchoalveolar lavage in these patients. It can be clearly seen that in some reports TBBx is not pursued in a vast majority of immunocompromised patients due to safety concerns [83–85].

Furthermore, nonspecific inflammatory and fibrosis are commonly reported on TBBx in immunocompromised patients with lung infiltrates. Clinicians need to interpret these nonspecific findings with caution. Some authors find nonspecific findings on TBBx to have a high negative predictive value for a treatable process. For example, in one study, specific diagnoses were obtained in 16 of 35 (48 %) patients undergoing TBBx [86]. The majority of remaining patient who had nonspecific histological findings either showed clinical and radiographic improvement, or had an untreatable disease. The authors reported 84 % sensitivity and 100 % specificity of TBBx for a treatable opportunistic infection in these patients. Nevertheless, others have experienced different results and have concluded that nonspecific findings on TBBx do not assure absence of a treatable lung infection or a correctable noninfectious disease process in immunocompromised patients with lung infiltrates [87]. Therefore, a thorough clinical review is essential if TBBx shows nonspecific findings in immunocompromised patients with pulmonary infiltrates. Surgical lung biopsy is often considered in this situation. The diagnostic yield of surgical lung biopsy is reported to vary from 46 to 85 % in immunocompromised patients with lung infiltrates [88–96]. Surgical lung biopsies in these patients have shown both noninfectious diseases such as malignancy, lymphoma, drug toxicity and cryptogenic organizing pneumonia, and infectious diseases such as pneumocystis carinii pneumonia, legionella pneumonia, CMV pneumonia, invasive aspergillosis, gram-negative pneumonia, nocardiosis, and pulmonary toxoplasmosis. Many of these disease entities are expected to resolve with institution of appropriate therapy. Therefore, surgical lung biopsy should be considered when TBBx is non-diagnostic and the patient fails to improve with empirical treatment [97].

Infections in HIV-Infected Patients

Pulmonary complications are very common in patients infected with human immunodeficiency virus (HIV). Flexible bronchoscopy has played a critical role in the diagnosis and appropriate management of pulmonary complications of HIV infection [98]. In recent times, with advances in antiretroviral therapy, there is a clear decrease in the incidence of pulmonary complications and need for diagnostic bronchoscopy. Nonetheless, in resource poor areas, pulmonary complications continue to pose a serious threat to patients with HIV infection. A large retrospective study early in AIDS epidemic reported that 91 % of all pulmonary infections could be diagnosed by a combination of BAL and TBBx [99]. Subsequent studies have reported 65–96 % diagnostic yields when both BAL and TBBx are performed [100–104]. Stover and associates performed BAL and TBBx in 72 patients with acquired immunodeficiency syndrome [100]. Overall, the bronchoscopy provided diagnosis in 65 % of patients. The diagnostic yield of FB was 94 % for Pneumocystis pneumonia (PCP), 67 % for Cytomegalovirus pneumonia, and 62 % for Mycobacterium avium-intercellulare infection. The main value of TBBx over and above BAL in this series was for the diagnosis of PCP. Broaddus and associates reported results of FB with BAL and TBB in 171 patients with acquired immunodeficiency syndrome [102]. The overall diagnostic yield of bronchoscopy was 96 %. BAL and TBBx had diagnostic yields of 86 % and 87 % respectively. BAL had a diagnostic yield of 89 % and TBB had a diagnostic yield of 93 % in patients with PCP. TBBx was the sole mean of diagnosis in 11 % of these patients. Pneumothorax developed after 9 % of procedures and chest tube was needed in 6 % of patients. Because BAL had high yield and TBBx was associated with complications, the authors concluded that TBBx could be avoided in patients at high risk of complications after bronchoscopy. Somewhat different results have been reported in a study from Rwanda in which FB with BAL and TBBx were performed in 111 HIV patients with lung infiltrates of unclear etiology [103]. In this study, BAL provided diagnosis in 26 % of patients, whereas TBBx provided diagnosis in 82 % of patients. Final diagnoses were nonspecific interstitial pneumonitis (NSIP) in 38 %, tuberculosis in 23 % cryptococcosis in 13 %, Kaposi sarcoma in 9 % and PCP in 5 % of study patients. Diagnosis remains unclear in 16 % of patients. TBBx and BAL were the only source of diagnosis in 74 % and 18 % respectively. Complications were encountered in 13 % of patients, including hemorrhage in 5 % and pneumothorax in 8 % of patients. The low yield of BAL in this series was clearly due to low incidence of PCP in the study patients.

TBBx has provided diagnostic material in as many as 58 % of patients with AIDS-related non-Hodgkin's lymphoma [105]. In contrast, TBBx has limited in pulmonary Kaposi's sarcoma and surgical lung biopsy is frequently needed for diagnosis [100, 106, 107]. In some reports, a diagnosis of NSIP has been made on the basis of TBBx in HIV infected patients with lung infiltrates [108, 109]. NSIP is diagnosed on the basis of histologic evidence of diffuse alveolar damage in association with chronic inflammation in the interalveolar septa in the absence of microbial pathogens on BAL stains, or cultures and on histopathological examination. Many of these patients show clinical and radiological improvement with empirical treatment.

Some investigators have questioned the value of routine TBBx in HIV infected patients with lung infiltrates [110]. This conclusion is largely based on studies in which the majority of patients had pneumocystis carinii pneumonia. On the contrary, when the role of FB in HIV-infected patients with a wider spectrum of pulmonary complications is analyzed, TBBx clearly improves the overall diagnostic yield. Even in PCP, some authors have found a significant improvement in diagnostic yield of FB when TBBx is performed with BAL as a routine. For example, in a recent study, BAL had a diagnostic yield of 74 %, whereas TBBx and BAL had a yield of 95 % in patients with PCP infection [111]. TBBx also seems to increases the diagnostic yield of FB for the patients receiving aerosolized pentamidine prophylaxis as the diagnostic yield of BAL is significantly lower in these patients [112]. We recommend both TBBx and BAL during FB for HIV infected patients with pulmonary infiltrates whenever feasible.

The usefulness of surgical lung biopsy in face of a non-diagnostic BAL and TBBx in HIV-infected patient is a debatable issue. Surgical biopsy is usually considered in these patients whenever the cause of lung infiltrate remains unclear and when the patient fails to respond to the treatment directed towards the diagnosis established with flexible bronchoscopy. In one study, the management was altered in only 1 of 66 patients who underwent surgical lung biopsy for these indications [113]. More favorable results are reported in other studies in which management was changed in a substantial proportion of carefully selected patients subjected to surgical lung biopsy [114, 115]. In one series, of

42 surgical lung biopsies, useful diagnosis was obtained in all 4 patients who had no preceding bronchoscopy, 13 of 18 patients who had non-diagnostic TBBx and BAL, 8 of 11 patients who had non-diagnostic BAL, but only 1 of 9 patients who had deterioration despite appropriate treatment for diagnosis established by bronchoscopy [116]. Based on these results, the authors did not support surgical lung biopsy on patients whose condition continued to worsen despite receiving appropriate therapy. We strongly recommend involvement of an expert in the field of HIV medicine before a decision is made to request surgical lung biopsy in these patients.

Lung Transplantation

TBBx plays a crucial role in the long-term management of lung transplant patients. A detailed discussion on the role of TBBx in lung transplant recipients is beyond the scope of this chapter and readers are referred to recent reviews for details [117, 118]. We briefly highlight a few important points.

In many centers, routine TBBx are performed for surveillance in asymptomatic lung transplant recipients, but their role for this purpose is controversial. Several studies have found surveillance bronchoscopy with TBBx to be a high-yield procedure. In an early study, 90 surveillance transbronchial biopsies were performed in 43 lung transplant recipients. Specific histological features of rejection or infection were found in 57 % of procedures [119]. In another study, 836 TBBx procedures were performed in 230 lung transplant recipients over a 5-year period [120]. Histological features of acute rejection, lymphocytic bronchiolitis, or infection were detected with 19 % of procedures. The yield of surveillance TBBx between 4 and 12 months post lung transplant was 6.1 % for acute graft rejection. In another study, clinical utility of 353 surveillance bronchoscopy procedures was studied in 124 lung transplant recipients [121]. High incidence of clinically important acute rejection was reported up to 1 year after the lung transplantation in these patients.

In contrast, others have found no benefits of surveillance bronchoscopy and TBBx in lung transplant recipients [122–124]. For example, in one study the outcome of 24 lung transplant recipients undergoing surveillance bronchoscopy was compared with 23 patients who underwent bronchoscopy for specific clinical indications [125]. A total of 240 TBBx were performed in 47 study patients. No acute rejection episode needing therapeutic intervention was detected with true surveillance bronchoscopy. No significant differences in respiratory infection, acute rejection, bronchiolitis obliterans syndrome (BOS) or survival were found in two groups.

More favorable results have been reported with FB and TBBx in assessment of clinically suspected acute rejection or pulmonary infection in lung transplant recipients. In fact, TBBx is the diagnostic procedure of choice for suspected acute allograft rejection [126]. TBBx has a sensitivity and specificity of 94 % and 90 % respectively for this indication [127]. Most transplant centers obtain at least 6–10 satisfactory transbronchial biopsies in these patients [128].

The clinical reasons for performing bronchoscopy with TBBx are >10 % decline in forced expiratory volume in 1 s (FEV1), >20 % decline in forced expiratory flow between 25 and 75 % of vital capacity, radiographic infiltrates, clinical suspicion for infection and symptoms referable to respiratory tract. FB with TBBx has high diagnostic yield in these patients. The diagnostic yield of FB with TBBx is close to 70 % when the procedure is performed for clinical indications [119, 129]. Apart from detecting acute rejection, FB with BAL and TBBx is the premier investigation for lung transplant patients for the diagnosis and surveillance of respiratory infections. For example, in one study, infection was diagnosed by bronchoscopy samples in 51 % of clinically indicated FB and 12 % of surveillance bronchoscopies [130]. It must be noted that the majority of infections in this study were diagnosed with analysis of BAL sample.

TBBx is also performed for follow-up of patient after treatment of acute rejection. Several studies have shown persistence of ongoing rejection despite appropriate initial treatment in a significant proportion of patients [119, 129, 131]. In one study, persistence of acute rejection was detected in as many as 26 % of patients on follow-up TBBx [132]. Bronchoscopy with BAL and TBBx is also reported to have a diagnostic yield of 74 % in lung transplant patients with solitary or multiple lung nodules [133].

Flexible bronchoscopy with TBBx is also performed for suspected chronic allograft rejection but TBBx has low sensitivity for detecting obliterative bronchiolitis, the characteristic histologic findings in chronic rejection [134, 135]. The main value of FB in these cases is exclusion of airway complications, lung infections and acute graft rejection. Another value of TBBx is in predicting the future risk of bronchiolitis obliterans syndrome (BOS). Acute rejection is an established risk factor for BOS [136]. Recent studies seem to indicate that presence of minimal acute rejection (grade A_1) on multiple transbronchial biopsies is also associated with higher future risk of developing BOS [137]. A recent study has also established lymphocytic bronchiolitis on TBBx as a risk factor for BOS and mortality independent of acute rejection in lung transplant recipients [138]. Lymphocytic bronchiolitis on TBBx has also been linked to the occurrence and severity of acute cellular rejection in lung transplant recipients [139].

TBB in Mechanically Ventilated Patients

Flexible bronchoscopy with BAL is commonly performed in mechanically ventilated patients with diffuse pulmonary infiltrates. The procedure is safe and provides useful diagnostic information in a significant proportion of these patients. TBBx is seldom performed in mechanically ventilated patients due to safety concerns. For example, in a prospective study TBBx was performed in only 7 of 147 bronchoscopy procedures in mechanically ventilated patients [140]. Few data are available on precise clinical usefulness of TBBx in mechanically ventilated patients. Papin and associates performed TBBx in 15 patients requiring mechanical ventilation [141]. Transbronchial lung biopsies provided diagnosis in 5 of 15 (33 %) of patients and altered management in seven patients. Three patients had self limiting bleeding and 1 patient developed delayed pneumothorax. Pincus and associates performed TBBx in 13 mechanically ventilated patients [142]. TBBx established specific diagnoses in 6 of 13 (46 %) of patients. The procedure was thought to have therapeutic implications in all 13 patients. Two patients developed pneumothorax after the procedure. Bulpa and associates performed FB with BAL and TBB in 38 mechanically ventilated patients [143]. All of the study subjects had unexplained pulmonary infiltrates. Diagnosis was established with TBB in 74 % of cases and management was altered in 63 % of patients. The procedure was complicated by pneumothorax in 9 (23 %) patients and self-limiting bleeding in 4 (11 %) of patients. In the largest series till date, O'Brien and associates reported the results of TBBx in 71 mechanically ventilated patients [144]. Specific histological diagnoses were made in 35 % of cases and the management was changed in 41 % of patients. Findings on TBBx also led to an important management change in 26 % of lung transplant recipients. The results of TBBx were similar to those found on surgical lung biopsy or autopsy in 11 of 13 study patients. Pneumothorax developed in 14 % of patients.

Traditionally, surgical lung biopsies are performed in critically ill patients with undiagnosed lung infiltrates. Surgical lung biopsy provides diagnostic information in 45–65 % of these patients [145, 146]. The results lead to an important management change in up to 70 % of patients. However, surgical lung biopsy is more invasive than TBBx with a complication rate of at least 20 %. In one study, surgical lung biopsy carried a mortality rate of 8.4 % in mechanically ventilated patients. TBBx may be safer but several important issues need further clarification. Should TBBx be performed as a routine or should it be done if the initial FB with BAL is non-diagnostic? Do the results of TBBx alter patient outcome? Only well designed prospective studies can answer some of these questions.

Diffuse Lung Diseases

Sarcoidosis

Bronchoscopy with TBBx is very useful for patients with suspected sarcoidosis. In some reports, TBBx have provided diagnosis in 90–95 % of patients with sarcoidosis [26, 147]. The diagnostic yield of TBBx in sarcoidosis depends on the radiological stage varying from 50 to 65 % in stage I, 63 to 82 % for stage II, and 80 to 85 % for stage III disease [148–150]. Ten biopsy specimens in stage I disease [27] and four to six TBBx in stage II and III sarcoidosis [26] are required to achieve optimal diagnostic yield from flexible bronchoscopy. Bronchial mucosa is frequently involved in sarcoidosis and endobronchial biopsies increase the diagnostic yield by as much as 20 % over and above the diagnostic yield of TBBx [148, 151]. Addition of TBNA [148, 150, 152] or EBUS-TBNA [153] to TBBx also increases the diagnostic yield of bronchoscopy for sarcoidosis.

Pulmonary Langerhans' Cell Histiocytosis

Although clinical features and HRCT findings may strongly suggest the diagnosis, histological confirmation is often needed in patients with suspected PLCH. Surgical lung biopsy remains the gold-standard of diagnosis. However, distinctive histological features allow the diagnosis to be established with TBBx in some cases. The diagnostic yield of TBB for PLCH is reported to vary from 10 to 40 % [154, 155] Low yield of TBBx is due sampling error secondary to patchy distribution of lung pathology in PLCH. Thus, absence of typical histological features on TBBx should not be considered conclusive and surgical biopsy should be performed for further evaluation. The presence of Langerhans' cells staining for CD1a and S100 protein on immunocytochemistry of TBBx specimen further supports the diagnosis. False positive immunocytochemistry results can be observed in smokers. Therefore, stains for these markers should only be performed in the biopsy specimens with histological findings consistent with PLHC [156]. Increased number (>5 %) of Langerhans' cells staining with antibodies to CD1a in bronchoalveolar lavage also support the bronchoscopic diagnosis of PLCH [157].

Lymphangioleiomyomtosis

Surgical lung biopsy is usually performed for a definitive diagnosis of LAM [158]. Transbronchial biopsies may be sufficient for diagnosis in some cases of LAM but caution is needed because LAM cells in the lung parenchyma on TBBx can be misinterpreted as fibrosis. Immunohistochemical studies show positive staining of LAM cells for HMB-45 monoclonal antibodies. Positive staining for estrogen receptors and HMB-45 in the TBBx specimen strongly supports the diagnosis of LAM [159, 160].

Cryptogenic Organizing Pneumonia

The pathologic hallmarks of cryptogenic organizing pneumonia (COP) are proliferation of granulation tissue in the terminal and respiratory bronchioles and alveolar ducts along with extension of organization into alveoli and chronic inflammatory changes in the surrounding interstitial space [161]. Large specimen of lung tissue obtained by thoracoscopic or surgical lung biopsy is needed to confirm the diagnosis and to exclude other conditions that mimic COP [162]. In some instances, TBBx is found to be adequate for diagnosis [163–165]. Poletti and associates performed TBBx in 32 patients with suspected COP [165]. The sensitivity, specificity, positive predictive value and negative predictive values of TBBx were 64 %, 86 %, 94 % and 40 % respectively. Although the ideal approach remains open to debate, some leading experts in this area recommend TBBx before subjecting the patients to more invasive approach [166]. However, surgical lung biopsy must be performed if the diagnosis remains uncertain after TBBx and when there is inadequate response to oral corticosteroids.

Hypersensitivity Pneumonitis

Hypersensitivity pneumonitis (HP) is fundamentally a clinical diagnosis and routine histological confirmation is unnecessary. Lung biopsy is occasionally indicated when diagnosis is uncertain despite a thorough clinical evaluation. The histologic triad of cellular bronchiolitis, diffuse interstitial infiltrates of chronic inflammatory cells and loosely formed scattered noncaseting granuloma is the usual finding in subacute HP.

These findings are best demonstrated on surgical lung biopsy [167]. However, TBBx is reported to provide adequate specimen in some cases of acute [168] and subacute HP [169]. Chronic HP is less likely to be diagnosed with TBBx [156].

Others

Transbronchial biopsy is the diagnostic procedure of choice for suspected lymphangitic carcinomatosis [41, 42, 170]. In patients with pulmonary alveolar proteinosis, TBBx may demonstrate typical PAS-positive alveolar infiltrates [171]. Similarly, TBBx is a useful initial step for the diagnosis of diffuse pulmonary amyloidosis [172]. TBBx may provide diagnostic material in patients with suspected lipoid pneumonia and pulmonary alveolar microlithiasis [173].

Limitations of Transbronchial Lung Biopsy

Low Yield in Diffuse Lung Diseases

In a large number of diffuse lung diseases, nonspecific findings on TBBx do not allow a confident pathological diagnosis [174]. A common example is idiopathic pulmonary fibrosis (IPF) where the pathological diagnosis is mainly based on low-power architecture of the biopsy specimen that cannot be established with TBBx. In one study, transbronchial lung biopsies from 22 patients with idiopathic pulmonary fibrosis were retrospectively examined to determine if a diagnosis of UIP could be established [175]. All except one of the study patients had already undergone surgical lung biopsy that showed usual interstitial pneumonia (UIP). After examining several TBBx specimens from individual patients, the investigators reported that diagnosis of UIP was possible on TBBx in 7 of 22 (30 %) of patients. However, this study was seriously flawed because the interpreting pathologists were not blinded to the findings of surgical lung biopsy. In an earlier study, Wall and associates performed surgical lung biopsies in 33 patients who had diffuse infiltrative disease with nonspecific or non-diagnostic transbronchial biopsies [176]. Surgical lung biopsy provided specific diagnosis in 92 % of patients. The findings on surgical biopsy specimen had little relationship to the TBBx results. For example, 9 of 21 patients reported to have normal lung or nonspecific findings on TBBx had idiopathic interstitial pneumonia on surgical lung biopsy. Out of 9 patients thought to have idiopathic interstitial pneumonia on TBBx the diagnosis was confirmed in only 2 patients on surgical lung biopsy. Furthermore, TBBx missed diagnosis of pulmonary Langerhans cell histiocytosis and sarcoidosis in 9 patients. In another study, the majority of patient with nonspecific chronic interstitial inflammation and fibrosis on TBBx had the disease process stabilized or regressed contrary to the natural history expected on the basis of the TBBx findings [177]. Taken together, TBBx cannot be used to diagnose UIP or differentiate it from other histological subtypes of idiopathic interstitial pneumonia such as NSIP [178]. Current evidence based guidelines do not recommend TBBx in patients with idiopathic interstitial pneumonia [179].

Transbronchial biopsy has occasionally provided the diagnostic material in Goodpasture's syndrome, Wegener's granulomatosis (WG), and Churg-Strauss syndrome (CSS) [180, 181]. However, in majority of patients, these diagnoses cannot be confirmed with TBBx. For example, in one study, even though adequate alveolar could be obtained in 17 of 19 patients, the histological diagnosis could be confirmed with TBBx in only 2 of 19 patients with WG [182]. Nonspecific findings were reported in majority of patients. Accordingly, surgical lung biopsy is usually recommended for the diagnosis of pulmonary vasculitis. Similarly, diffuse lung infiltrates due to occupational lung disease such as silicosis and asbestosis, collagen vascular diseases, and pulmonary drug toxicity also require surgical lung biopsy whenever the tissue diagnosis is deemed necessary.

Small biopsy size and the tissue artifacts in the TBBx specimen [183] create considerable diagnostic problems for the interpreting pathologists. In order to obtain larger tissue samples, some investigators have recently used flexible cryoprobe to obtain TBBx. In one study, 41 patients with diffuse lung disease underwent standard TBBx, followed by cryobiopsies from the same pulmonary segment [184]. All patients undergoing the procedure in this study had an endotracheal tube placed prior to bronchoscopy. The investigators used 2.4 mm flexible cryoprobe to obtain the biopsy. The cryoprobe was introduced via the working channel of flexible bronchoscope and was advanced to the area of interest under fluoroscopic guidance to a distance of 10 mm from thoracic wall. The probe was cooled for about 4 s and was retracted along with the frozen lung tissue. The median area of tissue specimen on the histologic slide was 15.22 mm^2 for the cryobiopsies compared to 5.82 mm^2 for standard transbronchial biopsies. The investigators found no artifacts in the cryobiopsy specimens. A confident diagnosis of NSIP could be made in ten patients with cryobiopsies. However, confirmatory surgical lung biopsies were not performed in any of the patient in this study. There was no significant bleeding after cryobiopsies. Similar results have been reported by another group of investigators in 15 patients with diffuse lung disease [185]. These studies have provided useful preliminary data on safety and feasibility of obtaining larger tissue specimens free of crush artifacts with the flexible cryoprobes. Prospective studies are now warranted to investigate the diagnostic accuracy of cryobiopsies in diffuse lung diseases using surgical lung biopsies as the reference criteria.

Low Yield in Solitary Lung Nodule

Establishing a tissue diagnosis of solitary lung nodule is one of the most difficult challenges in pulmonary medicine. Traditional flexible bronchoscopy with TBBx has a low diagnostic yield in these patients. For the lung nodules <2 cm, the data from ten studies shows the average diagnostic yield of FB to vary from 11 to 76 % with an average of 34 % [37]. On multivariate analysis, the independent predictors of obtaining diagnostic tissue sample from lung nodules with flexible bronchoscopy in a recent study were malignant etiology (odds ratio [OR] 4.8), diameter >2 cm (OR 3.6), and a positive bronchus sign (OR 2.4), again reinforcing the importance of size and bronchus sign as important determinants of diagnostic yield of conventional bronchoscopy in these patients [186]. Benign etiology of SPN is seldom established with transbronchial biopsies. Malignant etiology of SPN cannot be ruled out on the basis of negative bronchoscopy and transbronchial biopsies. The low yield of TBBx in SPN is mainly due to (1) inability to visualize the lesion on fluoroscopy, [187] and (2) inability to maneuver the biopsy forceps to its target in the absence of a favorable tumor–bronchus relationship.

Several attempts have been made in recent years to offset some of the limitations of traditional bronchoscopic methods to obtain biopsy specimen from SPN. The advanced techniques have been designed specifically to address the difficulties encountered in obtaining biopsy specimen from a small lung nodule. For example, CT-fluoroscopy and radial probe EBUS have been used to improve the likelihood of visualizing the lesion before obtaining the biopsy specimen. Virtual bronchoscopy navigation and electromagnetic navigation bronchoscopy (ENB) have been used to help the bronchoscopist to select the most appropriate path to reach the target for biopsy. Improved maneuverability is made possible with the use of ultrathin bronchoscope that can be advanced to seventh to ninth generation bronchi under direct operator control, steerable probe used with electromagnetic navigation, and double-hinged curette used with radial probe EBUS. In many instances, combinations of aforementioned techniques have been used to maximize the chances of obtaining diagnostic tissue from peripheral lesions smaller than 2–3 cm in diameter.

Several studies have looked into the feasibility of using CT-fluoroscopic guidance to obtain biopsy specimens from peripheral lung nodules. The main advantage is ability to localize the forceps in axial plane and visually confirm the contact between the forceps and the lesion [188]. In one study, a correct diagnosis could be established in 8 of 12 (67 %) of peripheral lesions with an average diameter of 2.2 cm with TBBx under CT-fluoroscopy guidance [189]. In another study, for the lesions <15 mm diameter, diagnosis could be established in 22 of 45 (49 %) patients with TBBx under CT-fluoroscopy guidance compared to only 3 of 26 (12 %) under conventional fluoroscopy guidance [190]. In contrast, in a recent randomized study, no difference was found in the diagnostic sensitivity of TBBx performed under CT versus conventional fluoroscopic guidance [191]. Overall, only 33 % of lesions ≤3 cm in size could be diagnosed with TBBx under CT or conventional fluoroscopic guidance in this study.

There are several problems with the use of CT-fluoroscopy with conventional bronchoscopy. The ability to visualize the lesion does not guarantee that the operator will be able to advance the biopsy instrument to the target. Also, performing bronchoscopy in CT room poses major scheduling and logistic difficulties. Bronchoscopy is often an awkward experience both for the patient and the operator, and the CT room may be ill-equipped to manage a serious bronchoscopy-related complication. Perhaps the most important drawback is the risk associated with excessive radiation exposure to the patients and the operators. According to current estimates, the radiation exposure to the patients with CT-fluoroscopy is 2–5 times that of conventional fluoroscopy [189, 191]. With the emergence of radiation neutral alternatives such as radial probe endobronchial ultrasound with guide sheath (EBUS-GS) and virtual bronchoscopy navigation (VBN), excessive use of diagnostic radiation with CT-fluoroscopy for this purpose is a direct contradiction to the principle of justification, and optimization- the guiding principles of radiation use in clinical practice [192].

Several studies have recently established usefulness of EBUS-GS to localize small lung nodules prior to biopsy (Chap. 4). In one study, diagnostic tissue could be obtained from 116 of 150 (77 %) of peripheral lesions using EBUS-GS technique [193]. Although the diagnostic yield for lesions >3 cm in size (92 %) was significantly higher than that for lesions ≤3 cm in size (74 %), the investigators could establish diagnosis in 59 of 81 (73 %) of lesions ≤2 cm in size. Further, the investigators could obtain diagnosis in 40 of 54 (74 %) lesions ≤2 cm in size that could not be located on fluoroscopy. In a prospective randomized study, the diagnostic yield of EBUS-GS directed TBBx was compared with that of standard fluoroscopically guided TBBx in 221 patients [194]. For patients with lung cancer, the diagnostic sensitivity in EBUS group (79 %) was significantly higher than that in standard TBBx group (55 %). On sub-group analysis, the diagnostic sensitivity was similar with either technique for lesions >3 cm. However, the diagnostic sensitivity was higher with EBUS-GS technique for lesions <3 cm in diameter (75 % vs. 31 %) as well as for lesions <2 cm in diameter (71 % vs. 23 %) than with the standard TBB technique.

A major advantage of EBUS-GS is in biopsy of those lesions that are not visible on conventional fluoroscopy. For example, in a prospective study, the investigators could obtain tissue diagnosis in 38 of 54 (70 %) of lesions with an average diameter of 2.2 cm that were not visible on fluoroscopy [187]. A additional advantage of this technique is better ability to navigate the biopsy instruments to the target lesions using the double-hinged curette introduced through the guide sheath [193]. It is typically used in those cases in which the lesion cannot be located with the EBUS.

Some limitations of this technique must also be noted. First, a high diagnostic yield for solitary lung nodules <2 cm has not been reproduced in every study. For example, in one study, TBBx using EBUS-GS technique was performed in 100 consecutive patients with lung nodules <2 cm in diameter [195]. The investigators could locate the lesions in 67 (67 %) patients with EBUS and obtain diagnostic tissue in 46 (46 %) of patients. Similarly, in another study, the diagnostic yield of TBBx with EBUS-GS technique for peripheral lesions >2 cm in diameter was 76 % but the diagnostic yield for lesions ≤2 cm in diameter was only 30 % [196]. Moreover, a recent randomized trial that enrolled 246 patients failed to show any difference in the detection rate of cancer between the EBUS-GS group (36 %) and the conventional bronchoscopy group (44 %) [197]. In fact, for lesions <3 cm in diameter, the diagnostic yield was higher with conventional TBBx under fluoroscopic guidance than with EBUS-GS directed biopsies in this study. Some of the variation in reported results with this technique may be related to experience and training of the operators performing the procedure.

Electromagnetic navigation bronchoscopy (ENB) is an image-guided localization system that allows real time navigation of the biopsy instruments to small peripheral lesions during flexible bronchoscopy (Chap. 6). Several studies have reported encouraging initial results in obtaining biopsy from small peripheral lesions with this technique. In a prospective study, investigators from The Cleveland Clinic Foundation have reported a diagnostic yield of 74 % in 54 peripheral lesions with an average diameter of 2.28 cm [198]. The diagnosis was established in 23 of 31 (74 %) of lesions ≤2 cm in diameter in this study. The overall diagnostic yield has ranged from 63 % to 84 % for lesions of all sizes and from 50 to 76 % for lesions ≤2 cm in diameter in several other studies [199–203]. The diagnostic yield of ENB is significantly higher for lesions with a CT bronchus sign than for those without a discernible CT-bronchus sign [202]. The technique appears to have a steep learning curve [203]. One disadvantage of the technique is that there is no real time confirmation that the biopsy is actually obtained from the lesion. The other disadvantages are high initial cost of the equipment and high cost of the disposable accessories used during the procedure.

Virtual bronchoscopy navigation is emerging as an important method to facilitate accurate navigation of bronchoscope and biopsy instruments to small peripheral lesions (Chap. 7). In this technique, virtual images of endobronchial tree are reconstructed from the CT data to simulate actual bronchoscopy. The display of most appropriate endobronchial route to the target lesion on virtual bronchoscopy images helps the operator to navigate the bronchoscope to the correct airways leading to the target lesion. Apart from navigational capabilities, the current VBN systems allow the images to be rotated and to go forward and backwards to emulate the actual bronchoscopy images. In most case series, the investigators have combined VBN with ultrathin bronchoscope in order to come as close to the lesion as possible. In some studies, biopsies have been performed under CT-fluoroscopy [204] and in others, under standard fluoroscopy guidance [205]. The overall diagnostic yield of TBBx using VBN with ultrathin bronchoscope have varied from 63 to 82 % and the diagnostic yield for peripheral lesions ≤2 cm in diameter has varied from 62 to 82 % in different studies [206–209]. The application of this technique during bronchoscopy does not need additional radiation exposure or costly accessories. However, the best results are achieved with the use of ultrathin bronchoscope which is not universally available. Further, the majority of data on application of VBN comes from investigators who are highly familiar with this technique.

To further improve the diagnostic yield of bronchoscopy for small peripheral lung nodules, several recent studies have combined ENB or VBN to navigate the bronchoscope and the accessory instruments bringing them close to the target and radial probe EBUS to confirm that the target is reached before obtaining the biopsy specimen. Very encouraging results have been reported with this multi-modality approach. Eberhardt and associates studied the usefulness of combining ENB and EBUS-GS in a prospective randomized study [210]. Biopsies were performed using EBUS-GS alone in 39 patients, ENB alone in 39 patients and combination of EBUS-GS and ENB in 40 patients. The diagnostic yield of EBUS-GS + ENB guided procedures (88 %) was significantly greater than the diagnostic yield of EBUS-GS guided procedures (69 %) or ENB-guided procedures (52 %). In another study, Asano and associates studied the usefulness of combining VBN, ultrathin bronchoscope (BF-type P260F, external diameter 4.0 mm, working channel 2.0 mm, Olympus Corporation), and EBUS-GS to obtain specimens from 32 peripheral lesions [211]. Diagnostic specimens could be obtained in 27 of 32 (84 %) of all lesions and 22 of 24 (79 %) of lesions ≤3 cm in diameter. The preliminary results from this study were confirmed in a recent randomized trial in which the 199 patients with peripheral lesions ≤3 cm in diameter were randomized to undergo biopsy with assistance of VBN+EBUS-GS ($n=102$) or EBUS-GS alone ($n=97$) [212]. The diagnostic yield in VBN+EBUS-GS group (80 %) was significantly higher than that in EBUS-GS group (67 %). The diagnostic yield with the combined approach was 76 % and that with EBUS-GS alone was 59 % for lesions <2 cm in diameter. There can be no doubt that application of multiple advanced techniques is increasing the ability to obtain biopsy specimen from lesions that cannot be diagnosed with conventional TBBx under fluoroscopic guidance. Unfortunately, many of these techniques are expensive and vigorous cost-effectiveness studies are needed before they can be incorporated in routine clinical practice.

CT-guided fine needle aspiration (CT-FNA) remains in common use for diagnosis of peripheral lung nodules. It has a diagnostic sensitivity of 90 % (range 65–94 %) but is associated with pneumothorax in 15–43 % (median 27 %) needing chest tube in 4–18 % (median 5 %) [213]. The diagnostic sensitivity of CT-FNA depends on the size of the lesion. For the lesions <2.0 mm in diameter, the diagnostic sensitivity of CT-FNA has varied from 74 to 77 % with 22–28 % risk of pneumothorax after the procedure [214, 215]. In these patients, advanced bronchoscopic techniques discussed above offer a safer alternative with a lower risk of pneumothorax and a similar or higher diagnostic yield compared to CT-FNA.

Complications of Transbronchial Biopsies

TBBx is generally safe, although severe and life-threatening procedure-related complications are occasionally encountered. According to a recent nationwide survey from Japan, the complication rate after forceps biopsy for a peripheral pulmonary lesion was 1.79 % [216]. In comparison, a review of 173 procedures from a university hospital has reported a complication rate of 6.8 % after TBBx [217]. Two most common complications of TBBx are bleeding and pneumothorax.

The reported incidence of bleeding after transbronchial biopsy has varied from 0 to 26 % in different series. Serious bleeding occurs in 1–2 % of patients undergoing transbronchial biopsies [1, 218]. The risk of bleeding is significantly higher in immunocompromised patients and in patients with underlying renal insufficiency [6, 8, 81]. Reports of deaths due to uncontrolled bleeding after TBBx are exceedingly uncommon, but it is plausible that it is under-reported. In the Japanese survey mentioned above, 0.85 % of 57,199 patients experienced significant bleeding after TBBx, but there were no deaths [216].

A major bleeding complication after transbronchial biopsy is unnerving, but the bleeding can be controlled in the majority of cases in the bronchoscopy room without adverse patient outcome [219]. The main danger of bleeding after transbronchial biopsy is aspiration of blood into non-bleeding segments rather than risk of exsanguination. Therefore, the top priority is to prevent the flooding of airways with large amounts of blood. As soon as significant bleeding is detected, tilt the bronchoscopy table so that bleeding side is dependent. The most effective way to control bleeding is to maintain the bronchoscope in wedged position into the bleeding segment till a blood clot is formed. Sometimes, the wedged position is compromised while pulling back the biopsy forceps. In these cases, the bronchoscopist should make every effort to immediately place the bronchoscope back into the bronchus. Fluoroscopic guidance may be needed in some cases as presence of blood may obscure the endoscopic view. After maintaining bronchoscope in wedged position for about 5 min, the bronchoscope is gently withdrawn. Bronchoscopist should be ready to re-wedge the bronchoscope if sudden gush of blood is seen. Cold saline lavage and topical application of dilute epinephrine are usually unsuccessful in controlling bleeding after the TBBx due to diluting effect of blood and distal bleeding site. If significant bleeding continues despite local measures and if the bronchoscope has slipped out of the bleeding segment, it is best to secure the airway with endotracheal tube and consider either balloon tamponade or selective intubation of contralateral lung. The facilities for rigid bronchoscopy must be held in readiness to manage a bleeding episode that cannot be controlled with the flexible bronchoscope. Management of hemoptysis is further discussed in Chap. 14.

Pneumothorax is reported in 1–6 % of patients after transbronchial biopsies [1, 24, 220]. Failure to control coughing during transbronchial biopsies greatly increases the risk of pneumothorax. Patients receiving positive pressure ventilation are also more likely to develop pneumothorax after transbronchial biopsies. Risk may also be higher in presence of bullous emphysema and in patients with pneumocystis pneumonia [102]. Appropriate fluoroscopic guidance during transbronchial biopsies reduces the risk of pneumothorax. Fluoroscopic examination detects pneumothorax immediately after the biopsies but in some case, slowly developing delayed pneumothorax can manifest several hours after completion of procedure [1]. Tension pneumothorax is very uncommon after transbronchial biopsies. Nonetheless, mild to moderate pneumothorax may cause disproportionate symptoms due to underlying pulmonary limitation in some patients undergoing flexible bronchoscopy. If no symptoms develop for 4 h after completion of procedure, a clinically significant pneumothorax is unlikely. Chest roentgenogram should be performed after ½ to 1 h after completion of biopsies when the pneumothorax is clinically suspected despite normal findings on immediate post-bronchoscopy fluoroscopy. Severity of symptoms and the extent on chest roentgenogram dictate the management of pneumothorax after bronchoscopy. Supplemental oxygen and observation in the hospital is sufficient in most cases. Moderately symptomatic patients with significant pneumothorax may be managed with Heimlich's valve placed in the bronchoscopy suite. These patients can be discharged with Heimlich's valve after 4–6 h of observation if repeat chest roentgenogram shows no further increase in pneumothorax. Patients who develop severe symptoms or tension pneumothorax, and those who fail to show resolution of pneumothorax with Heimlich's valve require chest tube placement. Chest tube should also be placed without further delay when pneumothorax develops in patients on mechanical ventilation.

Conclusions

Transbronchial biopsy is an essential skill for every bronchoscopist. Transbronchial biopsy is usually performed in outpatient setting under conscious sedation. A successful TBB may obviate need for surgical lung biopsy, which is more invasive and needs general anesthesia. The most common indication of TBBx is to obtain biopsy specimen from peripheral lung masses. The diagnostic yield of TBBx for peripheral lung cancer depends on the size of the tumor and the presence or absence of bronchus sign. TBBx is also useful in evaluation of patients with suspected tuberculosis, fungal infection, unexplained lung infiltrates in immunocompromised hosts and in post-lung transplant patients, both for surveillance as well as evaluation of rejection or opportunistic infections. Among noninfectious diseases, TBBx is most useful in diagnosis of sarcoidosis, lymphangitic carcinomatosis, and in some cases of PLCH and LAM. Transbronchial biopsy is not useful for histological diagnosis of idiopathic pulmonary fibrosis or for distinguishing histological subtypes of idiopathic interstitial pneumonia. The diagnostic yield is also suboptimal in lung nodules smaller than 2–3 cm in diameter. Several recent techniques such as radial probe endobronchial ultrasound with guide sheath, electromagnetic navigation bronchoscopy and virtual bronchoscopy navigation have been used to improve the diagnostic yield of TBBx for solitary lung nodule. Hemoptysis and pneumothorax are the two leading complications of TBBx, occurring in less than 2 % of cases. We believe that all bronchoscopists must develop proficiency in performing TBBx and managing complications that can arise after the procedure.

References

1. Ahmad M, Livingston DR, Golish JA, Mehta AC, Wiedemann HP. The safety of outpatient bronchoscopy. Chest. 1986;90:403–5.
2. Blasco LH, Hernandez IMS, Garrido VV, et al. Safety of the transbronchial biopsy in outpatients. Chest. 1991;99:562–5.

3. Herth FJF, Becker HD, Ernst A. Aspirin does not increase bleeding complications after transbronchial biopsy. Chest. 2002;12q2:1461–4.
4. Ernst A, Eberhardt R, Wahidi M, Becker HD, Herth FJF. Effect of routine clopidogrel use on bleeding complications after transbronchial biopsy in humans. Chest. 2006;129:734–7.
5. Wahidi MM, Rocha AT, Hollingsworth JW, Govert JA, Feller-Kopman D, Ernst A. Contraindications and safety of transbronchial biopsy via flexible bronchoscopy. Respiration. 2005;72:285–95.
6. Cunningham JH, Zavala DC, Corry RJ, Keim LW. Trephine air drill, bronchial brush, and fiberoptic transbronchial lung biopsies in immunosuppressed patients. Am Rev Respir Dis. 1977;115:213–20.
7. Mehta NL, Harkin TJ, Rom WN, Graap W, Addrizzo-Harris DJ. Should renal insufficiency be a relative contraindication to bronchoscopy biopsy? J Bronchol. 2005;12:81–3.
8. Jain P, Sandur S, Meli Y, Arroliga AC, Stoller JK, Mehta AC. Role of flexible bronchoscopy in immunocompromised patients with lung infiltrates. Chest. 2004;125:712–22.
9. Morris MJ, Peacock MD, Mego DM, Johnson JE, Anders GT. The risk of hemorrhage from bronchoscopic lung biopsy due to pulmonary hypertension in interstitial lung disease. J Bronchol. 1998;5: 117–21.
10. Diaz-Guzman E, Vadi S, Minai OA, Gildea TR, Mehta AC. Safety of diagnostic bronchoscopy in patients with pulmonary hypertension. Respiration. 2009;77:292–7.
11. Naidich DP, Harkin TJ. Airway and lung: correlation of CT with fiberoptic bronchoscopy. Radiology. 1995;197:1–12.
12. Cadranel J, Gillet-Juvin K, Antoine M, et al. Site directed bronchoalveolar lavage and transbronchial biopsy in HIV-infected patients with pneumonia. Am J Respir Crit Care Med. 1995;152:1103–6.
13. Loube DI, Johnson JE, Weiner D, Andres GT, Blanton HM, Hayes JA. The effect of forceps size on the adequacy of specimens obtained by transbronchial biopsy. Am Rev Respir Dis. 1993;148: 1411–3.
14. Wang KP, Wise RA, Terry PB, et al. Comparison of standard and large forceps for transbronchial lung biopsy in the diagnosis of lung infiltrates. Endoscopy. 1980;12:151–4.
15. Smith LS, Seaquist M, Schillaci RF. Comparison of forceps used for transbronchial lung biopsy. Bigger may not be better. Chest. 1985;87:574–6.
16. Milligan SA, Luce JM, Golden J, Stulbarg M, Hopewell PC. Transbronchial biopsy without fluoroscopy in patients with diffuse roentgenographic infiltrates and the acquired immunodeficiency syndrome. Am Rev Respir Dis. 1988;137:486–8.
17. Cox ID, Bagg LR, Russell NJ, et al. Relationship of radiologic position to the diagnostic yield of fiberoptic bronchoscopy in bronchial carcinoma. Chest. 1984;85:519–22.
18. Jain P, Fleming P, Mehta AC. Radiation safety for the health care workers in bronchoscopy suite. Clin Chest Med. 1999;20:33–8.
19. Ernst A, Smith L, Gryniuk L, et al. A simple teaching intervention significantly decreases radiation exposure during transbronchial biopsy. J Bronchol. 2004;11:109–11.
20. Jain P, Mehta AC. Infection control and radiation safety in the bronchoscopy suite. In: Wang KP, Mehta AC, Turner JF editors. Flexible bronchoscopy. 3rd ed. Oxford: Wiley-Blackwell, 2012. p. 6–31.
21. Kvale PA. Bronchoscopic lung biopsy. How I do it. J Bronchol. 1994;1:321–6.
22. Zavala DC. Transbronchial biopsy in diffuse lung disease. Chest. 1978;73:727S–33.
23. Frazier WD, Pope TL, Findley LJ. Pneumothorax following transbronchial biopsy. Low diagnostic yield with routine chest roentgenograms. Chest. 1990;97:539–40.
24. Descombes E, Gardiol D, Leuenberger P. Transbronchial lung biopsy: an analysis of 530 cases with reference to the number of samples. Monaldi Arch Chest Dis. 1997;52:324–9.
25. Curley FJ, Johal JS, Burke ME, Fraire AE. Transbronchial lung biopsy. Can specimen quality be predicted at the time of biopsy? Chest. 1998; 113:1037–41.
26. Gilman MF, Wang KP. Transbronchial biopsy in sarcoidosis. An approach to determine the optimal number of biopsies. Am Rev Respir Dis. 1980;122: 721–4.
27. Rothe RA, Fuller PB, Byrd RB, et al. Transbronchial lung biopsy in sarcoidosis. Optimal numbers and sites for biopsy. Chest. 1980;77:400–2.
28. Popovich Jr J, Kvale PA, Eichenhorn MS, Radke JR, Ohorodnik JM, Fine G. Diagnostic accuracy of multiple biopsies from flexible fiberoptic bronchoscopy. A comparison of central versus peripheral carcinoma. Am Rev Respir Dis. 1982;125:521–3.
29. Anders GT, Linville KC, Johnson JE, Blanton HM. Evaluation of float sign for determining adequacy of specimens obtained with transbronchial biopsy. Am Rev Respir Dis. 1991;144:1406–7.
30. Fraire AE, Cooper SP, Greenberg SD, Rowland LP, Langston C. Transbronchial lung biopsy. Histopathologic and morphometeric assessment of diagnostic utility. Chest. 1992;102:748–52.
31. Wu CC, Maher MM, Shepard JA. Complications of CT-guided percutaneous needle biopsy of the chest: prevention and management. AJR Am J Roentgenol. 2011;196:678–82.
32. Andersen HA. Transbronchial lung biopsy for diffuse pulmonary disease. Results in 939 patients. Chest. 1978;73:734S–6.
33. Ellis JH. Transbronchial lung biopsy via the fiberoptic bronchoscope. Experience with 107 consecutive cases and comparison with bronchial brushing. Chest. 1975;68:524–32.
34. Hanson RR, Zavala DC, Rhodes ML, Keim LW, Smith JD. Transbronchial biopsy via flexible bronchoscope: results in 164 patients. Am Rev Respir Dis. 1976;114:67–72.

35. Mitchell DM, Emerson CJ, Collins JV, Stableforth DE. Transbronchial lung biopsy with the fiberoptic bronchoscope: analysis of results in 433 patients. Br J Dis Chest. 1981;75:258–62.
36. Zellweger JP, Leuenberger PJ. Cytologic and histologic examination of transbronchial lung biopsy. Eur J Respir Dis. 1982;63:94–101.
37. Rivera MP, Mehta AC. Initial diagnosis of lung cancer. ACCP evidence-based clinical practice guidelines. 2nd edition. Chest. 2007;132:131S–48.
38. Mazzone P, Jain P, Arroliga AC, Matthay RA. Bronchoscopic and needle biopsy techniques for diagnosis and staging of lung cancer. Clin Chest Med. 2002;23:137–58.
39. Maxfield RA, Aranda CP. The role of fiberoptic bronchoscopy and transbronchial biopsy in the diagnosis of Pancoast's tumor. NY State J Med. 1987; 87:326–9.
40. Miller JI, Mansour KA, Hatcher Jr CR. Carcinoma of the superior pulmonary sulcus. Ann Thorac Surg. 1979;28:44–7.
41. Torrington KG, Hooper RG. Diagnosis of lymphangitic carcinomatosis with transbronchial biopsy. South Med J. 1978;71:1487–8.
42. Aranda C, Sidhu G, Sasso LA, Adams FV. Transbronchial lung biopsy in the diagnosis of lymphangitic carcinomatosis. Cancer. 1978; 42:1995–8.
43. Mohsenifar Z, Chopra SK, Simmons DH. Diagnostic value of fiberoptic bronchoscopy in metastatic pulmonary tumors. Chest. 1978;74:369–71.
44. Baaklini WA, Reinoso MA, Gorin AB, Sharafkaneh A, Manian P. Diagnostic yield of fiberoptic bronchoscopy in evaluating solitary pulmonary nodules. Chest. 2000;117:1049–54.
45. Tsuboi E, Ikeda S, Tajima M, et al. Transbronchial biopsy smear for diagnosis of peripheral pulmonary carcinomas. Cancer. 1967;20:687–98.
46. Gaeta M, Barone M, Russi EG, et al. Carcinomatous solitary pulmonary nodule: evaluation of tumor bronchi relationship with thin-section CT. Radiology. 1993;187:535–9.
47. Naidich DP, Sussman R, Kutcher WL, Aranda CP, Garay SM, Ettenger NA. Solitary pulmonary nodules. CT-Bronchoscopic correlation. Chest. 1988;93: 595–8.
48. Bilaceroglu S, Kumcuoglu Z, Alper H, et al. CT-bronchus sign guided bronchoscopic multiple diagnostic procedures in carcinomatous pulmonary nodules and masses. Respiration. 1998;65:49–55.
49. Gaeta M, Pandolfo I, Volta S, et al. Bronchus sign on CT in peripheral carcinoma of the lung. Value in predicting results of transbronchial biopsy. AJR Am J Roengenol. 1991;157:1181–5.
50. Gaeta M, Russi EG, La Spada F, et al. Small bronchogenic carcinomas presenting as solitary pulmonary nodules. Bioptic approach guided by CT-positive bronchus sign. Chest. 1992;102:1167–70.
51. Shure D, Fedullo PF. Transbronchial needle aspiration of peripheral masses. Am Rev Respir Dis. 1983;128:1090–3.
52. Feinsilver SH, Fein AM, Niederman MS, Schultz DE, Faegenburg DH. Utility of fiberoptic bronchoscopy in nonresolving pneumonia. Chest. 1990;98: 1322–6.
53. Arancibia F, Ewig S, Martinez JA, et al. Antimicrobial treatment failures in patients with community acquired pneumonia: causes and prognostic implications. Am J Respir Crit Care Med. 2000;162:154–60.
54. Wallace JM, Deutsch AL, Harrell JH, Moser KM. Bronchoscopy and transbronchial biopsy in evaluation of patients with suspected active tuberculosis. Am J Med. 1981;70:1189–94.
55. Danek SJ, Bower JS. Diagnosis of pulmonary tuberculosis by flexible fiberoptic bronchoscopy. Am Rev Respir Dis. 1979;119:677–9.
56. Charoenratanakul S, Dejsomritrutai W, Chaiprasert A. Diagnostic role of fiberoptic bronchoscopy in suspected smear negative pulmonary tuberculosis. Respir Med. 1995;89:621–3.
57. Tamura A, Shimada M, Matsui Y, et al. The value of fiberoptic bronchoscopy in culture positive pulmonary tuberculosis patients whose pre-bronchoscopic sputum specimen were negative both for smear and PCR analyses. Intern Med. 2010;49:95–102.
58. Kennedy DJ, Lewis WP, Barnes PF. Yield of bronchoscopy for the diagnosis of tuberculosis in patients with human immunodeficiency virus infection. Chest. 1992;102:1040–4.
59. Chan CHS, Chan RCY, Arnold M, Cheung H, Cheung SW, Cheng AFB. Bronchoscopy and tuberculostearic acid assay in the diagnosis of sputum negative pulmonary tuberculosis: a retrospective study with the addition of transbronchial biopsy. Q J Med. 1992;82:15–23.
60. Salzman SH, Schindel ML, Aranda CP, Smith RL, Lewis ML. Role of bronchoscopy in the diagnosis of pulmonary tuberculosis in patients at risk for HIV infection. Chest. 1992;102:143–6.
61. Jett JR, Cortese DA, Dines DE. The value of bronchoscopy in the diagnosis of mycobacterial disease. A five-year experience. Chest. 1981;80:575–8.
62. Griffith DE, Aksamit T, Brown-Elliot BA, et al. An official ATS/IDSA statement: diagnosis, treatment and prevention of nontuberculous mycobacterial diseases. Am J Respir Crit Care Med. 2007;175: 367–416.
63. Sabonya RE, Barber RA, Wiens J, et al. Detection of fungi and other pathogens in immunocompromised patients by bronchoalveolar lavage in an area endemic for coccidioidomycosis. Chest. 1990;97: 1349–55.
64. Patel RG, Patel B, Petrini MF, Carter RR, Griffith J. Clinical presentation, radiographic findings, and diagnostic methods of pulmonary blastomycosis: a review of 100 consecutive cases. South Med J. 1999; 92:289–95.

65. Martynowicz MA, Prakash. Pulmonary blastomycosis: an appraisal of diagnostic techniques. Chest. 2002;121:768–73.
66. Malabonga VM, Basti J, Kamholz SL. Utility of bronchoscopic sampling techniques for cryptococcal disease in AIDS. Chest. 1991;99:370–2.
67. Wallace JM, Catanzaro A, Moser KM, Harrell JH. Flexible fiberoptic bronchoscopy for diagnosing pulmonary coccidioidomycosis. Am Rev Respir Dis. 1981;123:286–90.
68. Salzman SH, Smith RL, Aranda CP. Histoplasmosis in patients at risk for the acquired immunodeficiency syndrome in a nonendemic setting. Chest. 1988;93: 916–21.
69. DiTomasso JP, Ampel NM, Sobonya RE, Bloom JW. Bronchoscopic diagnosis of pulmonary coccidioidomycosis. Comparison of cytology, culture, and transbronchial biopsy. Diagn Microbiol Infect Dis. 1994;18:83–7.
70. Stover DE, Zaman MB, Hajdu SI, et al. Bronchoalveolar lavage in the diagnosis of diffuse pulmonary infiltrates in the immunosuppressed host. Ann Intern Med. 1984;101:1–7.
71. Eriksson B-M, Dahl H, Wang F-Z, et al. Diagnosis of pulmonary infections in immunocompromised patients by fiberoptic bronchoscopy with bronchoalveolar lavage and serology. Scand J Infect Dis. 1996;28:479–85.
72. Cazzadori A, Di Perri G, Todeschini G, et al. Transbronchial biopsy in the diagnosis of pulmonary infiltrates in immunocompromised patients. Chest. 1995;107:101–6.
73. Matthay RA, Farmer WC, Odero D. Diagnostic fiberoptic bronchoscopy in the immunocompromised host with pulmonary infiltrates. Thorax. 1977; 32:539–45.
74. Puska S, Hutcheon MA, Hyland RH. Usefulness of transbronchial biopsy in immunosuppressed patients with pulmonary infiltrates. Thorax. 1983;38: 146–50.
75. Springmeyer SC, Silvestri RC, Sale GE, et al. The role of transbronchial biopsy for the diagnosis of diffuse pneumonias in immunocompromised marrow transplant recipients. Am Rev Respir Dis. 1982;126: 763–5.
76. Feldman NT, Pennington JE, Ehrie MG. Transbronchial lung biopsy in the compromised host. JAMA. 1977;238:1377–9.
77. Nishio JN, Lynch III JP. Fiberoptic bronchoscopy in the immunocompromised host: the significance of a nonspecific transbronchial biopsy. Am Rev Respir Dis. 1980;121:307–12.
78. Pennington JE, Feldman NT. Pulmonary infiltrates and fever in patients with hematologic malignancy. Assessment of transbronchial biopsy. Am J Med. 1977;62:581–7.
79. Shelhamer JH, Towes GB, Masur H, et al. Respiratory disease in the immunosuppressed patient. Ann Intern Med. 1992;117:415–31.
80. Mulabecirovic A, Gaulhofer P, Auner HW, et al. Pulmonary infiltrates in patients with hematological malignancies: transbronchial lung biopsy increases the diagnostic yield with respect to neoplastic and toxic pneumonitis. Ann Hematol. 2004; 83:420–2.
81. White P, Bonacum JT, Miller CB. Utility of fiberoptic bronchoscopy in bone marrow transplant patients. Bone Marrow Transplant. 1997;20:681–7.
82. Patel NR, Lee PS, Kim JH, Weinhouse GL, Koziel H. The influence of diagnostic bronchoscopy on clinical outcomes comparing adult autologous and allogenic bone marrow transplant patients. Chest. 2005;127:1388–96.
83. Peikert T, Rana S, Edell ES. Safety, diagnostic yield and therapeutic implications of flexible bronchoscopy in patients with febrile neutropenia and pulmonary infiltrates. Mayo Clin Proc. 2005;80:1414–20.
84. Shannon VR, Andersson BS, Lei X, Champlin RE, Kontoyiannis DP. Utility of early versus late fiberoptic bronchoscopy in the evaluation of new pulmonary infiltrates following hemopoietic stem cell transplantation. Bone Marrow Transplant. 2010; 45:647–55.
85. Dunagan DP, Baker AM, Hurd DD, Haponik EF. Bronchoscopic evaluation of pulmonary infiltrates following bone marrow transplantation. Chest. 1997; 111:135–41.
86. Poe RH, Utell MJ, Israel RH, Hall WJ, Eshleman JD. Sensitivity and specificity of non-specific transbronchial lung biopsy. Am Rev Respir Dis. 1979; 119:25–31.
87. Nisho JN, Lynch JP. Fiberoptic bronchoscopy in the immunocompromised host: the significance of a non-specific transbronchial biopsy. Am Rev Respir Dis. 1980;121:307–12.
88. Canham EM, Kennedy TC, Merrick TA. Unexplained pulmonary infiltrates in the compromised patient. An invasive investigation in a consecutive series. Cancer. 1983;52:325–9.
89. Kramer MR, Berkman N, Mintz B, et al. The role of open lung biopsy in the management and outcome of patients with diffuse lung disease. Ann Thorac Surg. 1998;65:198–202.
90. White DA, Wong PW, Downey R. The utility of open lung biopsy in patients with hematologic malignancies. Am J Respir Crit Care Med. 2000; 161:723–9.
91. Jaffe JP, Maki DG. Lung biopsy in immunocompromised patients: one institution's experience and an approach to management of pulmonary disease in the compromised host. Cancer. 1981;48:1144–53.
92. Catterall JR, Mccabe RE, Brooks RG, et al. Open lung biopsy in patients with Hodgkin's disease and pulmonary infiltrates. Am Rev Respir Dis. 1989; 139:1274–9.
93. Cockerill III FR, Wilson WR, Carpenter HA, et al. Open lung biopsy in immunocompromised patients. Arch Intern Med. 1985;145:1398–404.

94. Leight Jr GS, Michaelis LL. Open lung biopsy for the diagnosis of acute, diffuse pulmonary infiltrates in the immunosuppressed patient. Chest. 1978;73: 477–82.
95. Ellis ME, Spence D, Bouchama A, et al. Open lung biopsy provides a higher and more specific yield compared to bronchoalveolar lavage in immunocompromised patients. Scand J Infect Dis. 1995;27: 157–62.
96. oledo-pereyra LH, DeMeester TR, Kinealey A, et al. The benefits of open lung biopsy in patients with previous non-diagnostic transbronchial lung biopsy. A guide to appropriate therapy. Chest. 1980;77: 647–50.
97. Santamauro JT, Mangino DA, Stover DE. The lung in immunocompromised host: diagnostic methods. Respiration. 1999;66:481–90.
98. Miller RF, Leigh TR, Collins JV, Mitchell DM. Tess giving an etiological diagnosis in pulmonary disease in patients infected with the human immunodeficiency virus. Thorax. 1990;45:62–5.
99. Murray JF, Felton CP, Garay SM, et al. Pulmonary complications of the acquired immunodeficiency syndrome. N Engl J Med. 1984;310:1682–8.
100. Stover DE, White DA, Romano PA, Gellene RA. Diagnosis of pulmonary disease in acquired immune deficiency syndrome (AIDS). Role of bronchoscopy and bronchoalveolar lavage. Am Rev Respir Dis. 1984;130:659–62.
101. Harcup C, Baier HJ, Pitchenik AE. Evaluation of patients with the acquired immunodeficiency syndrome (AIDS) by flexible bronchoscopy. Endoscopy. 1985;17:217–20.
102. Broddus C, Dake MD, Stulbarg MS, et al. Bronchoalveolar lavage and transbronchial biopsy for diagnosis of pulmonary infections in the acquired immunodeficiency syndrome. Ann Intern Med. 1985;102:747–52.
103. Batungwanayo J, Taelman H, Lucas S, et al. Pulmonary disease associated with the human immunodeficiency virus in Kigali, Rawanda. A fiberoptic bronchoscopy study of 111 cases of undetermined etiology. Am J Respir Crit Care Med. 1994;149:1591–6.
104. Rosen MJ, Tow TW, Teirstein AS, Chuang MT, Marchevsky A, Bottone EJ. Diagnosis of pulmonary complications of acquired immunodeficiency syndrome. Thorax. 1985;40:571–5.
105. Eisner MD, Kaplan LD, Herndier B, Stulbarg MS. The pulmonary manifestations of AIDS related non-Hodgkin's lymphoma. Chest. 1996;110:729–36.
106. Ognibene FP, Steis RG, Macher AM, et al. Kaposi's sarcoma causing pulmonary infiltrates and respiratory failure in the acquired immunodeficiency syndrome. Ann Intern Med. 1985;102:471–5.
107. Meduri GU, Stover DE, Lee M, Myskowski PL, Caravelli JF, Zaman MB. Pulmonary Kaposi's sarcoma in the acquired immunodeficiency syndrome. Clinical, radiological, and pathological manifestations. Am J Med. 1986;81:11–8.
108. Suffredini AF, Ognibene FP, Lack EE, et al. Nonspecific interstitial pneumonitis: a common cause of pulmonary disease in the acquired immunodeficiency syndrome. Ann Intern Med. 1987;107:7–13.
109. Sattiler F, Nichols L, Hirano L, et al. Non-specific interstitial pneumonitis mimicking Pneumocystis carinii pneumonia. Am J Respir Crit Care Med. 1997;156:912–7.
110. Golden JA, Hollander H, Stulbarg MS, Gamsu G. Bronchoalveolar lavage as the exclusive diagnostic modality for pneumocystis carinii pneumonia. A prospective study among patients with acquired immunodeficiency syndrome. Chest. 1986;90:18–22.
111. Menon L, Patel R, Varadarajalu L, Sy E, Fuentes GD. Role of transbronchioal lung biopsy in HIV positive patients suspected to have Pneumocystis jirovecii pneumonia. J Bronchol. 2007;14:165–8.
112. Jules-Elysee KM, Stover DE, Zaman MB, Bernard EM, White DA. Aerosolized pentamidine: effect on diagnosis and presentation of Pneumocystis carinii pneumonia. Ann Intern Med. 1990;112:750–7.
113. Bonfils-Roberts EA, Nickodem A, Nealon TF. Retrospective analysis of the efficacy of open lung biopsy in acquired immunodeficiency syndrome. Ann Thorac Surg. 1990;49:115–7.
114. Trachiotis GD, Hafner GH, Hix WR, Aaron BL. Role of open lung biopsy in diagnosing pulmonary complications of AIDS. Ann Thorac Surg. 1992;54: 898–902.
115. Miller RF, Pugsley WB, Griffith MH. Open lung biopsy for investigation of acute respiratory episodes in patients with HIV infection and AIDS. Genitourin Med. 1995;71:280–5.
116. Fitzgerald W, Bevelaqua FA, Garay SM, Aranda CP. The role of open lung biopsy in patients with the acquired immunodeficiency syndrome. Chest. 1987;91:659–61.
117. Chhajed PN, Tamm M, Granville A. Role of flexible bronchoscopy in lung transplantation. Semin Respir Crit Care Med. 2004;25:413–23.
118. Glanville AR. Bronchoscopic monitoring after lung transplantation. Semin Respir Crit Care Med. 2010; 31:208–21.
119. Trulock EP, Ettinger NA, Brunt EM, Pasque MK, Kaiser LR, Cooper JD. The role of transbronchial biopsy in the treatment of lung transplant recipients. An analysis of 200 consecutive procedures. Chest. 1992;102:1049–54.
120. Hopkins PM, Aboyoun CL, Chhajed PN, et al. Prospective analysis of 1235 transbronchial lung biopsies in lung transplant recipients. J Heart Lung Transplant. 2002;21:1062–7.
121. McWilliams TJ, Williams TJ, Whitford HM, Snell GI. Surveillance bronchoscopy in lung transplant recipients: risk versus benefit. J Heart Lung Transplant. 2008;27:1203–9.
122. Valentine VG, Taylor DE, Dhillon GS, et al. Success of lung transplantation without surveillance bronchoscopy. J Heart Lung Transplant. 2002;21: 319–26.

123. Kesten S, Chamberlain D, Maurer J. Yield of surveillance transbronchial biopsies performed beyond two years after lung transplantation. J Heart Lung Transplant. 1996;15:384–8.
124. Tamm M, Sharples LD, Higenbottom TW, Stewart S, Wallwork J. Bronchiolitis obliterans syndrome in heart-lung transplantation: surveillance bronchoscopies. Am J Respir Crit Care Med. 1997;155: 1705–10.
125. Valentine VG, Gupta MR, Weill D, et al. Single-institution study evaluating the utility of surveillance bronchoscopy after lung transplantation. J Heart Lung Transplant. 2009;28:14–20.
126. Higenbottom T, Stewart S, Penketh A, Wallwork J. Transbronchial lung biopsy for the diagnosis of rejection in heart-lung transplant patients. Transplantation. 1988;46:532–9.
127. Scott JP, Fradet G, Smyth RL, et al. Prospective study of transbronchial biopsies in the management of heart-lung and single lung transplant patients. J Heart Lung Transplant. 1991;10:626–37.
128. Kukafka DS, O'Brien GM, Furukawa S, Criner GJ. Surveillance bronchoscopy in lung transplant recipients. Chest. 1997;111:377–81.
129. Chan CC, Abi-Saleh WJ, Arroliga AC, et al. Diagnostic yield and therapeutic impact of flexible bronchoscopy in lung transplant recipients. J Heart Lung Transplant. 1996;15:196–205.
130. Lehto JT, Koskinen PK, Anttila VJ, et al. Bronchoscopy in the diagnosis and surveillance of respiratory infections in lung and heart-lung transplant recipients. Transpl Int. 2005;18:562–71.
131. Sibley RK, Berry GJ, Tazelaar HD, et al. The role of transbronchial biopsies in the management of lung transplant recipients. J Heart Lung Transplant. 1993;12:308–24.
132. Aboyoun CL, Tamm M, Chhajed PN, et al. Diagnostic value of follow-up transbronchial lung biopsy after lung rejection. Am J Respir Crit Care Med. 2001;164:460–3.
133. Lee P, Minai O, Mehta AC, et al. Lung nodules in lung transplant recipients etiology and outcome. Chest. 2004;125:165–72.
134. Yousem SA, Paradis IL, Dauber JH, Griffith BP. Efficacy of transbronchial biopsy in the diagnosis of bronchiolitis obliterans in heart lung transplant recipients. Transplantation. 1989;47:893–5.
135. Kramer MR, Stoehr C, Whang JL, et al. The diagnosis of obliterative bronchiolitis after heart lung and lung transplantation: low yield of transbronchial biopsy. J Heart Lung Transplant. 1993;12:676–81.
136. Heng D, Sharples L, McNeil K, Stewart S, Wrenghitt T, Wallwork J. Bronchiolitis obliterans syndrome: incidence, natural history, prognosis and risk factors. J Heart Lung Transplant. 1998;17:1255–63.
137. Hopkins PM, Aboyoun CL, Chhajed PN, et al. Association of minimal rejection in lung transplant recipients with obliterative bronchiolitis. Am J Respir Crit Care Med. 2004;170:1022–6.
138. Glanville AR, Aboyoun CL, Havryk A, Plit M, Rainer S, Malouf M. Severity of lymphocytic bronchiolitis predicts long-term outcome after lung transplantation. Am J Respir Crit Care Med. 2008; 177:1033–40.
139. Burton CM, Iversen M, Scheike T, Carlsen J, Andersen CB. Is lymphocytic bronchiolitis a marker of acute rejection? An analysis of 2697 transbronchial biopsies after lung transplantation. J Heart Lung Transplant. 2008;27:1128–34.
140. Turner JS, Wilcox PA, Hayhurst MD, Potgieter PD. Fiberoptic bronchoscopy in the intensive care unit-a prospective study of 147 procedures in 107 patients. Crit Care Med. 1994;22:259–64.
141. Papin TA, Grum CM, Weg JG. Transbronchial biopsy during mechanical ventilation. Chest. 1986; 89:168–70.
142. Pincus PS, Kallenbach JM, Hurwitz MD, et al. Transbronchial biopsies during mechanical ventilation. Crit Care Med. 1987;15:1136–9.
143. Bulpa PA, Dive AM, Mertens L, et al. Combined bronchoalveolar lavage and transbronchial lung biopsy: safety and yield in ventilated patients. Eur Respir J. 2003;21:489–94.
144. O'Brien JD, Ettinger NA, Shevlin D, Kollef MH. Safety and yield of transbronchial biopsy in mechanically ventilated patients. Crit Care Med. 1997; 25:440–6.
145. Flabouris A, Myburgh J. The utility of open lung biopsy in patients requiring mechanical ventilation. Chest. 1999;115:811–7.
146. Warner DO, Warner MA, Divertie MB. Open lung biopsy in patients with diffuse pulmonary infiltrates and acute respiratory failure. Am Rev Respir Dis. 1988;137:90–4.
147. Koerner SK, Sakowitz AJ, Appelman RI, Becker NH, Schoenbaum SW. Transbronchial lung biopsies for the diagnosis of sarcoidosis. N Engl J Med. 1975;293:268–70.
148. Bilaceroglu S, Perim K, Gunel O, Cagirici U, Buyuksirin M. Combining transbronchial aspiration with endobronchial and transbronchial biopsy in sarcoidosis. Monaldi Arch Chest Dis. 1999;54:217–23.
149. Koontz CH. Lung biopsy in sarcoidosis. Chest. 1978;74:120–1.
150. Trisolini R, Lazzari AL, Cancellieri A, et al. Transbronchial needle aspiration improves the diagnostic yield of bronchoscopy in sarcoidosis. Sarcoidosis Vasc Diffuse Lung Dis. 2004;21: 147–51.
151. Shorr AF, Torrington KG, Hnatiuk OW. Endobronchial biopsy for sarcoidosis. A prospective study. Chest. 2001;120:109–14.
152. Leonard C, Tormey VJ, O'Keane C, Burke CM. Bronchoscopic diagnosis of sarcoidosis. Eur Respir J. 1997;10:2722–4.
153. Navani N, Booth HL, Kocjan G, et al. Combination of endobronchial ultrasound-guided transbronchial needle aspiration with standard bronchoscopic

techniques for the diagnosis of stage I and stage II pulmonary sarcoidosis. Respirology. 2011;16: 467–72.
154. Travis WD, Borok Z, Roum JH, et al. Pulmonary Langerhans cell granulomatosis (histiocytosis-X). A clinicopathological study of 48 cases. Am J Surg Pathol. 1993;17:971–86.
155. Housini I, Tomashefski JF, Cohen A, Crass A, Kleinerman J. Transbronchial biopsy in patients with pulmonary eosinophilic granuloma. Comparison with findings on open lung biopsy. Arch Pathol Lab Med. 1994;118:523–30.
156. Leslie KO, Gruden JF, Parish JM, Scholand MB. Transbronchial biopsy interpretation in the patient with diffuse parenchymal lung disease. Arch Pathol Lab Med. 2007;131:407–23.
157. Auerswald U, Barth J, Magnussen H. Value of CD-1 positive cells in bronchoalveolar lavage fluid for the diagnosis of pulmonary histiocytosis-X. Lung. 1991; 169:305–9.
158. Urban T, Lazor R, Lacronique J, et al. Pulmonary lymphangioleiomyomatosis. A study of 69 patients. Medicine. 1999;78:321–37.
159. Bonetti F, Chiodera PL, Pea M, et al. Transbronchial biopsy in lymphangiomyomatosis of the lung. HMB 45 for diagnosis. Am J Surg Pathol. 1993;17: 1092–102.
160. Torre O, Harari S. The diagnosis of cystic lung disease: a role for bronchoalveolar lavage and transbronchial biopsy? Respir Med. 2010;104: S81–5.
161. Epler GR, Colby TV, McLoud TC, Carrington CB, Gaensler EA. Bronchiolitis obliterans organizing pneumonia. N Engl J Med. 1985;312:152–8.
162. Cordier J-F. Cryptogenic organizing pneumonia. Clin Chest Med. 1993;14:677–92.
163. Bartter T, Irwin RS, Nash G, Balikian JP, Hollingsworth HH. Idiopathic bronchiolitis obliterans organizing pneumonia with peripheral infiltrates on chest roentgenogram. Arch Intern Med. 1989;149:273–9.
164. Azzam ZS, Bentur L, Rubin AH, Ben-Izhak O, Alroy G. Bronchiolitis obliterans organizing pneumonia. Diagnosis by transbronchial biopsy. Chest. 1993 ;104:1899–901.
165. Polpetti V, Cazzato S, Minicuci N, Zompatori M, Burzi M, Schiattone ML. The diagnostic value of bronchoalveolar lavage and transbronchial biopsy in cryptogenic organizing pneumonia. Eur Respir J. 1996;9:2513–6.
166. Cordier JF. Cryptogenic organizing pneumonia. Eur Respir J. 2006;28:422–46.
167. Coleman A, Colby TV. Histologic diagnosis of extrinsic allergic alveolitis. Am J Surg Pathol. 1988; 12:514–8.
168. Lacasse Y, Fraser RS, Fournier M, Cormier Y. Diagnostic accuracy of transbronchial biopsy in acute farmer's lung disease. Chest. 1997;112: 1459–65.
169. Gruden JF, Webb WR, Naidich DP, McGuinness G. Multinofdular disease: anatomic localization at thin section CT-multireader evaluation of a simple algorithm. Radiology. 1999;210:711–20.
170. Munk PL, Muller NL, Miller RR, Ostrow DN. Pulmonary lymphangitic carcinomatosis: CT and pathologic findings. Radiology. 1988;166:705–9.
171. Goldstein LS, Kavuru MS, Curtis-McCarthy P, Christie HA, Farver C, Stoller JK. Pulmonary alveolar proteinosis: clinical features and outcomes. Chest. 1998;114:1357–62.
172. Kim CH, Kim S, Kwon OJ, Han SK, Lee JS, Kim KY. Pulmonary diffuse alveolar septal amyloidosis–diagnosed by transbronchial lung biopsy. Korean J Intern Med. 1990;5:63–8.
173. Cale WF, Petsonk EL, Boyd CB. Transbronchial biopsy of pulmonary alveolar microlithiasis. Arch Intern Med. 1983;143:358–9.
174. Churg A. Transbronchial biopsy. Nothing to fear. Am J Surg Pathol. 2001;25:820–2.
175. Berbescue EA, Katzenstein AL, Snow JL, Zisman DA. Transbronchial biopsy in usual interstitial pneumonia. Chest. 2006;129:1126–31.
176. Wall CP, Gaensler EA, Carrington CB, Hayes JA. Comparison of transbronchial and open biopsies in chronic infiltrative lung diseases. Am Rev Respir Dis. 1981;123:280–5.
177. Wilson RK, Fechner RE, Greenberg SD, et al. Clinical implications of a non-specific transbronchial biopsy. Am J Med. 1978;65:252–6.
178. Churg A, Schwarz M. Transbronchial biopsy and usual interstitial pneumonia. A new paradigm? Chest. 2006;129:1117–8.
179. Raghu G, Collard HR, Egan JJ, et al. An official ATS/ERS/JRS/ALAT statement: idiopathic pulmonary fibrosis: evidence-based guidelines for diagnosis and management. Am J Respir Crit Care Med. 2011;183:788–824.
180. Lombard CM, Duncan SR, Rizk NW, Colby TV. The diagnosis of Wegener's granulomatosis from transbronchial biopsy specimens. Hum Pathol. 1990;21: 838–42.
181. Givens CD, Newman JH, McCurley TL. Diagnosis of Wegener's granulomatosis by trsnbronchial biopsy. Chest. 1985;88:794–6.
182. Schnabel A, Holl-Ulrich K, Dalhoff K, Reuter M, Gross WL. Efficacy of transbronchial biopsy in pulmonary vasculitides. Eur Respir J. 1997;10: 2738–43.
183. Kendell DM, Gal AA. Interpretation of tissue artifacts in transbronchial lung biopsy specimen. Ann Diagn Pathol. 2003;7:20–4.
184. Babiak A, Hetzel J, Krishna G, et al. Transbronchial cryobiopsy: a new tool for lung biopsies. Respiration. 2009;78:203–8.
185. Griff S, Ammenwerth W, Schonfeld N, et al. Morphometrical analysis of transbronchial cryobiopsies. Diagn Pathol. 2011;6:53.
186. Rial MB, Delgado MN, Sanmartin AP, et al. Multivariate study of predictive factors for clearly defined lesions without visible endobronchial lesions in transbronchial biopsies. Surg Endosc. 2010;24: 3031–6.

187. Herth FJH, Eberhardt R, Brcker HD, Ernst A. Endoscopic ultrasound guided transbronchial lung biopsy in fluoroscopically invisible solitary pulmonary nodules. A prospective study. Chest. 2006;129:147–50.
188. Wagner U, Walthers EM, Gelmetti W, Klose KJ, von Wichert P. Computer-tomograpghically guided fiberbronchoscopic transbronchial biopsy of small pulmonary lesions: a feasibility study. Respiration. 1996;63:181–6.
189. White CS, Weiner EA, Patel P, Britt J. Transbronchial needle aspiration. Guidance with CT fluoroscopy. Chest. 2000;118:1630–8.
190. Tsushima K, Sone S, Hanaoka T, Takayama F, Honda T, Kubo K. Comparison of bronchoscopic diagnosis for peripheral pulmonary nodule under fluoroscopic guidance with CT guidance. Respir Med. 2006; 100:737–45.
191. Ost D, Shah R, Anasco E, et al. A randomized trial of CT-fluoroscopic guided bronchoscopy vs conventional bronchoscopy in patients with suspected lung cancer. Chest. 2008;134:507–13.
192. Wrixon AD. New ICRP recommendations. J Radiol Prot. 2008;28:161–8.
193. Kurimoto N, Miyazawa T, Okimasa S, et al. Endobronchial ultrasound using a guide sheath increases the ability to diagnose peripheral lesions endoscopically. Chest. 2004;126:959–65.
194. Paone G, Nicastri E, Lucantoni G, et al. Endobronchial ultrasound-driven biopsy in the diagnosis of peripheral lung lesions. Chest. 2005;128:3551–7.
195. Eberhardt R, Ernst A, Herth FJF. Ultrasound-guided transbronchial biopsy of solitary pulmonary nodules less than 20 mm. Eur Respir J. 2009;34:1284–7.
196. Yoshikawa M, Sukoh N, Yamazaki K, et al. Diagnostic value of endobronchial ultrasonography with a guide sheath for peripheral pulmonary lesions without x-ray fluoroscopy. Chest. 2007;131:1788–93.
197. Roth K, Eagan TM, Andreassen AH, Leh F, Hardie JA. A randomized trial of endobronchial ultrasound guided sampling in peripheral lung lesions. Lung Cancer. 2011;74:219–25.
198. Gildea TR, Mazzone PJ, Karnak D, Meziane M, Mehta AC. Electromagnetic navigation bronchoscopy. A prospective study. Am J Respir Crit Care Med. 2006;174:982–9.
199. Eberhardt R, Anantham D, Herth F, Feller-Kopman D, Ernst A. Electromagnetic navigation diagnostic bronchoscopy in peripheral lung lesions. Chest. 2007;131:1800–5.
200. Makris D, Scherpereel A, Leroy S, et al. Electromagnetic navigation diagnostic bronchoscopy for small peripheral lung lesions. Eur Respir J. 2007;29:1187–92.
201. Mahajan AK, Patel S, Hogarth DK, Wightman R. Electromagnetic navigational bronchoscopy. An effective and safe approach to diagnose peripheral lung lesions unreachable by conventional bronchoscopy in high-risk patients. J Bronchology Interv Pulmonol. 2011;18:133–7.
202. Seijo LM, de Torres J, Lozano MD, et al. Diagnostic yield of electromagnetic navigation bronchoscopy is highly dependent on the presence of bronchus sign on CT imaging. Results from a prospective study. Chest. 2010;138:1316–21.
203. Lamprecht B, Porsch P, Wegleitner B, Strasser G, Kaiser B, Studnicka M. Electromagnetic navigation bronchoscopy (ENB): increasing diagnostic yield. Respir Med. 2012;106(5):710–5.
204. Shinagawa N, Yamazaki K, Onodera Y, et al. Virtual bronchoscopy navigation system shortens the examination time-feasibility study of virtual bronchoscopic navigation system. Lung Cancer. 2007;56: 201–6.
205. Tachihara M, Ishida T, Kanazawa K, et al. A virtual bronchoscopic navigation system under x-ray fluoroscopy for transbronchial diagnosis of small peripheral pulmonary lesions. Lung Cancer. 2007;2007:322–7.
206. Shinagawa N, Yamazaki K, Onodera Y, et al. CT-guided transbronchial biopsy using an ultrathin bronchoscope with virtual bronchoscopic navigation. Chest. 2004;125:1138–43.
207. Asano F, Matsuno Y, Shinagawa N, et al. A virtual bronchoscopic navigation system for pulmonary peripheral lesions. Chest. 2006;130:559–66.
208. Iwano S, Imaizumi K, Okada T, Hasegawa Y, Naganawa S. Virtual bronchoscopy-guided transbronchial biopsy for aiding the diagnosis of peripheral lung cancer. Eur J Cancer. 2011;79:155–9.
209. Omiya H, Kikuyama A, Kubo A, et al. A feasibility and efficacy study on bronchoscopy with a virtual navigation system. J Bronchology Interv Pulmonol. 2010;17:11–8.
210. Eberhardt R, Anantham D, Ernst A, Feller-Kopman D, Herth F. Multimodality bronchoscopic diagnosis of peripheral lung lesions. A randomized controlled trial. Am J Respir Crit Care Med. 2007;176: 36–41.
211. Asano F, Matsuno Y, Tsuzuku A, et al. Diagnosis of peripheral pulmonary lesions using a bronchoscope insertion guidance system combined with endobronchial ultrasonography with a guide sheath. Lung Cancer. 2008;60:366–73.
212. Ishida T, Asano F, Yamazaki K, et al. Virtual bronchoscopic navigation combined with endobronchial ultrasound to diagnose small peripheral pulmonary lesions: a randomized trial. Thorax. 2011;66: 1072–7.
213. Wahidi MM, Govert JA, Goudar RK, GouldMK MCDC. Evidence for the treatment of patients with pulmonary nodules: when is it lung cancer? ACCP evidence-based clinical practice guidelines (2nd edition). Chest. 2007;132:94S–107.
214. Huanqi L, Boiselle PM, Shepard JO, Trotman-Dickenson B, McCloud TC. Diagnostic accuracy and safety of CT-guided percutaneous needle aspiration biopsy of the lung: comparison of small and large pulmonary nodules. AJR Am J Roentgenol. 1996;167:105–9.

215. Ohano Y, Hatabu H, Takenaka D, et al. CT-guided transthoracic needle aspiration biopsy of small (≤20 mm) solitary pulmonary nodules. AJR Am J Roentgenol. 2003;180:1665–9.
216. Asano F, Aoe M, Ohsaki Y, et al. Deaths and complications associated with respiratory endoscopy: a survey by the Japan Society for respiratory endoscopy in 2010. Respirology. 2012;17(3): 478–85.
217. Pue CA, Pacht ER. Complications of fiberoptic bronchoscopy at a university hospital. Chest. 1995; 107:430–2.
218. Milman N, Fourschou P, Munch EP, Grode G. Trsnbronchial lung biopsy through fiberoptic bronchoscope. Results and complications in 452 examinations. Respir Med. 1994;88:749–53.
219. Cordasco EM, Mehta AC, Ahmad M. Bronchoscopically induced bleeding. A summary of nine years' Cleveland Clinic experience and review of literature. Chest. 1991;100:1141–7.
220. Pereira W, Kovnat DM, Snider GL. A prospective cooperative study of complications following flexible fiberoptic bronchoscopy. Chest. 1978;73: 813–6.

Transbronchial Needle Aspiration

3

Prasoon Jain, Edward F. Haponik,
A. Lukas Loschner, and Atul C. Mehta

Abstract

Transbronchial needle aspiration (TBNA) is a technique in which a cytology or histology specimen is obtained during flexible bronchoscopy from beyond the confines of the endobronchial tree. Mediastinal staging of lung cancer is the most common indication for TBNA. The procedure is also useful in diagnosis of sarcoidosis and tuberculosis as the cause of mediastinal lymph node enlargement. The procedure is performed under conscious sedation and does not need expensive guiding or tracking devices. The procedure is cost-effective, is easy to learn, and has an excellent safety record. Unfortunately, many bronchoscopists never adopted this technique in their practice due to lack of training and widespread misconceptions about the usefulness and safety issues. Endobronchial needle aspiration (EBNA) is a related technique in which the 22-gauge needle is used to obtain cytology specimen from endoscopically visible lesion. EBNA increases the diagnostic yield from submucosal and peribronchial lung tumors. Peripheral TBNA (P-TBNA) is a technique in which a cytology specimen is obtained from a suspected malignant peripheral lung nodule under fluoroscopic guidance. Addition of P-TBNA to conventional

P. Jain, M.B.B.S., M.D., F.C.C.P. (✉)
Pulmonary and Critical Care, Louis A Johnson
VA Medical Center, Clarksburg, WV 26301, USA
e-mail: prasoonjain.md@gmail.com

E.F. Haponik, M.D.
Pulmonary and Critical Care Medicine,
Wake-Forest School of Medicine, Winston-Salem,
NC, USA

A.L. Loschner, M.D.
Section of Pulmonary, Critical Care, Environmental
and Sleep, Carilion Clinic, Virginia Tech Carilion
School of Medicine, Roanoke, VA, USA

A.C. Mehta, M.B.B.S.
Respiratory Institute, Lerner College of Medicine,
Cleveland Clinic, Cleveland, OH 44195, USA

A.C. Mehta and P. Jain (eds.), *Interventional Bronchoscopy: A Clinical Guide*, Respiratory Medicine 10,
DOI 10.1007/978-1-62703-395-4_3, © Springer Science+Business Media New York 2013

sampling techniques improves diagnostic yield of bronchoscopy, especially in patients with Tsuboi type III or IV tumor bronchus relationship. The role of conventional TBNA has further become a topic of hot debates with the emergence of endobronchial ultrasound (EBUS)-guided TBNA. The authors believe that even in the era of EBUS-TBNA, the standard TBNA technique maintains an important position in the diagnosis and staging of lung cancer.

Keywords
Transbronchial needle aspiration • Mediastinal staging • Lung cancer staging • Endobronchial needle aspiration • Peripheral transbronchial needle aspiration

Introduction

Transbronchial needle aspiration (TBNA) is an important technique in which a cytology or histology specimen is obtained from beyond the confines of the endobronchial tree including mediastinal and hilar lymph nodes during flexible bronchoscopy [1]. Mediastinal staging of lung cancer is the most common indication for the procedure [2, 3]. In selected cases, it is also found useful in diagnosis of lung cancer, sarcoidosis, and tuberculosis [4, 5]. Although mediastinoscopy remains the gold standard for the mediastinal staging of lung cancer, TBNA staging has several intuitive advantages over the invasive surgical staging. Mediastinoscopy is performed under general anesthesia, whereas TBNA is performed under moderate sedation. TBNA is less costly, less invasive, and more comfortable for the patients than mediastinoscopy [6]. TBNA is an easy technique to learn and does not require any specialized equipment or guiding devices. A positive TBNA specimen obviates the need for mediastinoscopy or any additional invasive testing for staging of lung cancer.

Yet, several prior surveys have consistently shown considerable reluctance to embrace TBNA due to lack of training and unsubstantiated views regarding the safety and clinical usefulness of this technique [7, 8]. With recent availability of endobronchial ultrasound (EBUS)-TBNA, even those with a sound knowledge in this field have started to cast some doubts on the future of this technique.

In this chapter, we discuss the technique, clinical uses, and limitations of standard TBNA. One of our goals is to dispel some of the fears and hesitation that have prevented optimal clinical application of this technique. We discuss the current evidence on usefulness of TBNA in mediastinal staging of lung cancer, and its role in improving the diagnostic yield of bronchoscopy for visible lung cancers and peripheral lung nodules and masses. We also take this opportunity to highlight the circumstances in which EBUS-TBNA offers a clear advantage over the conventional TBNA technique.

Technique

Several reviews have addressed the technical aspects of TBNA procedure [9, 10]. In the following section, we briefly highlight the important aspects of the technique.

Chest Computed Tomography

TBNA involves sampling of an extra-luminal lymph node that is not visible to the operator. Therefore, it is essential for the operator to study the CT images for enlarged lymph nodes and their relationship to the airways and surrounding blood vessels before the procedure.

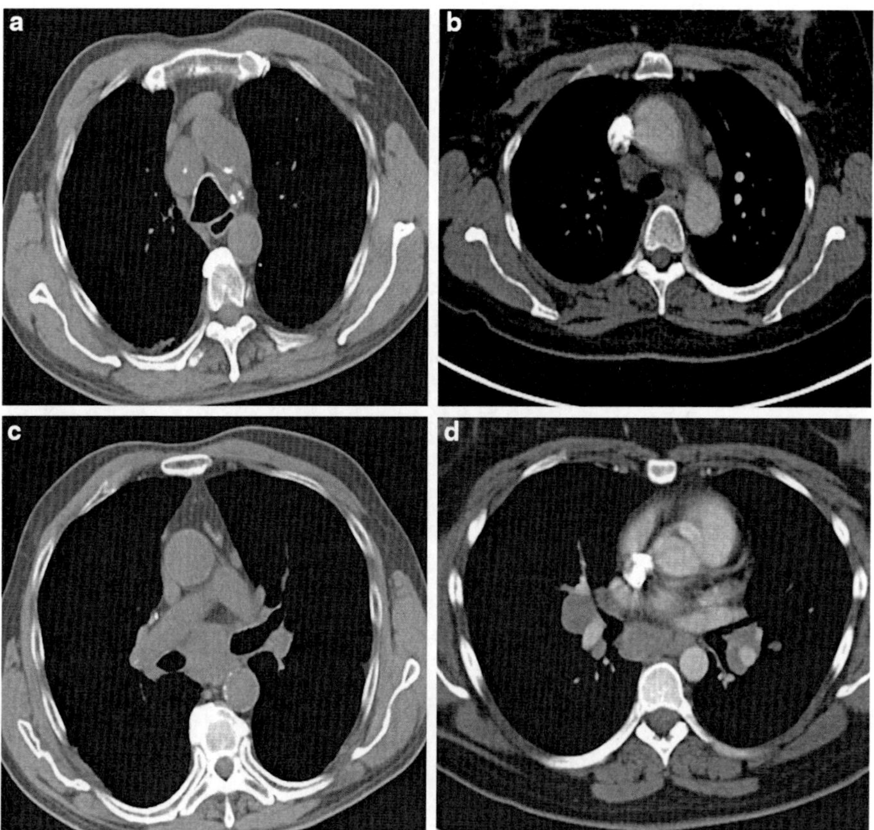

Fig. 3.1 CT images showing enlarged mediastinal lymph nodes. (**a**) Right paratracheal lymph node (station 4R). (**b**) Left paratracheal lymph node (station 4L). Aorto-pulmonary window lymph nodes (station 5) are also enlarged. Lymph nodes in station 5 cannot be accessed with TBNA. (**c**) Subcarinal lymph node (station 7). (**d**) Right interlobar lymph node (station 11R) and enlarged left interlobar lymph node (11L). Subcarinal lymph nodes are also enlarged

Once the lymph nodes are identified on the CT, the established anatomical endobronchial landmarks corresponding to the enlarged mediastinal and hilar lymph nodes guide the operator to select the appropriate site to puncture the airway. In this regard, carina is the most common landmark used to select the puncture site. Although a contrast-enhanced CT is more informative in this regard, a non-contrast CT is acceptable if contrast agent cannot be administered. In some studies PET/CT has been reported to improve the sensitivity and negative predictive value of TBNA for mediastinal staging of lung cancer [11, 12]. However, from technical standpoint, PET/CT has no advantage over chest CT in directing the operator to the target lymph nodes.

Traditionally, clinicians have used Mountain and Dressler's mapping system on CT to classify different groups of enlarged mediastinal and hilar lymph nodes [13]. Recently, International Association for Study of Lung Cancer (IASLC) has proposed modified lymph node definitions on the CT, which are adopted in the seventh edition of the TMN classification for lung cancer [14]. The clinicians should now follow IASLC definitions to identify the enlarged lymph node stations in lung cancer patients (see Fig. 5.1). Conventional TBNA method is most suitable for sampling of lymph nodes from 4R, 4L, and 7 that define N2 or N3 disease and 10R, 10L, 11R, and 11L stations that define N1 disease. Common lymph node stations that can be accessed by TBNA are illustrated in Fig. 3.1. One must note

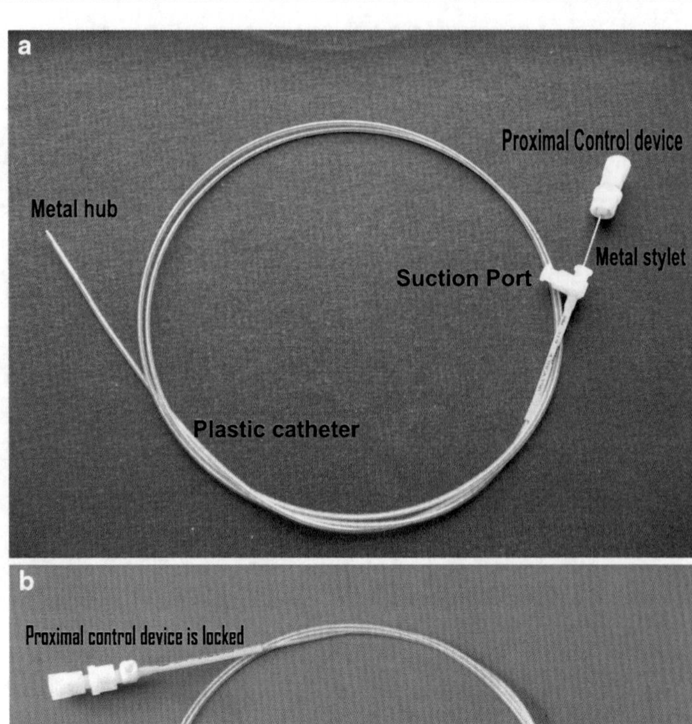

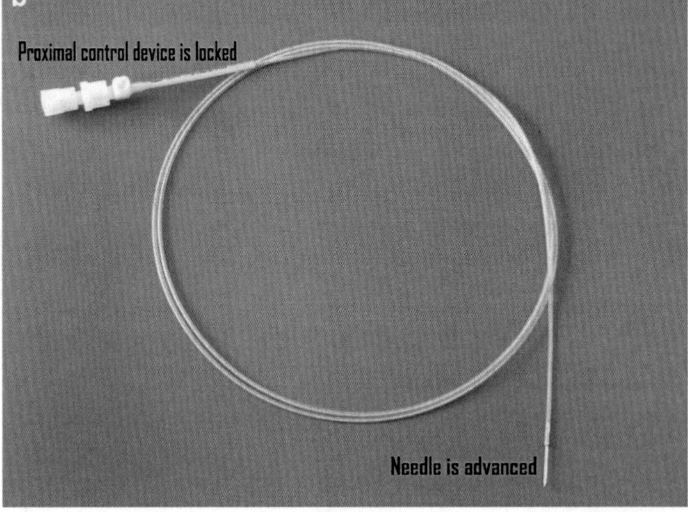

Fig. 3.2 (**a**) MW-222 needle with distal 22-g needle fully within metal hub. Make sure that the needle is fully housed within the metal hub as the catheter is passing through the working channel. (**b**) The proximal control device is advanced and locked in place to deploy the TBNA needle

that lymph nodes in aorto-pulmonary window (station 5) that are lateral to the ligamentum arteriosum and medial to the origin of first branch of the left pulmonary artery cannot be sampled through TBNA. Enlarged 2R and 2L lymph nodes are accessible with TBNA, but due to proximity of surrounding vessels, it is preferable to use EBUS-TBNA to obtain specimens from these stations. Besides, sampling of the abnormalities from this location may lead to over-staging by misinterpreting lung lesion with mediastinal lymph nodes.

TBNA Needles

Several types of TBNA needles are available. The choice of TBNA needle is a matter of personal preference. Of greater importance is familiarity with the needles used for the procedures. A 22-gauge TBNA needle (MW-222) is most commonly used for obtaining a cytology specimen (Fig. 3.2a, b). It has a distal, retractable, sharp beveled 13-mm needle. When fully retracted, the sharp end of the needle is housed within a metal hub. The needle can be advanced

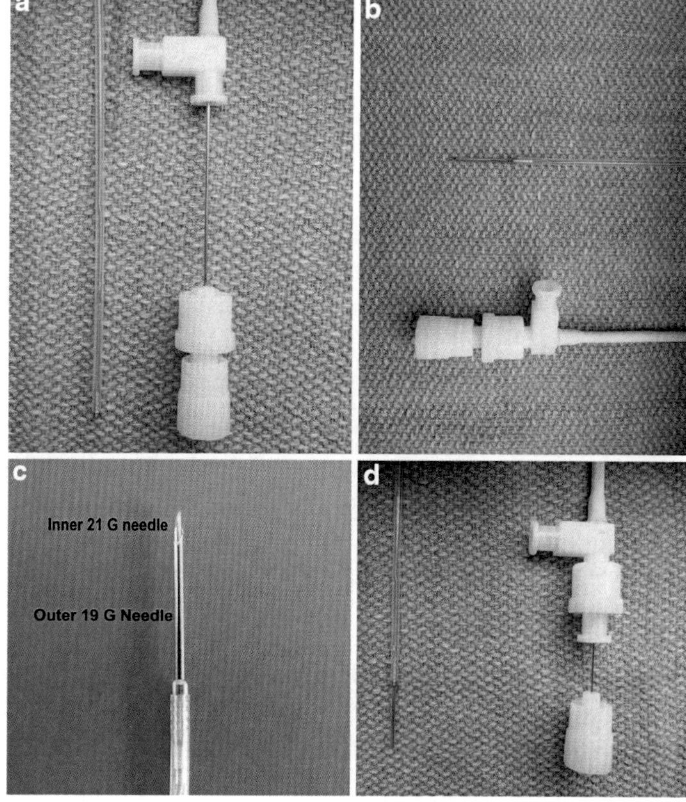

Fig. 3.3 MW-319 needle: (**a**) Both 19-gauge and 21-gauge needles within the catheter. (**b**) Both needles are advanced and locked. (**c**) Close-up of outer 19-gauge and inner 21-gauge needle. (**d**) 21-gauge needle is retracted back

and retracted by the proximal control device. The outer diameter of the clear plastic catheter is 1.9 mm. It can be passed through bronchoscopes with working channels of 2.2 mm or larger. The catheter is made stiff with a metal stylet that runs through the catheter. The stiffness of catheter prevents the plastic catheter from kinking and bending while trying to penetrate the needle through the tracheal wall. The suction is applied through the proximal suction port using a 20- or 50-cc syringe.

The histology specimen requires the use of a 19-gauge TBNA needle [15]. MW-319 is a commonly used needle for this purpose (Fig. 3.3a–d). It consists of a 19-gauge retractable, beveled needle, housed within a metal hub. When fully deployed, the 19-g needle projects 15 mm beyond the distal end of the metal hub. The proximal end of the needle is attached to a hollow spring, which runs through the length of the catheter and controls the movement of the 19-g needle. Another 21-gauge beveled needle is housed within the 19-gauge needle. It projects 3 mm beyond the distal end of 19-gauge needle when fully deployed. The proximal end of the 21-gauge needle is attached to a guide wire that lies inside the lumen of the hollow spring. The 21-gauge needle acts as a trocar for the larger 19-gauge needle and prevents its plugging by bronchial tissue and cartilage. To obtain a histology specimen, both 19-gauge and 21-gauge needles are advanced into the target site. The 21-gauge needle penetrates the airways and anchors the catheter into the intended lymph node. Suction is applied to confirm that catheter is not in a major vessel. At this time, the 21-gauge needle is drawn back and the core tissue is obtained by partially moving the 19-gauge needle in and out of the lymph node a few times while maintaining constant suction with the syringe. Both needles are then retracted and the TBNA catheter is withdrawn from the bronchoscope to retrieve the specimen. The operational aspects of this needle are somewhat cumbersome and complicated. Recent experience indicates that single-lumen 19-gauge TBNA

(MWF-319) needles are equally successful in obtaining a histology specimen and are easier to use than MW-319.

Planning

All TBNA procedures should be preceded by a thorough clinical evaluation. It is a common practice to obtain tissue sample from the mediastinal lymph nodes for staging prior to that from the primary tumor for the diagnosis during the initial diagnostic bronchoscopy. All sampling procedures and their sequence must be discussed with the assistant prior to bronchoscopy so that all accessory instruments needed during bronchoscopy are kept in readiness. For staging TBNA, it is useful to have slides labeled prior to the procedure to avoid any confusion as to the lymph node station from which the specimen is obtained. Nodes associated with the highest staging should be sampled before nodal stations associated with lower staging. Therefore, depending on the location of primary tumor, the N3 nodes should be sampled before N2 nodes, and the N2 nodes should be sampled before N1 nodes. This practice prevents contamination of higher stations from tumor cells obtained from the lower ones using a single needle for the entire procedure.

To avoid inadvertent damage to the working channel, the operator must make sure that the beveled end of the needle is housed fully within the distal metal hub before the TBNA catheter is introduced into the working channel of the bronchoscope. Proper and smooth deployment of needle must be ensured prior to every TBNA attempt. A kinked or damaged TBNA needle should be replaced.

Procedure

Nasal route is recommended for bronchoscopy as much as possible. Compared to oral route, the bronchoscope is held more firmly when it is introduced through the nose. Less movement during the TBNA procedure increases the accuracy with which the bronchoscopist is able to puncture the desired endobronchial site. The operator must keep the insertion tube and the bending section of the bronchoscope as straight as possible during insertion of TBNA catheter through the working channel to prevent any inadvertent damage to the scope. Suction through the working channel of the bronchoscope should be avoided prior to performing staging of TBNA to minimize the risk of false positive results from contamination with respiratory secretions. Secretions overlying the puncture site may be washed away using sterile saline solution. TBNA should always be performed before a detailed airway inspection or any other sampling procedure in order to avoid contamination of the working channel with malignant cells present in the endobronchial secretion. TBNA catheter should be advanced into the endobronchial tree while keeping the tip of the bronchoscope in the neutral forward-viewing position.

The puncture sites for common lymph node stations are illustrated in Fig. 3.4 a–e. Once the target site for puncture is identified, the TBNA catheter is advanced beyond the distal end of the bronchoscope. It is important to clearly visualize the distal metal hub before the TBNA needle is deployed. However, only a few millimeters of catheter should be advanced beyond the tip of the bronchoscope (Fig. 3.5). In this fashion working channel of the bronchoscope is used to splint the TBNA catheter. The catheter must be retracted if excessive length is seen to project beyond the distal end of the bronchoscope. Failure to do so will kink the catheter during the procedure. Penetration of the needle into the target area and aspiration of material from the lymph node may not be feasible once the distal end of TBNA catheter is kinked during the procedure.

The needle should be deployed through the inter-cartilaginous space. Several techniques used to insert the needle into the airway wall are described in Table 3.1 and illustrated in Fig. 3.6. In the absence of any comparative studies, the choice of technique is strictly a matter of personal choice. A combination of techniques may be needed in some cases. Regardless, one must maintain the TBNA needle as perpendicular, minimum at 45° angle to the airway wall as

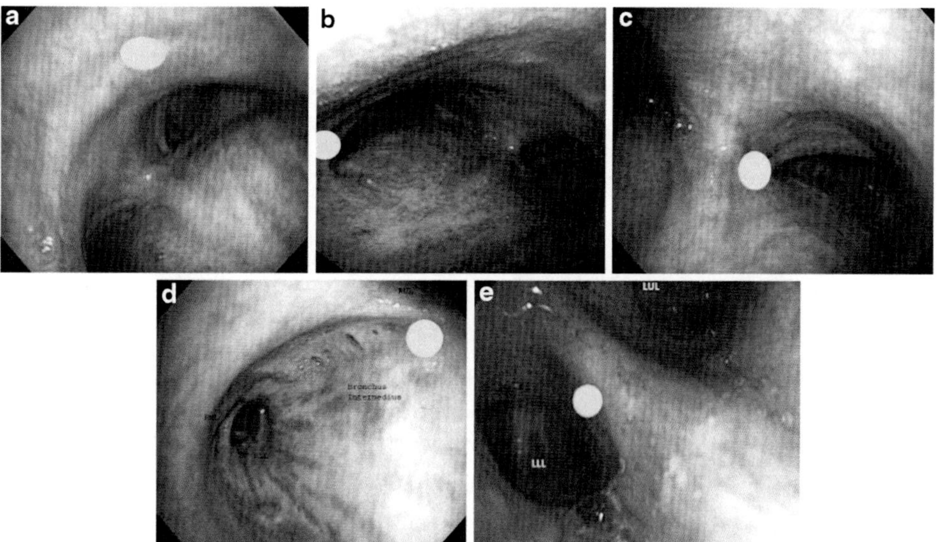

Fig. 3.4 (**a**) TBNA site for station 4R is about 2 cm above main carina in second or third intercartilaginous space between 1 and 2 o'clock position. Do not insert needle at 3 o'clock position to avoid azygos vein. (**b**) TBNA site for station 4L is at lateral wall of trachea and left main bronchus at the level of carina at 9 o'clock position. (**c**) TBNA site for station 7 lymph nodes is 3–5 mm below either side of the primary carina with the needle pointing in inferomedial direction. (**d**) TBNA site for the 11R lymph nodes is immediately below the origin of right upper lobe bronchus at 3 o'clock position on lateral wall of bronchus intermedius. (**e**) TBNA site for 11L lymph nodes is the secondary carina between *left upper* and *lower* lobe bronchus at 12–2 o'clock position

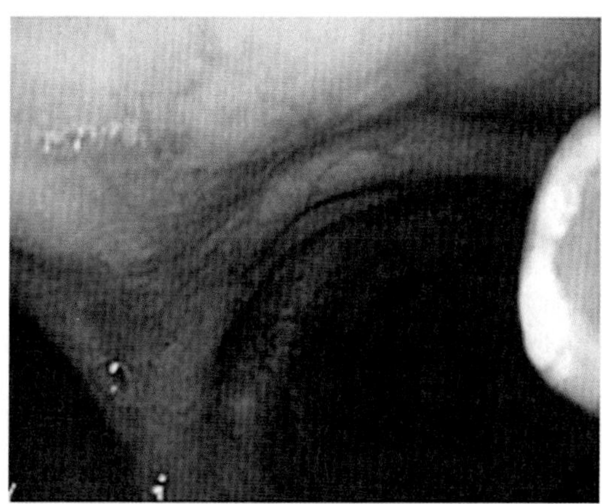

Fig. 3.5 The distal metal hub should be visible before the TBNA needle is deployed

possible to maximize the chances of needle reaching the core of the target lymph node (Fig. 3.7).

It is critical to make sure that the entire length of TBNA needle has penetrated the airway wall and the metal hub is flushed against the airway mucosa (Fig. 3.8). Once confirmed, the assistant is requested to apply the suction using the syringe. In some instances a pink-colored fluid may be seen to enter the clear plastic catheter. This usually represents material from the lymph node. With suction maintained, the operator vigorously moves the TBNA catheter to and fro into the lymph node while making sure that needle is not pulled out of the lymph node and the airway wall. After a few seconds, the assistant is instructed to release the suction and retract the needle back into the catheter. It is important to release the suction before the needle is withdrawn from the lymph node. Failure to do so may contaminate the TBNA sample with the airway secretions, thereby increasing the risk of false positive results. The distal end of the bronchoscope should be straightened as the TBNA catheter is withdrawn from the endobronchial tree.

Puncture of a blood vessel is implied if blood is seen to fill the catheter as soon as suction is applied. In this event, the bronchoscopy assistant should release the suction and withdraw the needle back into the catheter.

Table 3.1 Different techniques used for insertion of TBNA needle into airway wall

Jabbing method
• Once the tip of TBNA catheter is seen, advance the needle fully in the central airway
• Retract most of the catheter and part of needle back into working channel. Needle tip should be clearly visible
• Advance the bronchoscope and needle towards the intended puncture site
• Position the needle perpendicular to airway wall
• Hold bronchoscope stationary at nose or mouth
• Thrust the catheter forward into the target
Hub against the wall method
• With TBNA needle fully retracted, advance the metal hub through the distal end of bronchoscope
• Place the hub against the intended puncture site at a 90° angle
• Hold bronchoscope stationary at nose or mouth
• Instruct the assistant to deploy the TBNA needle
Piggyback method
• Position the bronchoscope close to the intended puncture site
• Advance the catheter till distal metal hub is seen
• Deploy the needle and lock it in place
• Stabilize the TBNA catheter at the biopsy port of the working channel using little finger
• Advance the bronchoscope and the TBNA needle en block into the target area at a 90° angle
Cough method
• Position the bronchoscope close to the intended puncture site
• Deploy the TBNA needle
• Stabilize the TBNA catheter at biopsy port
• Instruct the patient to cough. The inward movement of airway wall towards the needle facilitates the insertion

Number of Passes

The diagnostic yield of TBNA is related to the number of TBNA attempts made per lymph node station. In a prospective study, Chin and coworkers studied the number of passes on each lymph node station to achieve optimal yield from TBNA [16]. The authors found first sample to be diagnostic in 42% of patients. No further diagnoses were made after the seventh TBNA. Overall, 93% of diagnostic aspirates were obtained with 4 passes at a single nodal station. For lymph nodes larger than 2 cm in short axis, diagnosis of malignancy could be established in 92% of cases with initial two aspirates. The authors suggested at least 4 passes in a single nodal station and up to 7 passes to maximize yield in mediastinal staging of lung cancer. In another study, the diagnostic yields with the first, second, third, and fourth passes were 64, 85, 95, and 98%, respectively [17]. The authors suggested three TBNA passes to establish tissue diagnosis and 4–5 TBNA passes for mediastinal staging of lung cancer. We usually make 3–4 passes at every lymph node station to optimize our yield.

Specimen Collection and Interpretation

Proper handling of specimen by a trained assistant is a critical aspect of the procedure and is shown to improve diagnostic yield of TBNA. Direct method is the preferred method for submitting the cytology specimen. In this method the slides are prepared directly from the TBNA aspirate in the bronchoscopy room. Using air from the empty syringe used to aspirate the specimen, the TBNA aspirate is placed onto a slide, covered with a second slide and with gentle pressure, the slides are drawn apart. A thin smear forms on both the slides, which are immediately fixed in 95% alcohol solution or commercially available spray fixative. Any delay in this process leads to difficulties in interpretation due to development of drying artifacts.

Some bronchoscopists use fluid technique in which no slides are made and the TBNA aspirate is submitted to the cytology laboratory in 95% alcohol, to be processed in a standard fashion. In a prospective study the diagnostic yield was significantly lower with this method than with the direct technique of processing TBNA aspirate [18]. Based on these results, there is little reason to use fluid technique in preference to the direct method.

The specimen obtained with the histology needle should be submitted in formalin. Any visible tissue piece obtained with cytology needle should also be removed gently and placed in formalin solution. The leftover specimen within the

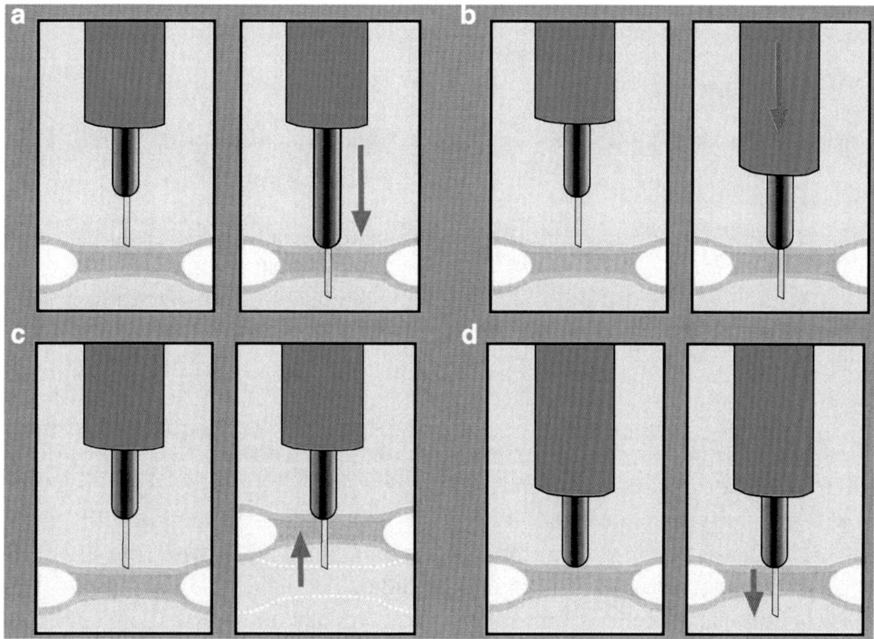

Fig. 3.6 Different techniques used for insertion of TBNA needle into the airway wall. (**a**) Jabbing method. (**b**) Piggyback method. (**c**) Cough method. (**d**) Hub against the wall method

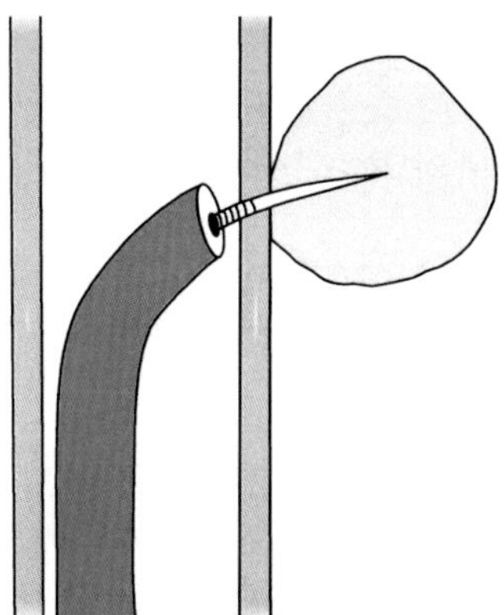

Fig. 3.7 TBNA needle should approach the airway wall close to a 90° angle

TBNA needle and catheter should be flushed into a container with normal saline, to be used in the laboratory for cell block preparation.

Careful interpretation of the specimen is mandatory for optimal application of TBNA technique. An adequate specimen obtained from the lymph node should have preponderance of lymphocytes and few if any bronchial epithelial cells.

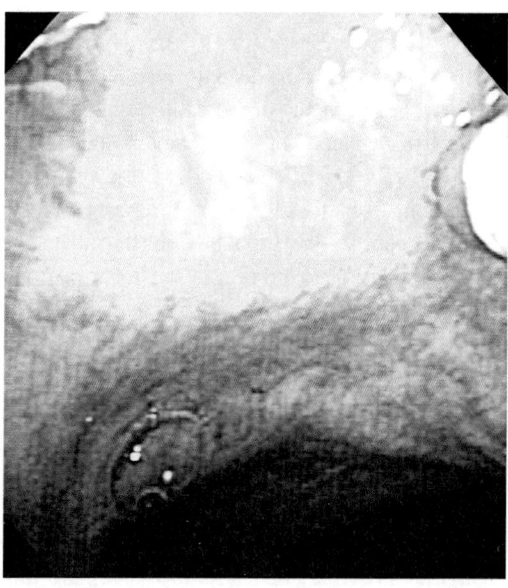

Fig. 3.8 The entire needle is seen to penetrate airway wall and metal hub is flushed against the wall

Even with lymphocytes present, it is critical to interpret both positive as well as negative TBNA results with utmost caution. TBNA has a low negative predictive value in staging of lung

Table 3.2 Measures to reduce chances of false positive results

• Perform TBNA before airway examination or other sampling procedure
• Do not apply suction until TBNA specimens are obtained
• Wash the target area with saline
• Obtain specimen from higher lymph node stations first. So, aspirate N3 before N2 and N2 before N1 stations
• Release suction before withdrawing the needle from the lymph node
• Obtain histology specimen as much as possible

Table 3.3 Factors associated with positive TBNA results

• Malignant disease
• Small-cell lung cancer
• Right paratracheal and subcarinal location
• Size of lymph node
• Use of histology needle
• Direct method of preparing slides
• High SUV value on PET scan
• Skills and experience of the operator and the assistant

cancer. Therefore, surgical staging is always indicated if a TBNA aspirate from mediastinal lymph nodes does not show malignant cells. On the other hand, a TBNA aspirate with clumps of malignant cells is diagnostic for lymph node metastasis and obviates the need for further staging procedures. However, the presence of an occasional malignant cell in the TBNA specimen is an insufficient evidence of lymph node metastasis. Any ambiguity in this regard needs further clarification with additional testing. Incorrect staging due to false positive TBNA has serious implications as it may lead to an inappropriate denial of lung cancer surgery. Although it is reassuring to note that most studies have found TBNA to have 100% specificity for detection of lymph node metastasis, there are a few reports of false positive results. The bronchoscopists must take every precaution to minimize the false positive TBNA results (Table 3.2).

Factors Associated with Positive Results

Studies have consistently reported a higher yield from TBNA for lung cancer as compared to a benign disorder such as sarcoidosis [2]. Among malignant diagnoses, TBNA has a higher sensitivity for small-cell lung cancer than for non-small-cell lung cancers [19]. The diagnostic yield of TBNA increases with increase in the size of the lymph nodes. Other factors associated with a higher TBNA yield are listed in Table 3.3 [20, 21].

Complications

TBNA is a safe technique with a complication rate of 0.3% [22]. Bleeding after TBNA procedure is usually minor and insignificant. Rarely, pneumothorax [23], pneumomediastinum, and hemomediastinum [24] have been reported after the procedure. A single case of purulent pericarditis has been reported after TBNA [25]. There are no reports of procedure-related deaths.

Clinical Applications

Staging of Lung Cancer

The principal use of TBNA is in mediastinal staging of lung cancer. Common lymph node stations such as 4R, 4L, and seven that frequently harbor the malignant cells and define N2 or N3 disease are easily accessible with TBNA. Identification of tumor cells in the TBNA specimen from these lymph nodes precludes the need for further invasive procedures, paving way for prompt initiation of nonoperative treatments. Sampling from hilar lymph nodes (stations 10, 11) is also feasible as discussed above but the presence of tumor in this location defines N1 disease that does not influence the decision to perform curative surgical resection.

In a meta-analysis, TBNA had a sensitivity of 39% and a specificity of 99% for mediastinal staging in patients with 34% prevalence of mediastinal metastasis. However, the sensitivity was

78% in studies in which the prevalence of mediastinal metastasis was 81% [22]. In another systemic review, the sensitivity and specificity of TBNA for lymph node staging were 76 and 96%, respectively, in patients with 70% prevalence of mediastinal metastasis [26]. TBNA is a convenient, cost-effective, and less invasive alternative to mediastinoscopy for staging of lung cancer [3, 27]. However, one must interpret the results with caution when the TBNA specimen does not show malignant cells and when insufficient material is obtained. The average negative predictive value of TBNA is 71% [26] but it depends on the prevalence of cancer in the lymph nodes. In one series, the negative predictive value of TBNA was only 40% for mediastinal lymph node metastasis [28]. Therefore, as a general rule, a negative TBNA does not exclude mediastinal spread of tumor and further testing is warranted before offering a curative lung cancer surgery to these patients. Although mediastinoscopy has been a traditional next step, recent studies indicate that EBUS-TBNA may be a reasonable alternative for this purpose.

Restaging of Lung Cancer

There is limited data on the usefulness of TBNA in restaging of mediastinal nodes after chemo-radiation therapy in stage IIIA NSCLC. In a small study, 14 patients with stage IIIA NSCLC had restaging of mediastinal lymph nodes with TBNA after chemotherapy or chemo-radiation therapy. The accuracy of TBNA was 71% and mediastinoscopy was avoided in 5 (36%) patients [29]. Recent experience appears to indicate that EBUS-TBNA is better than standard TBNA for this indication. For example, in one study, EBUS-TBNA had a sensitivity, specificity, and accuracy of 76, 100, and 77%, respectively, for restaging of mediastinum after induction chemotherapy. However, due to low negative predictive value, surgical staging is still indicated whenever EBUS-TBNA sample from mediastinal lymph nodes does not reveal malignant cells in these patients [30].

Diagnosis of Lung Cancer

In many instances, the tissue sampling from primary lung mass or nodule is non-diagnostic but the TBNA sample from the mediastinal or hilar lymph node provides the tissue diagnosis. In some reports, TBNA is found to be the sole method of tissue diagnosis in as many as 18–25% of patients with parenchymal lesions on initial bronchoscopy [3, 19, 27, 31]. TBNA obviates the need for further diagnostic as well as staging procedures in these patients.

TBNA is a suitable technique for tissue diagnosis in patients presenting with superior vena cava (SVC) syndrome secondary to lung cancer. In a prospective study, 27 patients with SVC syndrome underwent bronchoscopy with TBNA from right paratracheal and other accessible lymph nodes using a 22-gauge cytology needle [32]. Tissue diagnosis could be established in 96% of patients with the TBNA specimen. In 82% of patients with NSCLC and 47% of patients with small-cell lung cancer, TBNA was the exclusive source of diagnostic specimen. No procedure-related complications were encountered.

Sarcoidosis

The overall diagnostic yield of TBNA in sarcoidosis has varied from 53 to 94% in different series [33, 34]. For this indication, multiple EBB, TBBx, and TBNA samples should be obtained to maximize the diagnostic yield of bronchoscopy. With this approach, the diagnosis can be confirmed in >90% of sarcoidosis patients, with TBNA providing exclusive diagnosis in 20–60% of cases [33, 35]. TBNA sampling of two separate lymph node stations is shown to be associated with a higher likelihood of establishing this diagnosis [34]. The yield of TBNA is found to be higher for stage I sarcoidosis than for stage II sarcoidosis in some [33] but not in all studies [34]. Although some authors have achieved excellent results with Wang 22-gauge cytology needle [36], the majority of authors prefer a 19-gauge TBNA needle to obtain a histology core specimen for a more confident diagnosis.

EBUS-TBNA is emerging as an important diagnostic tool for sarcoidosis with a diagnostic sensitivity of 85% in stage I and II sarcoidosis in a recent report [37]. In a randomized study, the overall diagnostic yield of EBUS-TBNA for sarcoidosis was 83.3%, compared to 53.8% yield from conventional TBNA [38]. However, even though EBB and TBB were performed in <50% of patients in this study, the overall diagnostic yield of bronchoscopy and the exclusive yields of TBNA for sarcoidosis were similar in both groups. Based on these data, it is reasonable to conclude that EBUS-TBNA is preferable to conventional TBNA in suspected sarcoidosis if EBB and TBBx are not performed during bronchoscopy.

Tuberculosis

TBNA has a proven role in diagnosis of intrathoracic tuberculous lymphadenitis. In one study, 84 HIV-negative patients with mediastinal lymph node enlargement underwent TBNA with 19-gauge histology needle [39]. The pre-bronchoscopy sputum samples were negative for acid-fast bacilli in all subjects. The sensitivity, specificity, positive and negative predictive values, and accuracy for the diagnosis of tuberculosis were 83, 100, 100, 38 and 85% respectively. TBNA provided immediate diagnosis in 78% and was the exclusive source of diagnosis in 68% of patients. Furthermore, the acid-fast bacilli were isolated by culture of TBNA specimen in 27% of patients. In another study, the diagnosis of tuberculosis could be established in 65% of patients with the 22-gauge TBNA needle in 20 patients with tubercular mediastinal lymphadenitis [36].

TBNA is also useful in diagnosis of mediastinal lymph node tuberculosis in HIV-infected patients. The utility of TBNA with 19-gauge histology needle was studied in 41 HIV-infected patients with mediastinal and hilar lymphadenopathy [40]. Overall and exclusive diagnostic yields of TBNA were 52 and 32%, respectively. Mycobacterial disease was diagnosed with TBNA in 20 of 23 (87%) of the study patients. Immediate diagnosis was achieved in 74% of patients, culture was positive in 61% of patients, and exclusive diagnosis was achieved with TBNA in 48% of patients with lymph node tuberculosis.

Recent studies have also reported high diagnostic yield with EBUS-TBNA for patients with isolated tubercular mediastinal lymphadenitis [41, 42]. No comparison between standard TBNA and EBUS-TBNA has been reported in the medical literature for these patients.

Limitations and Controversies

"Blind Technique"

The most critical limitation of standard TBNA technique is the inability to visualize the mediastinal lymph node in real time during the procedure. Due to this reason, some authors have called conventional TBNA a "blind" technique. In reality, neither the operator nor the procedure is blind. The puncture site is chosen after a careful review of the chest CT and the operator is aware of the location of lymph nodes in relation to the airways. Certainly, a successful puncture of lymph node requires a thorough review of CT anatomy, technical skills, and confidence. Still, as tracheobronchial tree is surrounded by systemic and pulmonary vessels, many bronchoscopists have remained skeptical about the procedural safety even though the reports of bleeding and mediastinal hemorrhage after TBNA have been limited to a handful of case reports. Nevertheless, misconstrued view regarding its safety has played an important role in underutilization of this technique.

Blood vessels bear a fixed relationship to the airways. Safe landmarks to perform TBNA for various stations have already been established [43]. Station 7, one of the most common sites of TBNA, has no surrounding blood vessels. Similarly, TBNA from station 4R has an excellent safety record especially in the presence of large sized lymph nodes. One must concede that inability to visualize the targets does pose some difficulties in approaching small lymph nodes located in 2R, 2L, and some hilar stations.

Several options have been explored over the past two decades to circumvent this limitation of standard TBNA technique. Some investigators have used CT-fluoroscopy for real-time guidance during TBNA procedure. Although technical success could be achieved in nearly 80% of patients [44, 45], it was never adopted in mainstream bronchoscopy practice due to the radiation safety issues, logistic difficulties, and emergence of superior alternatives to achieve the same goal. Another approach is electromagnetic navigation bronchoscopy (ENB) to localize the lymph nodes for TBNA sampling. This technique is mainly employed for obtaining biopsy from small peripheral lung nodules [46–48]. However, it can also direct the operators to the mediastinal lymph nodes with a high degree of accuracy. Gildea and coworkers reported 100% success in obtaining adequate sample from 31 lymph node stations using this technique. The average lymph node size in this study was 2.8 cm. In another study, adequate sampling was possible with this technique in 94.3% of mediastinal lymph nodes with an average size of 1.8 cm [49]. Notwithstanding, in the absence of a control group, these data only establish the feasibility but not the superiority of EMN-guided TBNA over the conventional TBNA technique. An important but yet unanswered question of great importance is whether this technique is better than conventional TBNA in obtaining specimens from small mediastinal lymph nodes. High cost of equipment and accessories is another relevant issue surrounding this technique [50].

Another approach is to use data from pre-procedural multi-detector CT to develop virtual bronchoscopy images to guide TBNA procedure. In this technique, the virtual bronchoscopy images are displayed on the screen during actual bronchoscopy and the target is displayed through the semitransparent wall to guide the bronchoscopist during TBNA procedure. In one study, the diagnostic yield of TBNA from paratracheal and hilar nodes was increased from 69% with standard technique to 100% with virtual bronchoscopy-directed technique. The yield from subcarinal nodes was similar with either method [51]. Another CT bronchoscopic simulation software has been developed that not only displays the target lesion behind a transparent wall but also shows the most appropriate virtual needle path to the target in order to avoid the blood vessels and other vulnerable structures. In a prospective study, TBNA was performed sequentially without and with the assistance of this software in 28 patients with 50 lymph node targets [52]. The mean size of lymph nodes was 14 mm. The success rate of TBNA with CT bronchoscopic simulation was 58%, whereas the success rate was 30% with the conventional technique. Although CT-bronchoscopic simulation is not a real-time guidance system, it certainly has some appeal as there is no need for additional sensing and tracking devices or expensive accessories, and there is no additional radiation exposure. The preliminary results from these studies require independent validation by others.

EBUS is currently the most validated and clinically proven tool to visualize the extramural mediastinal and hilar lymph nodes for TBNA procedure [53]. The sensitivity of EBUS-TBNA has varied from 88 to 100% in different meta-analyses and systemic reviews [54–56]. The procedure is safe and has rapidly gained acceptance among the bronchoscopists across the globe. However, it requires dedicated bronchoscope, which cannot be used for other sampling procedures and the EBUS-TBNA needles are more cumbersome to use than Wang needles used with the standard technique. Further, the initial setup is expensive and is not universally available due to cost-constraints and lack of expertise. Nevertheless, with its ability to visualize lymph nodes and track the needle path in real time, EBUS-TBNA has provided most practical solution to the principal limitation of standard TBNA technique in approaching extramural structures.

Low Yield from Small Lymph Nodes

It is customary to consider all mediastinal nodes to be normal unless their size exceeds more than 1 cm in diameter on CT. However, unexpected metastases are detected in up to 15–20% of lung cancer patients on surgical dissection of <1-cm-sized mediastinal lymph nodes [57, 58]. It is crucial to detect N2 disease in these patients if a futile thoracotomy is to be avoided. The involvement of N1 nodes and the central location of tumor are associated with a higher chance of occult N2 disease [59]. In the absence of enlarged mediastinal lymph nodes, mediastinal staging is recommended for patients with central lung cancer and N1 disease prior to thoracotomy to detect occult N2 disease [60, 61]. Standard TBNA is not useful in mediastinal staging of these patients. Several studies have reported a low to negligible diagnostic yield from TBNA for lymph nodes smaller than 1 cm in short axis in patients with lung cancer. For example, in one TBNA series, none of the 54 aspirates from lymph nodes <5 mm, and only 15% of aspirates from 5 to 9 mm, were diagnostic of malignancy [19]. In another study, TBNA sample was diagnostic in only 1 of 75 patients with lymph nodes <10 mm in size [31]. There are several explanations for the low diagnostic yield of TBNA from small mediastinal lymph nodes. The absence of visual guidance is the most intuitive impediment to successful sampling of small-sized lymph nodes with standard TBNA procedure. Respiratory movement of lymph nodes during TBNA procedure is another important reason. Piet and associates have shown a significant movement of mediastinal lymph nodes in craniocaudal, mediolateral, and ventrodorsal directions with respiration on thoracic imaging with four-dimensional CT [62]. The mean displacement of center of lymph node in this study was 6.2 ± 2.9 mm, movement of carina was 6.5 ± 2.5 mm, and the lymph node movement relative to carina in craniocaudal direction was 5.3 ± 2.1 mm. Another factor limiting the yield of TBNA in these patients is the size of metastatic foci in CT/PET-negative mediastinal lymph nodes. For example, in one study, the mean size of the metastatic deposit in such lymph nodes was 3.7 ± 2.0 mm and 68% of foci were <4.0 mm on histological examination [63]. Taken together, a low yield from conventional TBNA is not entirely unexpected in these patients.

The ability to visualize the targets in real time is a clear advantage of EBUS-TBNA over standard TBNA in sampling of <1 cm mediastinal lymph nodes. Several recent studies have reported a high sensitivity, specificity, and accuracy with EBUS-TBNA for detecting the N2 disease in patients without any evidence of mediastinal involvement on CT or PET scan [64]. High success is also reported with a combination of EBUS-TBNA and EUS-FNA in these patients [65]. It now appears that EBUS-TBNA will have a stronger claim as a less invasive alternative to mediastinoscopy in future guidelines for staging of lung cancer patients with small mediastinal lymph nodes.

Other Misconceptions

Ever since the initial description, many concerns have been raised about the TBNA procedure which are not based on any firm grounds. Unsubstantiated safety concerns have already been addressed in prior sections. There is a widespread perception that TBNA is a complicated procedure and has a long learning curve. There is no truth to it. Many motivated investigators have reported achieving results similar to those reported in the literature through simple self-learning initiatives using books, teaching manuals, and videos, without going through any formal training [66, 67]. Furthermore, no evidence of a long curve for TBNA procedure was found in a recent study in which the TBNA yield of five operators proficient in basic bronchoscopy skills was followed over a 32-month period [68]. The diagnostic yield was 77% at the start of learning curve and 82% after 32 months of experience.

Although many of these studies serve to dispel the misconceptions regarding difficulties in learning this procedure, it must not be implied that formal education and quality improvement initiatives are unimportant. In fact studies have consistently shown that educational interventions and experience improve the diagnostic performance of TBNA. For example, in one study, comprehensive and multifaceted educational interventions directed towards bronchoscopists, technical support staff, and interpreting pathologists increased the TBNA yield from 21.4 to 47.6% over a 3-year period [69]. Several other studies have arrived at similar conclusions [70, 71]. A common theme that emerges from these studies is the importance of educating and training the bronchoscopy assistant in the TBNA techniques and proper handling of the specimen. Appropriate patient selection, consistency in TBNA technique, familiarity with the needle, and direct communication with the cytopathologist are also helpful. Failure to address some of these issues may explain why some bronchoscopists could never achieve the diagnostic yield similar to that reported in the literature and abandoned the procedure [8].

Concerns have also been raised regarding high risk of damage to the bronchoscope during TBNA procedure. Improper TBNA technique certainly has potential to damage the working channel needing expensive repair [72]. However, the damage to the bronchoscope is rare and can be avoided in nearly all cases if the following simple rules are followed. First, make sure that the beveled end of needle is fully inside the distal metal hub every time TBNA catheter is introduced into the bronchoscope. If it is projecting beyond the hub, it will damage the working channel during insertion. Also one must ascertain that the needle is not pulled back proximal to the metal hub where it can also perforate the overlying plastic catheter and damage the working channel during its forward thrust. Second, the proximal as well as the distal sections of the bronchoscope should be kept as straight as possible during passage of TBNA catheter through the bronchoscope. If resistance is met, never force the TBNA catheter through the distal end of the bronchoscope. The correct action is to keep the distal end of the bronchoscope in neutral, forward-viewing position. Third, never advance the needle unless the distal end of the TBNA catheter is clearly out of the bronchoscope and is seen within the airways. There is very high risk of damage to the scope if the needle is deployed while the TBNA catheter is still within the working channel. Finally, once the specimen is obtained, the bronchoscope should be straightened as much as possible to facilitate smooth withdrawal of needle.

Leak test must be performed after every TBNA procedure to make sure that the working channel is not damaged during the procedure.

Histology Versus Cytology Specimen

Several studies have established the feasibility of obtaining a histology sample from mediastinal lymph nodes with the TBNA technique [73, 74]. Because a histology specimen is better than a cytology specimen for benign diseases, it is probably wise to use 19-gauge needle for TBNA procedure as a routine, should sarcoidosis or tuberculosis feature strongly in the differential diagnosis. A histology specimen may also have some advantage over a cytology specimen in mediastinal staging of lung cancer. For instance, the presence of tumor in a TBNA histology specimen eliminates the risk of false positive results in staging of lung cancer. In some studies, TBNA histology specimen is also found to be more sensitive than TBNA cytology specimen in detection of lymph node metastasis. For example, in one study by Schenk and coworkers, the histology specimens had a sensitivity of 89.1% whereas the cytology specimens had a sensitivity of 52.7% in mediastinal staging of lung cancer [75]. Similar results were reported in a multicenter prospective study in which malignancy was detected in 57% of histology samples compared to 41% of the cytology samples [19]. Overall, a 14–35% increase in diagnostic yield with TBNA can be expected when histology sample is obtained in addition to cytology sample [76, 77]. Finally, switching from cytology to histology needle for routine TBNA procedures has also been shown to decrease the need for surgical procedures for mediastinal staging of lung cancer [2]. Nevertheless, there is some conflict in the literature in this regard, since in one study the increase in diagnostic yield for detection of lymph node metastasis did not reach statistical significance with the addition of 19-gauge needle to 22-gauge needle [78].

TBNA with 19-gauge needle has an excellent safety record. There is no evidence that a 19-gauge needle is associated with a higher risk of complications or a greater risk of damage to the bronchoscope than a 22-gauge TBNA needle. However, it is more difficult to pass a 19-gauge histology needle through the tracheal wall than a 22-gauge needle. As a result, it is not possible to obtain an adequate histology specimen with the 19-gauge TBNA needle in every patient [73, 79]. Since TBNA with 19-gauge needle is technically more challenging, switching to 19-gauge needles should be considered only after enough experience and proficiency in TBNA with a 22-gauge needle have been achieved [2, 71].

Rapid On-Site Evaluation

Rapid on-site evaluation (ROSE) is a strategy comparable to the intra-operative frozen section examination. Here, the cytopathologist and the technician are in attendance during the bronchoscopy and provide immediate feedback to the bronchoscopist on the quality and the preliminary findings of TBNA specimen. ROSE has an intuitive and obvious appeal to the bronchoscopists [80]. Further attempts of TBNA procedure can be stopped if the presence of malignant cells is confirmed with ROSE. The bronchoscopist may choose to forego further sampling procedures such as brushing and TBBx if a definite diagnosis is made with ROSE. On the contrary, the bronchoscopists may elect to continue further attempts, readdress the anatomical landmarks, choose alternative sites, and change TBNA needles if an adequate specimen is not obtained with the initial attempts. Immediate feedback could be a useful tool for those who are trying to improve their skills and diagnostic yield with this procedure. ROSE also gives opportunity to the pathology technician and the consultant to process and prepare the specimen in a manner that best suits their preference and the laboratory techniques. The most obvious impediment to ROSE is the added cost due to the extra time spent by cytopathologist in the bronchoscopy room. Due to time constraints and reimbursement issues, it is not unusual for the cytopathologists to decline the request for ROSE. Nevertheless, cost-analyses indicate that ROSE is a cost-effective strategy when used with TBNA procedures [81, 82].

Early studies on ROSE showed a significant increase in the overall diagnostic yield, a higher chance of detecting cancer on TBNA specimen, and a significant drop in the proportion of inadequate specimens [83, 84]. However, contrary to expectation, in many of these studies ROSE had no effect on the number of needle passes per lymph node site [81, 84].

However, the results of recent prospective randomized studies on ROSE are at odds with conclusions of the previous studies which were either retrospective or observational in design. In one such study, ROSE had no effect on TBNA diagnostic yield, cancer diagnoses, percent of adequate specimens, number of needle passes, procedure time, and the amount of sedatives used during the procedure [85]. However, the authors did notice a trend towards a reduction in the number of TBBx in the ROSE group. Similar findings were reported in another randomized study, but in this study, the complication rate was significantly lower in patients who were assigned to the ROSE group than those who had conventional TBNA (6% vs. 20%, $P=0.01$). Decrease in complication in the ROSE group resulted from avoidance of transbronchial biopsies once the diagnosis was confirmed with ROSE [86]. In light of these data, it now appears that a routine ROSE is unnecessary, especially when an experienced operator is performing the TBNA procedure. ROSE may still have an important role when a need is felt to secure the diagnosis with the TBNA technique that is less invasive than TBBx, especially in a high-risk patient.

Endobronchial Needle Aspiration

Endobronchial needle aspiration (EBNA) is the technique in which the transbronchial needle is used to obtain cytology specimen from endoscopically visible lesions. Several studies have shown a significant improvement in the diagnostic yield of bronchoscopy when EBNA is performed in

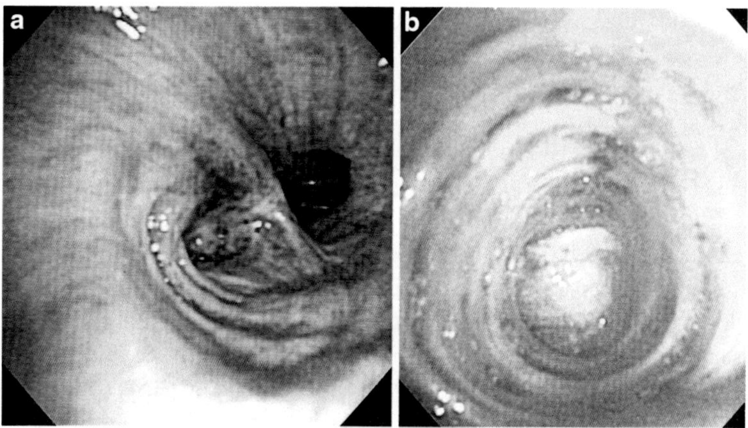

Fig. 3.9 (**a**) Submucosal and peribronchial tumor, (**b**) exophytic mass lesion

addition to conventional diagnostic procedures such as bronchial biopsies and brush. The added benefit of EBNA is greater in patients with submucosal and peribronchial disease (SPD) (Fig. 3.9a) than in those with exophytic mass lesion (EML) (Fig. 3.9b). A further advantage is in selected patients with underlying small-cell lung cancers in which the crush artifacts in the forceps biopsy specimens can obscure the histological details needed to make a confident diagnosis. EBNA has a clear advantage over conventional procedures in these cases, as there is no problem of crush artifact in EBNA cytology specimens [87].

Technique

The technique of EBNA is simple and depends on the type of endobronchial tumor from which sample is needed. The procedure is usually performed with a Wang's transbronchial 22-g cytology needle. To obtain specimen from SPD, the needle needs to be introduced into the submucosal tumor at an oblique angle of approximately 30–45° (Fig 3.10a). In case of EML, the needle should enter the tumor at 90° to ensure maximum depth of penetration because the goal in these cases is to obtain cytology specimen from the core of the tumor as much as possible (Fig. 3.10b). The optimal number of passes is not well defined, but 2–3 passes should be sufficient in most cases.

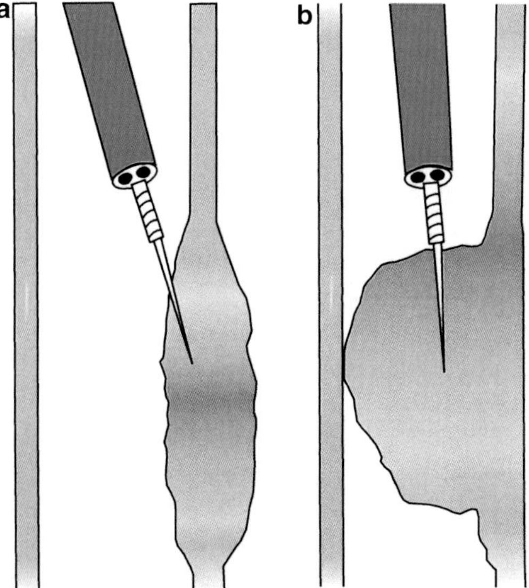

Fig. 3.10 (**a**) TBNA needle entering into the submucosal tumor at 30–45° angle. (**b**) TBNA needle entering into the exophytic tumor at 90° angle

Clinical Applications

EBNA is performed along with other sampling techniques to obtain a cytology specimen from endoscopically visible lung cancers. According to a review in 2002, the combined average diagnostic yield of EBNA from seven reported studies was 80% with a range of 68–91% [88]. Since then, several additional studies have reported similar results [89, 90]. In most of the studies, the individual diagnostic yield of EBNA has exceeded the individual diagnostic yields from conventional sampling techniques such as endobronchial biopsies and brushing [89, 91].

Addition of EBNA to conventional sampling procedures increases the overall diagnostic yield of bronchoscopy for endoscopically visible lung cancer [89–92]. For example, in a prospective study, our group reported an increase in the diagnostic yield of FB from 76% with conventional sampling procedures to 96% with EBNA and conventional procedures [91]. Govert and associates similarly reported increase in diagnostic sensitivity of bronchoscopy from 82 to 95% when EBNA was performed in addition to conventional sampling procedures [92].

EBNA is particularly useful for obtaining specimens from SPD where the tumor involvement is predominantly in the submucosal plane. Conventional procedures such as forceps biopsy and brushing tend to sample the superficial mucosal areas and can miss the submucosal tumors and certainly the tumor located outside the bronchial wall. Another difficulty in obtaining forceps biopsy in these patients is the tendency of the forceps to slip over the bronchial wall because in many instances, the overlying mucosa is hardened and thickened due to submucosal infiltration. It is also challenging to obtain good biopsy specimens when the biopsy forceps approaches tangentially towards the bronchial wall involved with the tumor. It is easier to introduce endobronchial needle into the deeper layers of bronchial wall to obtain the specimens from submucosal and peribronchial tumors in these situations. In fact, studies have consistently shown a larger benefit in diagnostic yield with EBNA in patients with SPD than in patients with EMLs. For example, an increase in the diagnostic yield from 65% with conventional diagnostic procedures to 96% with EBNA and conventional diagnostic procedures was found in patients with SPD in one [91] and from 64 to 94% in another study [89]. Based on these results, EBNA should be considered a standard technique for obtaining specimens from SPD, along with the conventional procedures.

The added benefit of EBNA in patients with EML is less impressive and although a trend of increased diagnostic yield is reported, it did not reach statistical significance in most of the studies [89, 91]. Therefore, routine EBNA in addition to conventional diagnostic procedures cannot be recommended in these patients. In our experience, EBNA improves the diagnostic yield of FB in patients with large EML that appear white and pallid on bronchoscopy. In these patients, surface biopsies and brush may only yield necrotic tissue that may not be sufficient to render a confident tissue diagnosis. The ability of endobronchial needles to penetrate the surface increases the likelihood of obtaining viable cells from the core of the tumor, thereby improving the diagnostic yield of bronchoscopy. EBNA is also preferred over conventional procedures for obtaining specimens from hemorrhagic tumors, since the risk of bleeding appears to be lower with EBNA than with forceps biopsies. Failure of the first bronchoscopic procedure that employed only conventional sampling techniques would be another indication to perform EBNA in patients with EML.

Limitations

EBNA adds to the overall duration and the upfront cost of procedure. However, according to a cost minimization analysis, the combination of biopsy, brushing, and EBNA is more economical than biopsy and brush alone when the cost of EBNA is below Euro 250 and the increase in diagnostic yield with it is more than 5.2% [93]. Routine EBNA appears to be a sound economic decision at least in patients with SPD, who are expected to incur a greater benefit in diagnostic yield with it. Another potential disadvantage is a greater risk of damage to the bronchoscope with EBNA procedure than with conventional procedures. Clearly, the importance of training and experience cannot be overstated in this regard. Finally, the cytology specimen from EBNA is less suitable than histology specimen for immunohistochemical and molecular studies to define the tumor characteristics further.

Peripheral Transbronchial Needle Aspiration

Peripheral transbronchial needle aspiration (P-TBNA) is a safe and simple technique to obtain the cytology specimen from solitary lung nodules and lung masses under fluoroscopic guidance. Even though its role in the diagnosis of peripheral lung cancers is widely accepted, this technique appears to be underutilized.

Technique

P-TBNA should be performed prior to other sampling procedure. The procedure is usually performed using 22-gauge cytology TBNA needle. First, the lesion is identified on fluoroscopic imaging. The bronchoscope is then introduced into the bronchus corresponding to lesion. The TBNA needle is passed through the biopsy channel of the bronchoscope making sure that the distal end of the needle is fully retracted within the metal hub. In some instances, the distal end of the bronchoscope needs to be straightened and pulled back into the proximal airway to facilitate the passage of TBNA needle into the airways. Once the hub is visualized, the TBNA needle is advanced towards the peripheral edge of the target lesion under fluoroscopic guidance. Resistance is felt as the metal hub approaches the periphery of the lesion. Excessive force should never be applied during this process to avoid kinking of TBNA catheter, which essentially makes the procedure ineffective. The placement of needle is confirmed by rotating the c-arm of the fluoroscope. The location of the TBNA needle is adequate when the hub and the mass lesion maintain a constant relation as c-arm is rotated.

Once adequate placement of hub is ensured, the assistant is instructed to deploy the 22-gauge needle that pushes the needle into peripheral mass (Fig. 3.11a, b). After the needle position is confirmed on fluoroscopy, the assistant is requested to apply suction with the syringe while the operator gently moves the needle back and forth within the lesion to shear off cells. After obtaining the specimen, the needle is pulled back into the hub and the distal section of the bronchoscope is straightened by removing the thumb from the angulation lever. Frequently, bronchoscope needs to be retracted towards central airways to straighten the distal segment of the bronchoscope. The needle is removed while keeping bronchoscope as straight as possible. The cytology specimen is collected using the standard methods. Two needle passes are sufficient for obtaining cytology specimens from the peripheral tumors. Fluoroscopy is advised at the termination of procedure to rule out the development of pneumothorax.

Clinical Applications

P-TBNA is mainly performed in patients suspected to have primary lung cancer. The

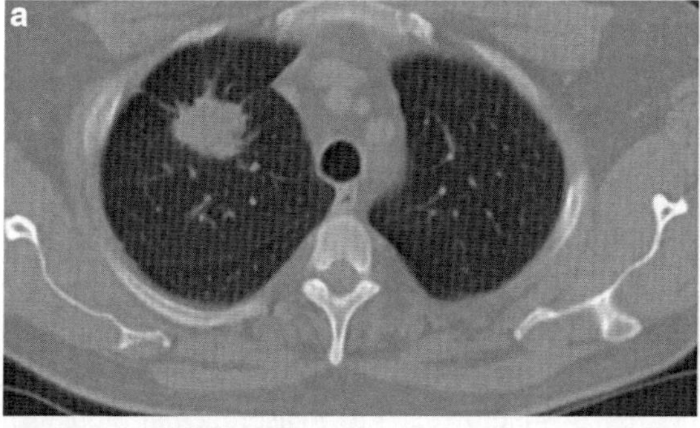

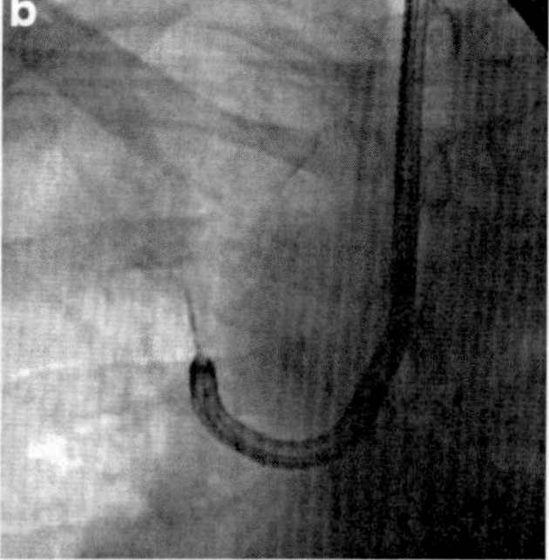

Fig. 3.11 (**a**) Chest CT showing a *right upper lobe* mass. (**b**) TBNA needle is seen within the mass. Pathological examination showed adenocarcinoma of lung

diagnostic yield of P-TBNA has varied from 36 to 69% with a combined average yield of 60% [88]. The majority of individual studies on this subject have shown a higher diagnostic yield from P-TBNA than from any other sampling technique such as brushing or biopsy. Being an exclusive source of diagnosis in 8–35% of patients, addition of P-TBNA to conventional diagnostic procedures is shown to increase the overall diagnostic yield from flexible bronchoscopy for peripheral lung cancers. For example, in one study, addition of P-TBNA to bronchial washings, brushing, and transbronchial biopsies increased the diagnostic yield of FB from 46 to 70% [94].

A large prospective study from Italy has recently reaffirmed the important role of P-TBNA in diagnosis of peripheral lung tumors [95]. In this study, 218 patients with peripheral nodules or lung masses underwent BW, TBB, and P-TBNA during the same examination. Nearly 60% of lesions in this study were <3 cm in size. The majority (88%) of lesions were malignant in etiology. The diagnostic yields were 65% from P-TBNA, 45% from TBB, and 22% from BW. P-TBNA was an exclusive source of diagnosis in 21% of the patients. Major complications were encountered in eight (3.7%) patients, including pneumothorax in four patients and major bleeding in four patients. It is uncertain as to which procedure led to the major complications in this study.

Size of the lesion is an important factor affecting the diagnostic yield of P-TBNA. In one study, the diagnostic yield of P-TBNA was 27.5% for <3 cm and 65.5% for >3 cm malignant tumors [96]. Similarly, the diagnostic yield was 46.7% for lesions <3 cm and 80% for lesions >3.0 cm in another study by Wang and associates [97]. The odds ratio of establishing diagnosis was 0.25 (95% CI 0.12 to 0.7) in lesions <2.0 cm than in lesions >2.0 cm in the study by Trisolini and associates [95]. In fact, there is no evidence that P-TBNA increases the diagnostic yield of bronchoscopy over and above the conventional diagnostic procedures in peripheral tumors that are smaller than 2 cm in diameter [95, 97, 98].

Tumor–bronchus relationship is another important factor affecting the diagnostic yield of different sampling procedures from peripheral lung tumors. For example, in one study, P-TBNA was diagnostic in 20 of 26 (77%) whereas TBB was positive in 5 of 26 (19%) of peripheral tumors with type 3 or 4 tumor–bronchus relationship as determined with high-resolution chest CT [99]. High success of P-TBNA in type 3 and 4 lesions appears to be due to the ability of TBNA needle to penetrate through the distorted or narrowed segment of the bronchus to reach deep into the tumor mass, whereas the biopsy forceps is either pushed away (in type 3 relation) or is unable to reach the intended target (in type 4 relation). Therefore, P-TBNA should be strongly considered when a type 3 or 4 tumor–bronchus relation is detected on pre-bronchoscopy chest CT.

Limitations of P-TBNA

Several limitations of P-TBNA should be noted. First, P-TBNA obtains a cytology specimen, which is less suitable than a histology specimen for the immunohistochemical studies or molecular studies. Second, the diagnostic value of P-TBNA is more or less limited to identification of malignant lesions [95]. Histology specimens obtained with TBB have a clear advantage over cytology specimens obtained with P-TBNA in diagnosis of benign pathology. Perhaps the most important limitation of P-TBNA is its inability to improve the diagnostic yield for peripheral lesions smaller than 2 cm in size. More widespread use of CT has resulted in a clear increase in detection of small lesions of uncertain significance with an attendant increase in referrals for obtaining tissue diagnosis with bronchoscopy. In these patients, conventional diagnostic procedures, including P-TBNA, have a low yield. Guidance with radial probe endobronchial ultrasound, virtual bronchoscopy navigation, and ENB to obtain tissue specimen is very helpful in these patients. With each of these techniques, the specimens from the peripheral lesions are obtained using standard bronchoscopic techniques such as transbronchial biopsy and brushing. In a randomized prospective trial, Chao and associates compared the diagnostic yields of radial probe EBUS-guided conventional diagnostic procedures with or without EBUS-guided P-TBNA in 202 patients with peripheral lesions [100]. The average size of the peripheral lesions in patients undergoing EBUS P-TBNA was 3.5 cm and the investigators did not use the guide sheath during the procedure. The diagnostic yield was significantly higher in patients who had P-TBNA plus conventional procedures than in those who only had conventional diagnostic procedures (78.4% vs. 60.6%). The diagnostic yield of EBUS-guided P-TBNA was 62.5% whereas that of EBUS-guided TBBx was 48.9%. Although a higher overall diagnostic yield was achieved with bronchoscopy when the EBUS probe was located within the lesion (78.3%) than when it was located adjacent to the lesion (47.2%), the diagnostic yield of EBUS-guided P-TBNA was not affected by the location of EBUS probe relative to the lesion. No procedure-related complications were experienced with EBUS P-TBNA.

The preliminary results from this study are encouraging, but more work is needed for independent validation of these findings. It would also be worthwhile to study the potential role of EBUS-guided P-TBNA in improving diagnostic yield from lung lesions smaller than 3 cm in size.

Current Status of TBNA

Increasing popularity of EBUS-TBNA has incited some discussion on the current value of standard TBNA in bronchoscopy practice [101]. We argue that a simple, safe, and inexpensive technique with proven clinical value should not be abandoned without an indisputable reason to do so. There are many reasons to learn standard TBNA technique and apply it effectively in everyday practice of bronchoscopy.

No study has directly compared the diagnostic yield of convex-probe EBUS-TBNA with the conventional TBNA technique in mediastinal staging of lung cancer. One must also point out that in a large number of studies, EBUS-TBNA has been performed under general anesthesia using an endotracheal tube or laryngeal mask airway, whereas the conventional TBNA is always performed under moderate sedation during initial bronchoscopy. EBUS-TBNA is more costly than standard TBNA and local availability of equipment and expertise are important issues that limit its widespread application. If diagnosis and staging are to be accomplished in a single session, the operator has to withdraw the EBUS scope after TBNA procedure and obtain other specimens using standard flexible bronchoscope, which increases the cost and duration of bronchoscopy.

Lung diseases including bronchogenic carcinoma are more prevalent in the Third World countries. Cost and required training for performing EBUS-TBNA remain quite prohibitive for pulmonologists from this part of the world. Besides, one has to acquire skills of using the convex-probe US bronchoscope, familiarize with complex design of EBUS-TBNA, gather the know-how of using the ultrasound system, and learn how to read the ultrasound images. It requires approximately 50 procedures to be confident with the technique. This may require as long as a year for a community bronchoscopist to overcome the learning curve. It also takes more than 25 procedures a year to maintain proper skills at the procedure. The latter may be possible mainly at the tertiary care centers or the so-called Centers of Excellences. In this respect conventional TBNA still remains a procedure of choice for conventional pulmonologists.

We hold a firm belief that conventional TBNA remains at the forefront of mediastinal staging in contemporary practice and will continue to remain so in the future. For bulky lymph nodes in TBNA-accessible stations such as 4R and 7, EBUS-TBNA offers no advantage over the standard technique. Staging with conventional TBNA would be sufficient in an overwhelming majority of these patients. To subject these patients to EBUS-TBNA as a habit is ill advised and would only increase the duration and the cost of procedure. Nevertheless, EBUS-TBNA would be a reasonable next step if the conventional TBNA fails to establish N2 or N3 disease in these patients.

On the other hand, in the presence of normal or minimally enlarged mediastinal nodes on CT or PET/CT, conventional TBNA is less likely to provide staging information. In this situation, it is prudent to forego conventional TBNA and perform EBUS-TBNA during initial bronchoscopy. EBUS-TBNA is also preferable to conventional TBNA for small lymph nodes located in 2R and 2L stations.

TBNA with the 19-gauge needle along with endobronchial and transbronchial biopsies is a reasonable approach in patients with suspected stage I or II sarcoidosis. However, EBUS-TBNA is preferable to conventional TBNA if the bronchoscopic lung biopsies cannot be performed. TBNA is also recommended for suspected tuberculous mediastinal lymphadenitis. EBUS-TBNA is also useful in these patients, but it is unclear if it is better than standard TBNA for this indication. The role of TBNA as a stand-alone test for lymphoma has not been validated.

EBNA has a proven role in improving the diagnostic yield of bronchoscopy for submucosal and peribronchial tumors. In EMLs, EBNA is useful when the bronchoscopy shows the presence of extensive necrosis on the surface. Routine application of EBNA in EML is not recommended.

P-TBNA improves the diagnostic yield of bronchoscopy in patients with peripheral lung tumors. It is recommended for all patients undergoing diagnostic bronchoscopy for peripheral lung tumors. The technique is most useful when the pre-bronchoscopy CT shows a type 3 or 4 tumor–bronchus relationship.

References

1. Dasgupta A, Mehta AC. Transbronchial needle aspiration. An underused diagnostic technique. Clin Chest Med. 1999;20:39–51.
2. Patel NM, Pohlman A, Husain A, Noth I, Hall JB, Kress JP. Conventional transbronchial needle aspiration decreases the rate of surgical sampling of intrathoracic lymphadenopathy. Chest. 2007;131:773–8.
3. Shah PL, Singh S, Bower M, Livni N, Padley S, Nicholson AG. The role of transbronchial fine needle aspiration in an integrated care pathway for the assessment of patients with suspected lung cancer. J Thorac Oncol. 2006;1:324–7.
4. Cetinkaya E, Yildiz P, Kadakal F, et al. Transbronchial needle aspiration in the diagnosis of intrathoracic lymphadenopathy. Respiration. 2002;69:335–8.
5. Khoo KL, Chua GSW, Mukhopadhyay A, Lim TK. Transbronchial needle aspiration: initial experience in routine diagnostic bronchoscopy. Respir Med. 2003;97:1200–4.
6. Jeune IL, Baldwin D. Measuring the success of transbronchial needle aspiration in everyday clinical practice. Respir Med. 2007;101:670–5.
7. Prakash UBS, Offord KP, Stubbs SE. Bronchoscopy in North America: the ACCP survey. Chest. 1991;100:1668–75.
8. Haponik EF, Shure D. Underutilization of transbronchial needle aspiration. Experience of current pulmonary fellows. Chest. 1997;112:251–3.
9. Rajamani S, Mehta AC. Transbronchial needle aspiration of central and peripheral nodules. Monaldi Arch Chest Dis. 2001;56:436–45.
10. Wang KP. Transbronchial needle aspiration. J Bronchol. 1994;1:63–8.
11. Bernasconi M, Chhajed PN, Gambazzi F, et al. Combined transbronchial needle aspiration and positron emission tomography for mediastinal staging of NSCLC. Eur Respir J. 2006;27:889–94.
12. Hsu LH, Ko JS, You DL, Liu CC, Chu NM. Transbronchial needle aspiration accurately diagnoses subcentimeter mediastinal and hilar lymph nodes detected by integrated positron emission tomography and computed tomography. Respirology. 2007;12:848–55.
13. Mountain CF, Dressler CM. Regional lymph node classification for lung cancer staging. Chest. 1997;111:1718–23.
14. Rusch VW, Asamura H, Watanabe H, et al. The IASCL lung cancer staging project. A proposal for a new international lymph node map in the forthcoming seventh edition of the TMN classification for lung cancer. J Thorac Oncol. 2009;4:568–77.
15. Wang KP. Transbronchial needle aspiration to obtain histology specimen. J Bronchol. 1994;1:116–22.
16. Chin R, McCain TW, Lucia MA, et al. Transbronchial needle aspiration in diagnosing and staging lung cancer. How many aspirates are needed? Am J Respir Crit Care Med. 2002;166:377–81.
17. Diacon AH, Schuurmans MM, Theron J, et al. Transbronchial needle aspirates: how many passes per target site? Eur Respir J. 2007;29:112–6.
18. Diacon AH, Shuurmans MM, Theron J, et al. Transbronchial needle aspirates. Comparison of two preparation methods. Chest. 2005;127:2015–8.
19. Harrow EM, Abi-Saleh W, Blum J, et al. The utility of transbronchial needle aspiration in the staging of bronchogenic carcinoma. Am J Respir Crit Care Med. 2000;161:601–7.
20. Seijo LM, Campo A, de Torres JP, et al. FDG uptake and the diagnostic yield of transbronchial needle aspiration. J Bronchology Interv Pulmonol. 2011;18:7–14.
21. Horrow E, Halber M, Hardy S, Halterman W. Bronchoscopic and roentgenographic correlates of a positive transbronchial needle aspiration in the staging of lung cancer. Chest. 1991;100:1592–6.

22. Holty JC, Kuschner WG, Gould MK. Accuracy of transbronchial needle aspiration for mediastinal staging of non-small cell lung cancer: a meta-analysis. Thorax. 2005;60:949–55.
23. Wang KP, Brower R, Haponik EF, Siegelman S. Flexible transbronchial needle aspiration for staging of bronchogenic carcinoma. Chest. 1983;84:571–6.
24. Kuchera RF, Wolfe GK, Perry ME. Hemomedidiastinum after transbronchial needle aspiration. Chest. 1986;90:466.
25. Epstein SK, Winslow CJ, Brecher SM, Faling LJ. Polymicrobial bacterial pericarditis after transbronchial needle aspiration. Case report with an investigation on the risk of bacterial contamination during fiberoptic bronchoscopy. Am Rev Respir Dis. 1992;146:523–5.
26. Toloza EM, Harpole L, Detterbeck F, McCrory DC. Invasive staging of non-small cell lung cancer. A review of current evidence. Chest. 2003;123: 157S–66S.
27. Medford ARL, Agrawal S, Free CN, Bennett JA. A prospective study of conventional transbronchial needle aspiration: performance and cost utility. Respiration. 2010;79:482–9.
28. Bilaceroglu S, Cagirici U, Gunel O, Bayol U, Perim K. Comparison of rigid and flexible transbronchial needle aspiration in the staging of bronchogenic carcinoma. Respiration. 1998;65:441–9.
29. Kunst PWA, Lee P, Paul MA, Senam S, Smit EF. Restaging of mediastinal nodes with transbronchial needle aspiration after induction chemoradiation for locally advanced non-small cell lung cancer. J Thorac Oncol. 2007;2:912–5.
30. Herth FJF, Annema JT, Eberhardt R, et al. Endobronchial ultrasound with transbronchial needle aspiration for restaging the mediastinum in lung cancer. J Clin Oncol. 2008;26:3346–50.
31. Oki M, Saka H, Kamazava A, Sako C, Ando M, Watanabe A. The role of transcranial needle aspiration in the diagnosis and staging of lung cancer: computed tomographic correlates of a positive result. Respiration. 2004;71:523–7.
32. Selcuk ZT, Firat P. The diagnostic yield of transbronchial needle aspiration in superior vena cava syndrome. Lung Cancer. 2003;42:183–8.
33. Bilacerglu S, Perin K, Gunel O, Cagirici U, Buyuksirin M. Combining transbronchial aspiration with endobronchial and transbronchial biopsy in sarcoidosis. Monaldi Arch Chest Dis. 1999;54:217–23.
34. Trisolini R, Tinelli C, Cancellieri A, et al. Transbronchial needle aspiration in sarcoidosis: yield and predictors of a positive aspirate. J Thorac Cardiovasc Surg. 2008;135:837–42.
35. Trisolini R, Lazzari L, Cancellieri A, et al. The value of flexible transbronchial needle aspiration in the diagnosis of stage I sarcoidosis. Chest. 2003;124: 2126–30.
36. Cetinkaya E, Yildiz P, Altin S, Yilmaz V. Diagnostic value of transbronchial needle aspiration by Wang 22-gauge cytology needle in intrathoracic lymphadenopathy. Chest. 2004;125:527–31.
37. Navani N, Booth HL, Kocjan G, et al. Combination of endobronchial ultrasound-guided transbronchial needle aspiration with standard bronchoscopic techniques for the diagnosis of stage I and stage II pulmonary sarcoidosis. Respirology. 2011;16:467–72.
38. Trembley A, Stather DR, MacEachern P, Khalil M, Field SK. A randomized controlled trial of standard vs endobronchial ultrasonography guided transbronchial needle aspiration in patients with suspected sarcoidosis. Chest. 2009;136:340–6.
39. Bilaceroglu S, Gunel O, Eris N, Cagirici U, Mehta AC. Transbronchial needle aspiration in diagnosing intrathoracic tuberculous lymphadenitis. Chest. 2004;126:259–67.
40. Harkin TJ, Ciotoli C, Addrizzo-Harris DJ, Naidich DP, Jagirdar J, Rom WN. Transbronchial needle aspiration (TBNA) in patients infected with HIV. Am J Respir Crit Care Med. 1998;157:1913–8.
41. Hassan T, McLaughlin AM, O'Connell F, Gibson N, Nicholson S, Keane J. EBUS-TBNA performs well in the diagnosis of isolated thoracic tuberculous lymphadenopathy. Am J Respir Crit Care Med. 2011;183:136–7.
42. Navani N, Molyneaux PL, Breen RA, et al. Utility of endobronchial ultrasound-guided transbronchial needle aspiration in patients with tuberculous intrathoracic lymphadenopathy: a multicenter study. Thorax. 2011;66:889–93.
43. Wang K-P. Staging of bronchogenic carcinoma by bronchoscopy. Chest. 1994;106:588–93.
44. Garpestad E, Goldberg SN, Herth F, et al. CT fluoroscopy guidance for tracheobronchial needle aspiration. An experience in 35 patients. Chest. 2001;119:329–32.
45. White CS, Weiner EA, Patel P, Britt EJ. Transbronchial needle aspiration. Guidance with CT fluoroscopy. Chest. 2000;118:1630–8.
46. Gildea TR, Mazzone PJ, Karnak D, Meziane M, Mehta AC. Electromagnetic navigation diagnostic bronchoscopy. A prospective study. Am J Respir Crit Care Med. 2006;174:982–9.
47. Makris D, Scherpereel A, Leroy S, et al. Electromagnetic navigation diagnostic bronchoscopy for small peripheral lung lesions. Eur Respir J. 2007;29:1187–92.
48. Mahajan AK, Patel S, Hogarth DK, Wightman R. Electromagnetic navigational bronchoscopy. An effective and safe approach to diagnose peripheral lung lesions unreachable by conventional bronchoscopy in high risk patients. J Bronchology Interv Pulmonol. 2011;18:133–7.
49. Wilson DS, Bartlett RJ. Improved diagnostic yield of bronchoscopy in a community practice: combination of electromagnetic navigation system and rapid on-site evaluation. J Bronchol. 2007;14:227–32.
50. Gildea TR. Electromagnetic navigation: a rosy picture. J Bronchol. 2007;14:221–2.

51. McLennan G, Ferguson JS, Thomas K, Delsing AS, Cook-Granroth J, Hoffman EA. The use of MDCT-based computer aided pathway finding for mediastinal and perihilar lymph node biopsy: a randomized controlled prospective trial. Respiration. 2007;74:423–31.
52. Weiner GM, Schulze K, Geiger B, Ebhardt H, Wolfe KJ, Albrecht T. CT bronchoscopic simulation for guiding transbronchial needle aspiration of extramural mediastinal and hilar lesions. Initial clinical results. Radiology. 2009;250:923–31.
53. Cameron SHE, Andrade RS, Pambuccian SE. Endobronchial ultrasound guided transbronchial needle aspiration cytology: a state of the art review. Cytopathology. 2010;21:6–26.
54. Gu P, Zhao YZ, Jiang LY, et al. Endobronchial ultrasound guided transbronchial needle aspiration for staging of lung cancer. Eur J Cancer. 2009;45:1389–96.
55. Adams K, Shah P, Edmonds L, et al. Test performance of endobronchial ultrasound and transbronchial needle aspiration biopsy for mediastinal staging in patients with lung cancer: systemic review and meta-analysis. Thorax. 2009;64:757–62.
56. Varela-Lema L, Fernandez-Villar A, Ruano-Ravina A. Effectiveness and safety of endobronchial ultrasound transbronchial needle aspiration: a systemic review. Eur Respir J. 2009;33:1156–64.
57. Kerr KM, Lamb D, Wathen CG, Walker WS, Douglas NJ. Pathological assessment of mediastinal lymph nodes in lung cancer: implications for non-invasive mediastinal staging. Thorax. 1992;47:337–41.
58. Gomez-Caro A, Garcia S, Reguart N, et al. Incidence of occult mediastinal nodal involvement in cN0 non-small cell lung cancer patients after negative uptake of positron emission tomography/computer tomography scan. Eur J Cardiothorac Surg. 2010;37:1168–74.
59. Verhagen AFT, Bootsma GP, Tjan-Heijnen VCG, et al. FDG-PET in staging lung cancer. How does it change the algorithm? Lung Cancer. 2004;44:175–81.
60. Detterbeck FC, Jantz MA, Wallace M, Vansteenkiste J, Silvestri GA. Invasive mediastinal staging of lung cancer. ACCP evidence-based clinical practice guidelines. Chest. 2007;132:202S–20S.
61. Leyn PD, Lardinois D, Van Schil PE, et al. ESTS guidelines for preoperative lymph node staging for non-small cell lung cancer. Eur J Cardiothorac Surg. 2007;32:1–8.
62. Piet AHM, Lagerwaard FJ, Kunst PWA, Van de Sornsen Koste JR, Slotman BJ, Senam S. Can mediastinal nodal mobility explain the low yield rates for transbronchial needle aspiration without real time imaging. Chest. 2007;131:1783–7.
63. Kanzaki R, Higashiyama M, Fugiwara A, et al. Occult mediastinal lymph node metastasis in NSCLC patients diagnosed as clinical N0-1by preoperative integrated FDG-PET/CT and CT: risk factors, pattern, and histopathological study. Lung Cancer. 2011;71:333–7.
64. Herth FJF, Eberhardt R, Krasnik M, Ernst A. Endobronchial ultrasound guided transbronchial needle aspiration of lymph nodes in the radiologically and positron emission tomography-normal mediastinum in patients with lung cancer. Chest. 2008;133:887–91.
65. Szlubowski A, Zielinski M, Soja J, et al. A combined approach of endobronchial and endoscopic ultrasound guided needle aspiration in the radiologically normal mediastinum in non-small cell lung cancer staging—a prospective trial. Eur J Cardiothorac Surg. 2010;37:1175–9.
66. Boonsarngsuk V, Pongtippan A. Self learning experience in transbronchial needle aspiration in diagnosis of intrathoracic lymphadenopathy. J Med Assoc Thai. 2009;92:175–89.
67. Kupeli E, Memis L, Ozdemirel TS, Ulubay G, Akcay S, Eyuboglu FO. Transbronchial needle aspiration by the book. Ann Thorac Med. 2011;6:85–90.
68. Herman FHW, Limonard GJM, Termeer R, et al. Learning curve of conventional transbronchial needle aspiration in pulmonologists experienced in bronchoscopy. Respiration. 2008;75:189–92.
69. Haponik EF, Cappellari JO, Chin R, et al. Education and experience improve transbronchial needle aspiration performance. Am J Respir Crit Care Med. 1995;151:1998–2002.
70. Hsu LH, Liu CC, Ko JS. Education and experience improve the performance of transbronchial needle aspiration. A learning curve at a cancer center. Chest. 2004;125:532–40.
71. Phua GC, Rhee KJ, Koh M, Loo CM, Lee P. A strategy to improve the yield of transbronchial needle aspiration. Surg Endosc. 2010;24:2105–9.
72. Mehta AC, Curtis PS, Scalzitti ML, et al. The high price of bronchoscopy. Maintenance and repair of the flexible fiberoptic bronchoscope. Chest. 1990;98:448–54.
73. Mehta AC, Kavuru MS, Meeker DP, Gephardt GN, Nunez C. Transbronchial needle aspiration for histology specimens. Chest. 1989;96:1228–32.
74. Schenk DA, Strollo PJ, Pickard JS, et al. Utility of Wang 18-gauge transbronchial histology needle in the staging of lung cancer. Chest. 1989;96:272–4.
75. Schenk DA, Chambers SL, Derdak S, et al. Comparison of Wang 19-gauge and 22-gauge needles in the mediastinal staging of lung cancer. Am Rev Respir Dis. 1993;147:1251–8.
76. Hermens FHW, Limonard GJM, Hoevenaars BM, de Kievit I, Janssen JP. Diagnostic value of histology compared with cytology in transbronchial aspiration samples obtained by histology needle. J Bronchol. 2010;17:19–21.
77. Stratakos G, Porfyridis I, Papas V, et al. Exclusive diagnostic contribution of the histology specimens obtained by 19-gauge transbronchial aspiration needle in suspected malignant intrathoracic lymphadenopathy. Chest. 2008;133:131–6.
78. Patelli M, Agli LL, Poletti V, et al. Role of fiberoptic transbronchial needle aspiration in the staging of N2 disease due to non-small cell lung cancer. Ann Thorac Surg. 2002;73:407–11.

79. Herman FHW, van Engelenburg TCA, Visser FJ, Thunnissen FBMJ, Termeer R, Janssen JP. Diagnostic yield of transbronchial histology needle aspiration in patients with mediastinal lymph node enlargement. Respiration. 2003;70:631–5.
80. Gasparino S. It is time for this ROSE to flower. Respiration. 2005;72:129–31.
81. Baram D, Garcia RB, Richman PS. Impact of rapid onsite cytologic evaluation during transbronchial needle aspiration. Chest. 2005;128:869–75.
82. Diacon AH, Schuurmans MM, Theron J, et al. Utility of on-site evaluation of transbronchial needle aspirates. Respiration. 2005;72:182–8.
83. Davenport RD. Rapid on-site evaluation of transbronchial aspirates. Chest. 1990;98:59–61.
84. Diette GB, White P, Terry P, Jenckes M, Rosenthal D, Runin HR. Utility of onsite cytopathology assessment for the bronchoscopic evaluation of lung masses and adenopathy. Chest. 2000;117:1186–90.
85. Yarmus L, van der Kloot T, Lechtzin N, Napier M, Dressel D, Feller-Kopman D. A randomized prospective trial of the utility of rapid on-site evaluation of transbronchial needle aspirate specimen. J Bronchology Interv Pulmonol. 2011;18:121–7.
86. Trisolini R, Cancellieri A, Tinelli C, et al. Rapid on-site evaluation of transbronchial aspirates in the diagnosis of hilar and mediastinal adenopathy: a randomized trial. Chest. 2011;139:395–401.
87. Jones DF, Chin R, Cappellari JO, Haponik EF. Endobronchial needle aspiration in the diagnosis of small cell carcinoma. Chest. 1994;105:1151–4.
88. Mazzone P, Jain P, Arroliga AC, Matthay RA. Bronchoscopy and needle biopsy techniques for diagnosis and staging of lung cancer. Clin Chest Med. 2002;23:137–58.
89. Kacar N, Tuksavul F, Edipoglu O, Sulun E, Guclu SZ. Effectiveness of transbronchial needle aspiration in the diagnosis of exophytic endobronchial lesions and submucosal/peribronchial disease of the lung. Respir Med. 2005;50:221–6.
90. Caglayan B, Akturk UA, Fidan A, et al. Transbronchial needle aspiration in the diagnosis of endobronchial malignant lesions. A 3-year experience. Chest. 2005;128:704–8.
91. Dasgupta A, Jain P, Minai OA, et al. Utility of transbronchial needle aspiration in the diagnosis of endobronchial lesions. Chest. 1999;115:1237–41.
92. Govert JA, Dodd LG, Kussin PS, Samuelson WM. A prospective comparison of fiberoptic transbronchial needle aspiration and bronchial biopsy for bronchoscopically visible lung tumors. Cancer. 1999;87: 129–34.
93. Roth K, Hardie JA, Andreassen AH, Leh F, Eagan TML. Cost-minimization analysis for combination of sampling techniques in bronchoscopy of endobronchial lesions. Respir Med. 2009;103:888–94.
94. Katis K, Inglesos E, Zachariadis E, et al. The role of transbronchial needle aspiration in the diadnosis of peripheral lung masses or nodules. Eur Respir J. 1995;8:963–6.
95. Trisolini R, Cancellieri A, Tinelli C, et al. Performance characteristics and predictors of yield from transbronchial needle aspiration in the diagnosis of peripheral pulmonary lesions. Respirology. 2011;16:1144–9.
96. Reichenberger F, Weber J, Tamm M, et al. The value of transbronchial needle aspiration in the diagnosis of peripheral pulmonary lesions. Chest. 1999;116: 704–8.
97. Wang KP, Haponik EF, Britt JB, Khouri N, Erozan Y. Transbronchial needle aspiration of peripheral pulmonary nodules. Chest. 1984;86:819–23.
98. Shure D, Fedullo PF. Transbronchial needle aspiration of peripheral masses. Am Rev Respir Dis. 1983; 128:1090–2.
99. Bilaceroglu S, Kumcuoglu Z, Alper H, et al. CT bronchus sign guided bronchoscopic multiple diagnostic procedures in carcinomatous solitary pulmonary nodules and masses. Respiration. 1889;65:49–55.
100. Chao TY, Chien MT, Lie CH, Chung YH, Wang JL, Lin MC. Endobronchial ultrasonography-guided transbronchial needle aspiration increases the diagnostic yield of peripheral pulmonary lesions. A randomized trial. Chest. 2009;136:229–36.
101. Yarmus L, Feller-Kopman D, Browning R, Wang K-P. TBNA: should EBUS be used on all lymph node aspirations? J Bronchology Interv Pulmonol. 2011;18:115–6.

Part II

Diagnostic Interventional Bronchoscopy

4 Radial Probe Endobronchial Ultrasound

Noriaki Kurimoto

Abstract

Radial probe endobronchial ultrasound is a technique in which a small ultrasound probe is introduced into the tracheobronchial lumen to obtain sonographic images of peribronchial tissues. Using a water-filled balloon around the probe, five-layered structure of the tracheal and bronchial wall can be identified with this technique in normal subjects. In the central airways, this technique is most useful in determination of the depth of invasion of endobronchial tumor into the airway wall. Endobronchial ultrasound with guide sheath is a modified technique in which the radial probe ultrasound is introduced via a guide sheath and is advanced into the peripheral pulmonary lesion. A diagnostic yield of 74 % has been reported with this technique for peripheral pulmonary lesion smaller than 3 cm in size. In recent years, efforts have been made to utilize electromagnetic navigation or virtual bronchoscopy navigation for more accurate placement of ultrasound probe and guide sheath into the tumor, in order to further improve diagnostic yield from peripheral pulmonary nodules using this technique.

Keywords

Endobronchial ultrasound • Radial probe endobronchial ultrasound • Peripheral pulmonary lesions

Introduction

Endobronchial ultrasonography (EBUS) is a diagnostic modality in which a miniature ultrasonic probe is introduced into the tracheobronchial lumen to provide the sonographic images of the peribronchial tissue.

Radial probe EBUS is most commonly used for localization of peripheral lung nodule before obtaining tissue sample during bronchoscopy. Our

N. Kurimoto, M.D., F.C.C.P. (✉)
Department of Chest Surgery, St. Marianna University, 2-16-1, Sugao Miyamae-ku, Kawasaki, Kanagawa 216-8511, Japan
e-mail: n.kurimoto@do7.enjoy.ne.jp

A.C. Mehta and P. Jain (eds.), *Interventional Bronchoscopy: A Clinical Guide*, Respiratory Medicine 10, DOI 10.1007/978-1-62703-395-4_4, © Springer Science+Business Media New York 2013

group started using radial probe EBUS in August 1994. Initially, we performed EBUS using a radial probe without a guide sheath for the diagnosis of peripheral pulmonary lesions. From 1996, we have been using guide sheaths to identify the accurate location of peripheral pulmonary lesions prior to biopsy. Another application of EBUS using a radial probe with a balloon is to visualize the structural layers of the tracheobronchial wall [1].

Scientific Basis

Ultrasound

There is a considerable variation in the range of frequencies audible to human ear. Ordinarily, the sounds with a frequency of 20–20,000 hertz (Hz) are audible to human ears. In general, *ultrasound* refers to sounds with frequency greater than 20 KHz that cannot be heard by human beings. Therefore, we often define sounds in terms of their purpose. Ultrasound is not intended for humans to hear. The *frequency* of a sound tells us whether it is high or low in pitch. The unit of frequency is hertz, which is defined as the number of oscillations per second. For example, a sound with a frequency of 20 KHz has 20×10^3 oscillations per second. A sound with a frequency of 1 megahertz (MHz) has 1×10^6 oscillations per second. Medical ultrasound equipment produces sounds with a frequency between 2 and 50 MHz. The *wavelength* is the distance between any successive identical part of the sound wave, and varies inversely with the frequency; so, the higher the frequency the shorter the wavelength. Sound can travel through a variety of materials such as air and water (hereafter media), and the speed at which it travels through each medium is the speed of sound for that medium. The speed of sound through the human body is generally considered to be 1,530 m/s, although the actual speed of passage varies for different organs and tissues. For example, the actual speed of sound in the fat tissues is 1,450 m/s.

Production of Ultrasound Images

Ultrasonic probes used in medical ultrasonography use a piezoelectric transducer that transforms electrical signals into ultrasound, and ultrasound into electrical signals. When an electric signal is applied to the electrode of the ultrasonic transducer (also oscillator/transformer), ultrasound waves are transmitted from the surface of the device, and when the returning ultrasound waves are received by the device surface, an electrical signal is generated. *Propagation* refers to the travel of the ultrasound waves produced by the ultrasonic transducer through a medium. As the sound wave is propagated, the energy of its oscillations is absorbed and scattered, and becomes steadily weaker. This phenomenon is called *attenuation*. In general, the higher the frequency of ultrasound waves, the greater is the attenuation rate.

As with light, a proportion of ultrasound waves are *reflected* at the boundary between different media, and a proportion penetrate the boundary and continue to travel forward. The ultrasonic transducer emits pulses of ultrasound, and receives the ultrasound pulses reflected from the boundaries between media. The ultrasonic processor analyzes these reflections to construct images. The ultrasonic processor calculates the positions (distance from the probe) of boundaries between media based on the time between transmitting and receiving ultrasound pulses, and converts the strength of the returning pulses into the brightness of the image.

Depth Penetration

As mentioned above, the ultrasound waves are attenuated as they propagate through a medium. As a consequence, these waves can only reach a certain distance from their source. Ultrasound images can therefore only be attained for a certain distance from the ultrasonic probe. This distance is called *the depth penetration*. For a given medium, the depth penetration depends on the frequency and the transducer size (aperture area). The attenuation rate of an ultrasound wave increases as its frequency increases, so depth penetration increases as the frequency decreases. As the aperture area of the ultrasonic transducer increases, it can emit a stronger pulse, and it can also convert weaker received pulses into electrical signals. Depth penetration therefore increases as the transducer size increases.

Clinical Applications

Based on many studies, the present applications of radial probe EBUS are as follows: (a) determination of the depth of tumor invasion of the tracheal/bronchial wall, (b) analysis of the structure of the bronchial wall for airway diseases such as tracheobronchomalacia, (c) identification of the location of a peripheral lung lesion during bronchoscopic examination. Radial probe EBUS is more accurate than fluoroscopy in determining contact between lesion and bronchus. Therefore it reduces the time to determine the biopsy sites and the duration of fluoroscopy, (d) qualitative analysis of peripheral lung lesions to differentiate between benign and malignant lesions, (e) guidance for transbronchial needle aspiration-radial probe EBUS is largely replaced by convex-probe EBUS for this indication.

Procedure

Balloon Probes for Central Lesions

Air interferes with the visualization of ultrasound images. Consequently, a saline-filled balloon that surrounds the EBUS probe is needed to obtain ultrasound images of central lesions located in relation to the trachea, main-stem bronchi, segmental bronchi, and sub-segmental bronchi. Beyond the sub-segmental bronchi, the outer surface of the ultrasonic probe usually fits snugly to the bronchial surface so that the ultrasound images of the bronchial wall and peribronchial structures can be obtained without needing saline-filled balloon around the EBUS probe.

Equipment

For some time, we employed a 20 MHz mechanical radial ultrasonic probe (UM-3R, Olympus Optical Co., Ltd, Tokyo, Japan) with a balloon-tip sheath (MH-246R, Olympus). The diameter of this sheath is 3.6 mm that can only be accommodated in a bronchoscope with a large working channel (BF-ST40, working channel diameter: 3.7 mm). In recent years, we have switched to a thinner 20 MHz mechanical radial ultrasonic probe (UM-BS-20-26R, Olympus) with a balloon-tip sheath (MH-676R, Olympus) that can be introduced through the 2.8 mm diameter working channel of a flexible bronchoscope (BF-1T260, Olympus) (Fig. 4.1). These probes are connected with the Endoscopic Ultrasound System (EU-ME1 and EU-M 2000, Olympus) to obtain EBUS images.

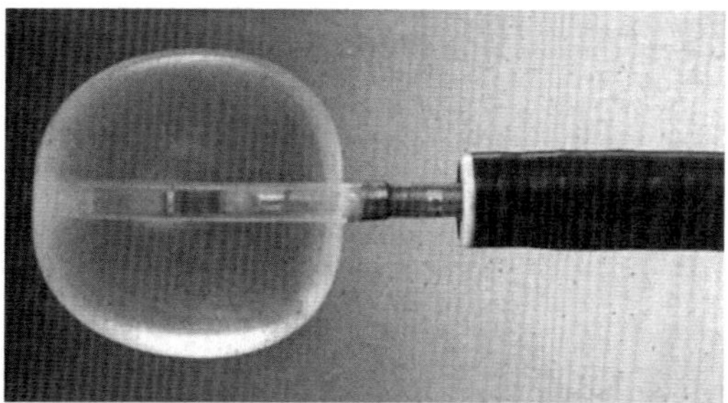

Fig. 4.1 Radial probes for EBUS. Balloon method for central lesions: We use a thinner 20 MHz mechanical radial ultrasonic probe (UM-BS-20-26R, Olympus) with a *balloon-tip* sheath (MH-676R, Olympus) through the 2.8 mm diameter working channel of a flexible bronchoscope (BF-1T260, Olympus)

Preparation of the Balloon Probe

The ultrasonic probe is inserted into the balloon sheath. The probe and sheath are fixed in place by the connecting unit. A 20 ml syringe containing about 15 ml of saline is connected to the injection port in the connecting unit. Most of the air between the inner surface of the sheath and the outer surface of the probe is removed in two or three aspirations using the same 20 ml syringe. Saline is injected from the syringe into the sheath and the balloon at its tip, inflating the balloon to a diameter of about 15 mm with saline. A small amount of air collected in the uppermost part of the balloon is flushed out of the open end of the balloon. The open end of the balloon is pushed back into the hollow portion of the ultrasonic probe.

Performing EBUS Using a Balloon Probe

We use flexible bronchoscopes (1T-40, 1T-240R, Olympus) with a working channel 2.8 mm in

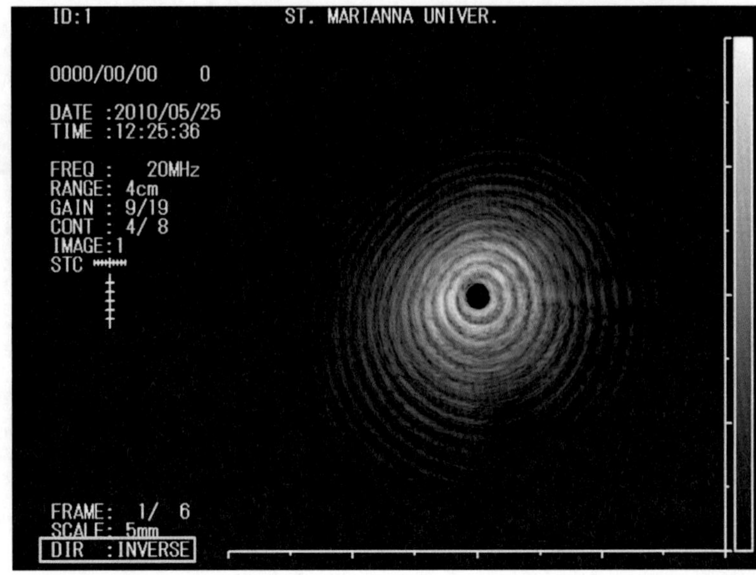

Fig. 4.2 Inverse image. We should press the "Image Direction" switch to change the monitor image from normal to inverse. This inverts the ultrasound image so that *left* and *right* are the same as the endoscopic image to an image seen from the rostral direction

diameter for all EBUS procedures using a balloon probe. We should press the "Image Direction" switch to change the monitor image from normal to inverse (Fig. 4.2). This inverts the ultrasonography image so that left and right are the same as the endoscopic image seen from the head end of the patient. In gastrointestinal endoscopic ultrasound (EUS), the normal ultrasonography image is seen from the caudal direction, for easy comparison with computer tomography (CT) scans, but in EBUS it is desirable for the directions in the ultrasound image to coincide with the image from the bronchoscope, for visualization of central lesions from the tracheobronchial lumen. The normal mode is only used in special situations, such as for comparison with CT images.

In order to avoid excessive coughing, sufficient local anesthetic must be applied to the bronchi with which the balloon probe will make contact during the procedure. The balloon probe is inserted into the working channel of the bronchoscope, advanced beyond the lesion, and then inflated with the minimum amount of saline required to obtain an EBUS image of the entire circumference of the bronchial wall. Scanning is performed while retracting the probe slowly. Advancing the probe from proximal to distal airways can cause damage to the probe, and should be avoided.

Orientation of the 12 o'clock position on EBUS images does not correspond to the bronchoscopic 12 o'clock orientation. Comparison of bronchoscopic images and the EBUS images makes it expedient to rotate the EBUS image. As we angulate the bronchoscope upwards, we should check the angle which the probe moves to. We routinely rotate the EBUS image to give the same orientation as the bronchoscopic image. The balloon probe should be withdrawn gradually to enable acquisition of EBUS images in the short axis of lesions and the tracheobronchial wall.

We offer the following two tips for successful EBUS using a balloon probe: (a) keep the probe in the center of the balloon, and (b) assess the depth of the tumor at a site where the first layer is thick and hyperechoic.

Using a 20 MHz probe, five layers can be identified on ultrasound images of the cartilaginous portion of extrapulmonary and intrapulmonary bronchi (Fig. 4.3) [1]. The first layer

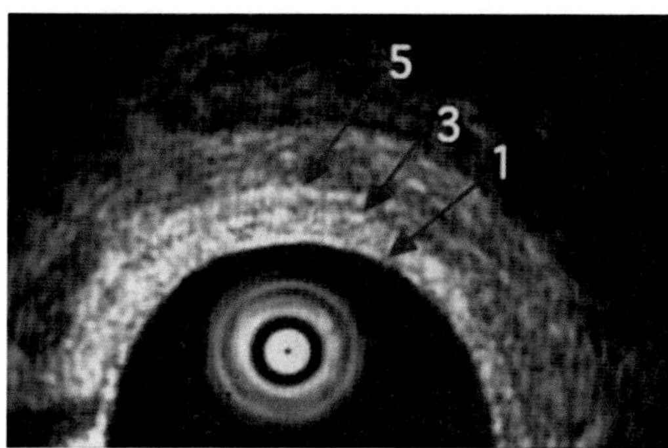

Fig. 4.3 Bronchial wall layers delineated by endobronchial ultrasonography. Extrapulmonary bronchus: The cartilaginous portion of the trachea and the extrapulmonary bronchi have five layers, and the membranous portion has three layers. The first layer (hyperechoic) is a marginal echo, the second layer (hypoechoic) represents submucosa, the third layer (hyperechoic) is the marginal echo on the inner side of the bronchial cartilage, the fourth layer (hypoechoic) represents bronchial cartilage, and the fifth layer (hyperechoic) is the marginal echo on the outer side of the cartilage. In the membranous portion of the extrapulmonary bronchi, the first layer (hyperechoic) is a marginal echo, the second layer (hypoechoic) represents the submucosa, and the third layer (hyperechoic) is the adventitia.

(hyperechoic) is a marginal echo, the second layer (hypoechoic) represents submucosal tissue, the third layer (hyperechoic) is the marginal echo on the inner aspect of the bronchial cartilage, the fourth layer (hypoechoic) represents bronchial cartilage, and the fifth layer (hyperechoic) is the marginal echo on the outer aspect of the bronchial cartilage. In the membranous portion, the first layer (hyperechoic) is a marginal echo, the second layer (hypoechoic) represents submucosal tissue, and the third layer (hyperechoic) is the adventitia.

For determination of the depth of tracheobronchial tumor invasion using EBUS, one must carefully examine the third and fourth layers that correspond to the bronchial cartilage. An important limitation of preoperative EBUS in determination of the depth of tumor invasion is difficulty in distinguishing lymphocytic infiltration from tumor invasion. As ultrasonography visualizes tissues according to the speed of propagation of ultrasound waves, it would appear that the speed of ultrasound waves from the 20 MHz probe passing through invasive cancer is similar to that through lymphocytic infiltrates and hypertrophied bronchial glands. Similar difficulty in differentiating fibrotic reaction and lymphoid hyperplasia from tumor invasion has also been reported with endoscopic ultrasonography (EUS) for patients with esophageal cancer [2, 3]. For example, Arima et al. noted that changes in the tissues such as hyperplasia of lymphoid follicles, cellular infiltration, and fibrosis in vicinity of esophageal cancer were often misinterpreted as tumor [2]. Similarly, Kikuchi et al. attributed misdiagnosis of the depth of invasion of colorectal cancers using EUS to attenuation of ultrasound waves related to tumor thickness, as well as difficulty in differentiating between cancer invasion and lymphocytic infiltration, lymphoid follicles, or submucosal fibrosis [4]. Menzel and Domschke [5] have reported that there is potential for ultrasonographic over-staging of esophageal cancers due to misinterpretation of submucosal inflammation as tumor. Thus, it is essential that operators realize this limitation of radial probe EBUS in assessment of the extent of involvement of airway wall with the tumor.

EBUS for Peripheral Lesions

In recent years, radial probe EBUS has become an important bronchoscopic technique in patients with solitary pulmonary nodules. Radial probe EBUS has been found useful in assessing the internal structure of the peripheral lung nodules and in localizing the lesions before obtaining biopsy specimens for the tissue diagnosis.

Analysis of the Internal Structures of Peripheral Pulmonary Lesions

Several investigators have used miniature ultrasound probes for assessment of peripheral pulmonary lesions. Hürter et al. reported successful visualization of peripheral lung lesions in 19 out of 26 cases [6], and Goldberg and colleagues reported that EBUS provided unique information that complemented other diagnostic modalities in 18 out of 25 cases that included 6 peripheral lesions and 19 hilar tumors [7].

We developed a classification system with the goal of distinguishing between benign and malignant lesions, identifying the type of lung carcinoma, and determining the degree of differentiation [8]. On ultrasound imaging of peripheral lung nodules, the lesions are classified on the basis of internal echo pattern (homogeneous or heterogeneous), vascular patency, and morphology of hyperechoic areas (reflecting the presence of air and the state of the bronchi). Type I lesions have homogeneous pattern, 92 % of which are benign; type II lesions have hyperechoic dots and linear arcs pattern, 99% of which are malignant, and type III lesions have a heterogeneous pattern, 99 % of which are malignant.

Hosokawa et al. reported that a typical EBUS pattern of neoplastic disease has the following features: (1) continuous marginal echo, (2) rough internal echoes, and (3) no hyperechoic spots representing bronchi, or no longitudinal continuity if present [9]. Kuo et al. assessed the feasibility of EBUS in differentiating between benign and malignant lesions using the following three characteristic ultrasonic features indicating malignancy: (1) continuous margin, (2) absence of a linear–discrete air bronchogram, and (3) heterogeneous echogenicity [10]. The negative predictive value for malignancy of a lesion when none of these three echoic features was present was 93.7 %. The positive predictive value for malignancy of a lesion with any two of these three echoic features was 89.2 %.

Although CT and MRI scans have been used for qualitative diagnosis of peripheral pulmonary lesions, bronchoscopic EBUS evaluation has several advantages. With EBUS, (1) patency of vasculature can be seen within the lesion, (2) the distribution of pneumatosis seen as small white dots within the lesion can be visualized, (3) the existence of anechoic areas corresponding to necrosis within the lesion can be seen, and (4) the echogenic strength within the lesion can be seen.

In particular, the echogenic strength within lesions visualized by 20 MHz high-frequency ultrasonography varies according to factors such as the distribution and density of tumor cells, presence of mucus, and interstitial hyperplasia within the lesion. The echo strength depends on the extent that ultrasound waves are reflected at interfaces between tissue types. Bronchioloalveolar carcinoma (mucinous type), which is difficult to distinguish from pneumonia using CT scanning, produces a stronger echo than pneumonia on high-frequency ultrasonography at 20 MHz. The reason for this is unclear, but is suspected to be due to viscous mucous, or increased reflection from neoplastic tissue in the alveolar septa.

Based on above, EBUS has provided an exciting new way to visualize the internal structure of peripheral pulmonary lesions. Although more work is needed, findings on the EBUS imaging may suggest the underlying pathology and histology.

Endobronchial Ultrasound with a Guide Sheath for Biopsy of Peripheral Lesions

Since 1996, we have deployed the ultrasonic probe through a guide sheath with the active part of the probe protruding from the tip to identify the location of the lesion on ultrasound imaging; remove the ultrasound probe, leaving the guide sheath in place; and then pass the instruments such as brushes and biopsy forceps down the guide sheath to collect cytology or tissue specimens [11] (Fig. 4.4). The technique is briefly discussed below.

Equipment

We use two miniature ultrasonic probes (UM-S20-20R, UM-S20-17R; 20 MHz, mechanical radial, Olympus) with outer diameters of 1.7 and 1.4 mm, respectively. Probes are connected to an Endoscopic Ultrasound System (EU-ME1,

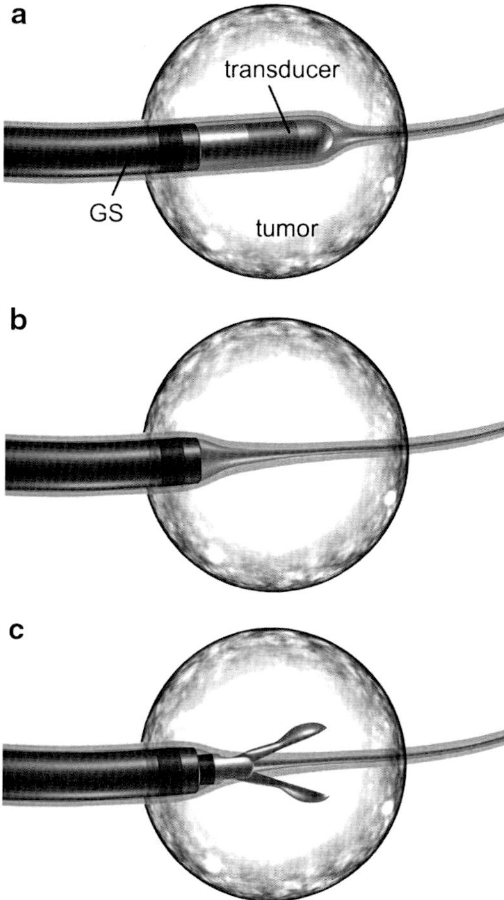

Fig. 4.4 Procedure for EBUS-GS. (**a**) The probe is advanced until it reaches a point where the operator feels resistance, and is then pulled back for scanning. (**b**) Once the location of the lesion has been identified precisely using EBUS, the probe is withdrawn, leaving the guide sheath in place. (**c**) Biopsy forceps or a bronchial brush is introduced into the sheath until the point marked by stopper reaches the proximal end of the sheath. A few vigorous back-and-forth movements of the brush are made under fluoroscopic guidance to collect a sample on the brush. Multiple biopsies are obtained from the tumor by passing biopsy forceps repeated through the guide sheath

EU-M2000, Olympus Optical Co., Ltd). The Guide Sheath Kit (K-201-202, K-203-204, Olympus Optical Co., Ltd.) contains a guide sheath (1.95 and 2.55 mm outer diameter, respectively), a disposable brush (BC-204D-2010, BC-202D-2010: 1.4 and 1.8 mm outer diameter, respectively), and disposable biopsy forceps (FB-233D, BC-231D-2010: 1.5 and 1.9 mm outer diameter, respectively).

Preparation for EBUS-GS

First, a bronchial brush (BC-202D-2010, BC-204D-2010, Olympus Optical Co., Ltd), or a biopsy forceps (FB-231D, FB-233D, Olympus Optical Co., Ltd) for transbronchial biopsy (TBBx), is introduced into the guide sheath so that the tip of the forceps reaches the far end of the sheath. At this time, the brush or the forceps are marked at the near end of the sheath using a stopper. This will facilitate insertion of appropriate length of the brush and the biopsy forceps through the guide sheath during bronchoscopy.

Then, a miniature ultrasound probe is introduced into the guide sheath (SG-201C, SG-200C, Olympus Optical Co., Ltd) until the tip of the probe protrudes about 2 mm from the far end of the guide sheath. At this time, the probe and the sheath are bound together at the proximal end of the sheath with the stopper so that the tip of the probe remains positioned beyond the far end of the sheath.

Performing EBUS-GS

We use a flexible bronchoscope (BF 1T-30, 40, 240R, 260, or P260F) for all procedures. In the recent years, our preference is to use a 4 mm bronchoscope with a working channel of 2 mm. After the bronchoscope is advanced beyond the vocal cords, all segments of the bronchial tree are visualized. Based on the radiographic findings, the miniature probe with the guide sheath is negotiated into the bronchus of interest. The subtending bronchus is chosen on the basis of careful study of the chest CT prior to bronchoscopy. With small lesions, choosing the correct bronchus can pose considerable difficulties. It is useful to make a list of possible fifth- or sixth-order candidate bronchi through which the lesion in question can be approached before the procedure.

The probe is advanced until it reaches a point where the operator feels resistance, and is then pulled back for scanning (Fig. 4.4a). Once an EBUS image of the lesion has been obtained and the location of the lesion has been identified precisely using EBUS, the probe is withdrawn, leaving the guide sheath in place (Fig. 4.4b).

Biopsy forceps or a bronchial brush is introduced into the sheath until the point marked by the stopper reaches the proximal end of the sheath (Fig. 4.4c). A few vigorous back-and-forth movements of the brush are made under fluoroscopic guidance to collect a sample on the brush.

After the brush is withdrawn, the biopsy forceps is introduced into the sheath until the stopper over the forceps reaches the end of the sheath. After the forceps cusps are opened, the forceps are advanced 2 or 3 mm into the lesion and the cusps closed under imaging guidance. After an adequate biopsy specimen is obtained, it is submitted to the laboratory in formalin for histological analysis.

The guide sheath is left in place for about 2 min that puts pressure on the biopsy site to control the bleeding. The procedure is concluded after it is confirmed that hemostasis has been achieved.

Diagnostic Yield

We previously reported the overall yield of EBUS using a thick guide sheath (EBUS-thick GS) to be 77 % (116/150), and the diagnostic yield of EBUS-GS in malignant and benign lesions to be 81 % (82/101) and 73 % (35/49), respectively [11]. Lesions in which the probe was advanced to within the lesion, as determined from the EBUS image, had a significantly higher overall diagnostic yield (105/121, 87 %) than when the probe was adjacent to the lesion on the EBUS image (8/19, 42 %). The diagnostic yield using TBBx for lesions in which the probe was located within the lesion (85/104, 82 %) was also significantly higher than when the probe was adjacent to the lesion (1/15, 7 %).

The diagnostic yield using EBUS-GS for lesions defined as a mass (>30 mm; 24/26, 92 %) was significantly higher than that for lesions defined as nodules (≤30 mm; 92/124, 74 %). However, the diagnostic yields using EBUS-GS for lesions ≤10 mm (16/21, 76 %), >10 and ≤15 mm (19/25, 76 %), >15 and ≤20 mm (24/35, 69 %), and >20 and ≤30 mm (33/43, 77 %) were similar. In other words, for lesions ≤30 mm, size did not affect the diagnostic yield using EBUS-GS, and the yield was not decreased for lesions ≤10 mm. It was impossible to confirm on fluoroscopy that biopsy forceps had reached the lesion in 54 out of 81 lesions ≤20 mm in size. Still, the diagnostic yield in these lesions was 74 % (40/54), which was similar to the yield when it was possible to determine fluoroscopically that the forceps had reached the lesion (18/27, 67 %). Moderate bleeding was seen in 2 (1 %) out of 150 patients. There were no deaths, pneumothorax, or other clinically significant morbidities.

Using EBUS-GS technique, it is now possible to obtain tissue specimens from lesions which could only be approached with CT-guided fine needle aspiration in the past. In one study, Fielding et al. [12] compared EBUS-GS to CT-guided percutaneous core biopsy. In lesions <2 cm, CT-guided biopsy had higher yield; however, EBUS-GS had better tolerability and fewer complications.

Tips for Successful EBUS-GS

These comprise tips for confirming that the guide sheath is placed within the lesion, and for moving the probe from adjacent location to within the lesion prior to the biopsy procedure.

1. *Use of signal attenuation caused by the guide sheath*

   As mentioned above, the diagnostic yield is higher when the guide sheath and the ultrasound probe are located within the lesion than when these are located adjacent to the tumor [11]. Signal attenuation method can be used to confirm that guide sheath is located within a peripheral pulmonary lesion. Once a peripheral lesion has been delineated using EBUS, at the point the lesion appears at its largest and clearest, the assistant should keep the guide sheath stationary and after undoing the connection of the ultrasound probe to the guide sheath withdraw the ultrasonic probe 2 mm at a time until the probe transducer enters the sheath. When the transducer completely enters the guide sheath, the ultrasonic pulse will be blocked by the guide sheath, and the ultrasound image will suddenly become darker. If the lesion can still be seen while the ultrasound probe is fully within the guide sheath, it indicates that the tip of the guide sheath is placed precisely within the peripheral pulmonary lesion.

2. *Moving the guide sheath from adjacent to the lesion to within the lesion*
If the guide sheath is located adjacent to the target lesion, efforts should be made to move it within the lesion prior to the biopsy procedures. However, moving the guide sheath from adjacent location to within the tumor can be challenging. Several techniques can be used to achieve this goal: (1) Another bronchus can be chosen for introduction of guide sheath on the basis of bronchoscopic findings. This is made possible with 4-mm-diameter bronchoscopes, which allow direct inspection of more distal branches of bronchi that cannot be seen with the standard sized flexible bronchoscopes. If the initial choice of bronchus leads the ultrasound transducer and the guide sheath to an adjacent location, the guide sheath may be withdrawn and the probe can be introduced into another sub-segmental bronchus under direct bronchoscopic vision in an attempt to place the probe within the lesion. (2) Fluoroscopic guidance can also be used to select a different bronchus to place the guide sheath within the lesion. When the probe is located adjacent to the lesion on EBUS image, the probe should be pulled back, and angulation lever of the bronchoscope should be used to push the probe towards the direction of the target lesion as seen on fluoroscopy. (3) Another simple technique to select a different bronchus is to use the up and down angle of the bronchoscope. When the probe is adjacent to the lesion on EBUS image, the probe should be moved using the up and down angle of the bronchoscope. For example, using up angle, if the probe is seen to move into the lesion on the EBUS image, the guide sheath and the probe should be pulled back, and reintroduced into the target lesion while continuing to use the up angle. (4) A different bronchus may also be selected using a guiding device called double-hinged curette. When a lesion cannot be delineated using EBUS, the ultrasonic probe should be removed without moving the guide sheath, and hinged curette should be introduced into the guide sheath until its tip is seen to protrude from the distal end of the guide sheath. The tip of the hinged curette is then bent in the direction of the lesion and the guiding device is then withdrawn slowly, till it moves slightly towards the lesion as seen under fluoroscopic guidance. The aim of this maneuver is to enter that branch of the bronchus that is directly leading to the target lesion. If the tip of the curette is advanced in this direction, the guide sheath will follow and will reach the lesion. Sometimes such a branch point is felt as a slight "crank" as the curette drops into a bronchial opening. This allows accurate placement of the guide sheath within the peripheral lung lesion. The curette is then removed, the ultrasonic probe is reintroduced, and the lesion is delineated and biopsied using standard technique as discussed above.

Advantages of EBUS-GS Technique

The main benefits of using EBUS-GS technique to obtain biopsy specimen from peripheral pulmonary lesion are as follows: (1) the position of lesions can be accurately determined prior to biopsy, which is not feasible for small lesions when biopsy is performed under fluoroscopy; (2) forceps can be introduced any number of times to the same bronchial segment; (3) the internal structure of lesions can be analyzed; and (4) there is very little post-transbronchial biopsy bleeding.

How to Identify the Bronchus Leading to the Target Lesion

An accurate identification of the bronchus that corresponds to the target lesion is a key determinant of successful tissue sampling using EBUS-GS technique. This can be accomplished by a review of pre-bronchoscopy CT or with the help of virtual bronchoscopy navigation or electromagnetic navigation system.

Using CT Imaging

On careful review of CT scan, it is feasible in many cases to identify the bronchus entering the lesion, and follow it backwards towards the hilum. With this information, the bronchial branch, its bronchial segment and subsegment, and subsequent branches that lead to the target lesion can be identified. The path constructed on CT images helps delineate the bronchial path to the target lesion during bronchoscopy. For example, if the candidate bronchus is the right B6c bronchus, and the B6c lesion is next to the region of segment B6b on the CT, at bronchoscopy we should introduce the ultrasonic probe into the bronchus branches of the right B6c bronchus which are closest to the B6b bronchi.

Using Navigation Systems

In recent years, two methods of navigation for PPLs have been developed. The electromagnetic navigation system is a localization device that assists in placing endobronchial equipment in the desired areas of the lung. This system uses low-frequency electromagnetic waves, which are emitted from an electromagnetic board placed under the bronchoscopy table mattress [13]. The system allows operator to navigate the probe sensor and extended working channel towards the lesion. Once the target is reached, radial probe EBUS can be performed to confirm the location of extended working channel within the lesion. Higher diagnostic yield has been reported with combined use of electromagnetic navigation and radial probe EBUS than with either technique alone [14]. Harms et al. [15] have proposed a new approach to the treatment of inoperable peripheral lung tumors combining an electromagnetic navigation system and EBUS for 3-D-planned endobronchial brachytherapy. Asano et al. [16–18] have developed a bronchoscope insertion guidance system that produces virtual images by extracting the bronchi by automatic threshold adjustment, and searching for the bronchial route to the determined target. They used this system in combination with a thin bronchoscope and EBUS-GS. This system automatically produced virtual images to fifth-order bronchi on average. EBUS visualized 93.8 % of cases successfully, providing a tissue diagnosis in 84.4 %. Using this bronchoscope insertion guidance system, virtual images can be readily produced, successfully guiding the bronchoscope to the target. This method shows promise as a routine part of PPL biopsy techniques.

Future Directions

At present, we use a 4 mm diameter endoscope with a 2 mm working channel, through which we pass a guide sheath and ultrasonic probe which is 1.4–1.7 mm in outer diameter. In the future, we hope to pass even thinner bronchoscopes into ever more peripheral bronchi, detecting early lesions using thinner gauge guide sheaths and ultrasonic probes.

Cytology and tissue biopsies are presently taken under fluoroscopic control, but it would be useful to watch the real-time EBUS image as we obtain the specimens using thinner bronchoscope with the convex probe.

Conclusions

EBUS using a high-frequency ultrasonic probe allows determination of the depth of invasion of tracheobronchial tumors, which is not possible with other diagnostic imaging methods. Preoperative EBUS using a 20 MHz probe clearly visualizes the presence of bronchial cartilage within the tumor mass when the adventitia has been invaded. Although this technique has shown great potential, some problems persist with the use of radial probe EBUS for the determination of the depth of tumor invasion. The main problem remains its inability to visualize carcinoma in situ and difficulty in distinguishing tumor invasion from lymphocytic infiltration and hypertrophied bronchial glands. EBUS-GS permits more accurate collection of samples from PPLs than other methods. This method facilitates multiple biopsies from the same site, protects against bleeding into the proximal bronchus from the biopsy site, and can delineate the inner structure of PPLs.

References

1. Kurimoto N, Murayama M, Yoshioka S, et al. Assessment of usefulness of endobronchial ultrasonography in determination of depth of tracheobronchial tumor invasion. Chest. 1999;115:1500–6.
2. Arima M, Tada M. Endosonographic assessment of the depth of tumor invasion by superficial esophageal cancer, using a high-frequency miniature US probe: difficulties in interpretation and misleading factors. Stomach Intest. 2004;39:901–13.
3. Kawano T, Nagai Y, Inoue H, et al. Endoscopic ultrasonography for patients with esophageal cancer. Stomach Intest. 2001;36:307–14.
4. Kikuchi Y, Tsuda S, Yurioka M, et al. Diagnosis of the depth infiltration in colorectal cancer-diagnosis and issues of the depth of infiltration investigated by endoscopic ultrasonography (EUS). Stomach Intest. 2001; 36:392–402.
5. Menzel J, Domschke W. Gastrointestinal miniprobe sonography: the current status. Am J Gastroenterol. 2000;95:605–16.
6. Hürter T, Hanarath P. Endobronchiale sonographie zur diagnostik pulmonaler und mediastinaler tumoren. Dtsch Med Wochenschr. 1990;115:1899–905.
7. Goldberg B, Steiner R, Liu J, et al. US-assisted bronchoscopy with use of miniature transducer-containing catheters. Radiology. 1994;190:233–7.
8. Kurimoto N, Murayama M, Yoshioka S, Nishisaka T. Analysis of the internal structure of peripheral pulmonary lesions using endobronchial ultrasonography. Chest 2002;122:1887–94.
9. Hosokawa S, Matsuo K, Watanabe Y, et al. Two cases of nodular lesions in the peripheral lung field, successfully diagnosed by endobronchial ultrasonography (EBUS). Kokyuu. 2004;23:57–60.
10. Kuo C, Lin S, Chen H, et al. Diagnosis of peripheral lung cancer with three echoic features via endobronchial ultrasound. Chest. 2007;132:922–9.
11. Kurimoto N, Miyazawa T, Okimasa S, et al. Endobronchial ultrasonography using a guide sheath increases the ability to diagnose peripheral pulmonary lesions endoscopically. Chest. 2004;126:959–65.
12. Fielding DI, Chia C, Nguyen P, et al. Prospective randomized trial of EBUS guide sheath versus CT guided percutaneous core biopsies for peripheral Lung Lesions. Intern Med J 2012;42:894–900.
13. Schwarz Y, Mehta AC, Ernst A, et al. Electromagnetic navigation during flexible bronchoscopy. Respiration. 2003;70:516–22.
14. Eberhardt R, Anantham D, Ernst A, Feller-Kopman D, Herth F. Multimodality bronchoscopic diagnosis of peripheral lung lesions. A randomized controlled trial. Am J Respir Crit Care Med. 2007;176:36–41.
15. Harms W, Krempien R, Grehn C, et al. Electromagetically navigated brachytherapy as a new treatment option for peripheral pulmonary tumors. Strahlenther Onkol. 2006;182:108–11.
16. Asano F, Matsuno Y, Matsushita T, et al. Transbronchial diagnosis of a pulmonary peripheral small lesion using an ultrathin bronchoscope with virtual bronchoscopic navigation. J Bronchol. 2002;9:108–11.
17. Asano F, Matsuno Y, Shinagawa N, et al. A virtual bronchoscopic navigation system for pulmonary peripheral lesions. Chest. 2006;130:559–66.
18. Asano F, Matsuno Y, Tsuzuku A, et al. Diagnosis of pulmonary peripheral lesions using a bronchoscope insertion guidance system combined with endobronchial ultrasonography with a guide sheath. Lung Cancer. 2008;60:366–73.

EBUS-TBNA Bronchoscopy

5

Sonali Sethi and Joseph Cicenia

Abstract

Endobronchial ultrasound (EBUS) is an evolving technology that has been used successfully to visualize structures adjacent to central airways that cannot be seen during bronchoscopy. EBUS-guided transbronchial needle aspiration (EBUS-TBNA) has been shown to be a well tolerated, minimally invasive, cost-effective, and accurate procedure in the sampling of mediastinal and hilar lymph nodes. Its major indications include diagnosis and staging of lung cancer, restaging after chemotherapy and/or radiation, diagnosis of metastasis from extrathoracic malignancy, diagnosis of sarcoidosis, tubercular mediastinal lymphadenitis, and other etiologies of mediastinal lymphadenopathy. In this chapter we discuss the technique, specimen handling, anesthesia issues, and diagnostic yield of EBUS-TBNA in various disease processes and compare its diagnostic yield with other methods of sampling lymph nodes. Complications and limitations of EBUS-TBNA are also discussed.

Keywords

Endobronchial ultrasound • Transbronchial needle aspiration • Bronchoscopy • Mediastinal lymphadenopathy • Lung cancer staging • EBUS-TBNA

Introduction

Over the past 20 years endobronchial ultrasound (EBUS) technology has become a major diagnostic modality in the workup and evaluation of diseases of the lung, specifically disorders of the mediastinum. From its first description in the early 1990s [1] its use and popularity have increased exponentially across the world. Initially EBUS was performed by placing radial

S. Sethi, M.D. (✉)
Respiratory Institute - Department of Interventional Pulmonary, Cleveland Clinic, Cleveland, OH 44114, USA
e-mail: sonasethi@gmail.com

J. Cicenia, M.D.
Respiratory Institute - Department of Advanced Diagnostic Bronchoscopy, Cleveland Clinic, Cleveland, OH 44114, USA

A.C. Mehta and P. Jain (eds.), *Interventional Bronchoscopy: A Clinical Guide*, Respiratory Medicine 10, DOI 10.1007/978-1-62703-395-4_5, © Springer Science+Business Media New York 2013

ultrasound probes through the working channel of a standard bronchoscope and making contact with the bronchial wall [1]. The radial probe EBUS has remained useful for a variety of purposes: to identify the location of mediastinal nodes before performing transbronchial needle aspiration (TBNA) procedures [2]; to evaluate the depth of tumor invasion into the tracheobronchial wall [3]; and to guide bronchoscopic tools to obtain tissue specimen from solitary pulmonary nodules and peripheral lesions [4]. Although radial probe EBUS allows the operator to visualize the structures outside the bronchial wall, real-time guidance for the biopsy of lesions beyond the airway wall is not feasible. To overcome this limitation, a convex probe EBUS which is built directly onto the distal tip of the bronchoscope has been developed that allows for real-time visualization and guided biopsy of mediastinal structures [5]. The development of this scope, classically called the "EBUS puncture scope," has led to broad application of this technology for sampling of mediastinal lymph nodes and masses both by pulmonologists and thoracic surgeons [6]. Owing to ease of use and low complication rate, this technology has been adopted rapidly in both academic as well as community health care settings. In this chapter, we discuss the technical aspects and current clinical status of EBUS-TBNA for staging of lung cancer. We also discuss the usefulness of EBUS-TBNA for diagnosis of a variety of other mediastinal disorders. Use of the radial probe EBUS in peripheral lesions is discussed in Chap. 4 and has been reviewed elsewhere [7–11].

Options for Mediastinal Sampling

Historically, mediastinoscopy has been the gold standard to evaluate disease within the mediastinum. However, it is an invasive procedure with a small but measurable complication rate [12, 13]. Moreover, mediastinoscopy cannot reach all areas of the mediastinum and is most suitable to approach the lymph nodes in paratracheal (stations 2, 3, and 4) and subcarinal regions (station 7) [14, 15]. The lymph nodes in the posterior subcarinal region are difficult to access with mediastinoscopy. The aortopulmonary window (station 5), para-aortic (station 6), para-esophageal (station 8), and pulmonary ligament (station 9) lymph nodes are beyond the reach of standard cervical mediastinoscopy. Indeed, in the setting of lung cancer staging, much of the reduced sensitivity of mediastinoscopy appears to be due to failure to detect involved lymph nodes in regions not accessible by the mediastinoscope [16]. Furthermore, even though this technique is readily available, in actual practice, it is not always performed for preoperative lung cancer staging, even when clinically indicated [17]. The yield of mediastinoscopy has varied in different studies, depending on the indications [16–22]. In lung cancer staging, cervical mediastinoscopy is reported to have an average pooled sensitivity of approximately 80 % [16]. Video-assisted mediastinoscopy may improve the sensitivity, with an average pooled sensitivity of approximately 90 %, as video-assisted mediastinoscopy allows for more diligent inspection of the mediastinum with more lymph nodes being able to be sampled compared to conventional mediastinoscopy [23].

Over the past three decades, several techniques that are less invasive than mediastinoscopy have emerged for mediastinal staging of lung cancer. Conventional TBNA is one of such techniques in which a needle is passed through the bronchial wall into a lymph node for aspiration (Chap. 3). The TBNA technique was first described by Eduardo Schieppati in 1949 [24], who performed transbronchial puncture of mediastinal lymph nodes using a rigid bronchoscope. The method was found to be safe and useful for staging of intrathoracic malignancies, and for obtaining tissue sample from mediastinal tumors, and other disease entities causing lymphadenopathy [25]. Following the same principle, Ko Pen Wang pioneered a TBNA technique using the flexible bronchoscope in the early 1980s [26]. Lymph nodes in stations 2, 4, 7, 10, and 11 are readily accessible via TBNA. Although the procedure is safe, it is limited by inability to visualize the target beyond the airway wall and therefore, the yield of this technique has been variable [27]. The success rate of TBNA is dependent upon several factors: the size of the nodes sampled, with higher yield occurring with nodes >20 mm in short axis diameter [27]; the lymph node station, with 4R and 7 being associated with the best yield [27]; malignant involvement of the node [16]; the number of aspirates performed [28, 29]; and the use of rapid on-site cytologic evaluation (ROSE) [29]. In the setting of malignant disease the TBNA has high specificity, but a relatively modest pooled sensitivity of 78 % [16, 27]. Low yield of TBNA in the setting of benign disease has also limited its use as a diagnostic modality. Furthermore, many pulmonologists never embraced this technique due to lack of training and many misconceptions surrounding the safety and clinical usefulness of this technique, as discussed in Chap. 3.

EBUS-TBNA has emerged as a technique that combined the high yield of mediastinoscopy with the minimal invasiveness of TBNA. The ability to locate lymph nodes and obtain the sample under direct visualization is the main advantage of EBUS-TBNA over the conventional TBNA technique. All mediastinal lymph node stations accessible via conventional TBNA are also suitable for EBUS-TBNA. However, EBUS-TBNA has a clear advantage over standard technique in obtaining specimens from mediastinal lymph nodes smaller than 1 cm in size, which are difficult to approach with the conventional TBNA technique. There are also some data in the literature to suggest that EBUS-TBNA is more sensitive than conventional TBNA for mediastinal staging, although no well-designed randomized study has directly compared the usefulness of these techniques in mediastinal staging of lung cancer.

EBUS-TBNA Technique

The EBUS scope is used to visualize and access structures within the mediastinum. When accessing lymph nodes within the mediastinum, it is conventional to describe these nodes as they pertain to the lymph node "station" in which they are located, as defined by the IASLC lymph node map. The proposed IASLC lymph node map and anatomic definitions for each of the lymph node stations are shown in Fig. 5.1. This includes the proposed grouping of lymph node stations into "zones" for the purposes of prognostic analyses [30].

The EBUS scope is generally larger and stiffer than a standard bronchoscope (Fig. 5.2). The external diameter of the Olympus EBUS scope is 6.2 mm and the tip of EBUS scope is 6.9 mm, as compared with the typical 5–6 mm uniform diameter of standard bronchoscopes. It has a 2.0 mm instrument channel for introducing a dedicated 22-gauge or 21-gauge TBNA needle for the procedure. The scope allows simultaneous display of two images: an ultrasound image and an airway image. The ultrasound image is at 90 degrees to the EBUS tip shaft, and encompasses a 50-degree slice of this region. The probe has a frequency of 7.5 MHz that can obtain images from a depth of penetration of up to 9 cm. Utilizing properties of ultrasound imaging, the new-generation scopes have Doppler image capability that allows differentiation of vascular structures from nonvascular structures. Doppler imaging comes in two modes: power Doppler and color Doppler. Power Doppler is sensitive for the detection of blood flow within the lymph node, although it does not detect directionality of the flow (Fig. 5.3). Color Doppler is less sensitive for detection of flow, but has the ability to determine directionality of flow in the lymph node when detected (Fig. 5.4). Use of power and color Doppler imaging has been reported to be useful in the evaluation of vascular patterns within the lymph node, which may have diagnostic utility [31]. The optical view of the EBUS scope is 30 degrees to the horizontal, not the typical 0-degree view of a standard scope. This has practical implications in that to obtain a forward 0-degree view, the scope must be flexed to −30 degrees; otherwise one can unknowingly injure the vocal cords or bronchial wall if the bronchoscope is advanced in neutral position. The size and vision of the scope may limit the evaluation of the airway only to the segmental or subsegmental level, and therefore a standard bronchoscope must be used for a thorough endobronchial inspection. The needle channel is built such that the EBUS-TBNA needle placed through the scope extends at an angle of 20 degrees to its axis

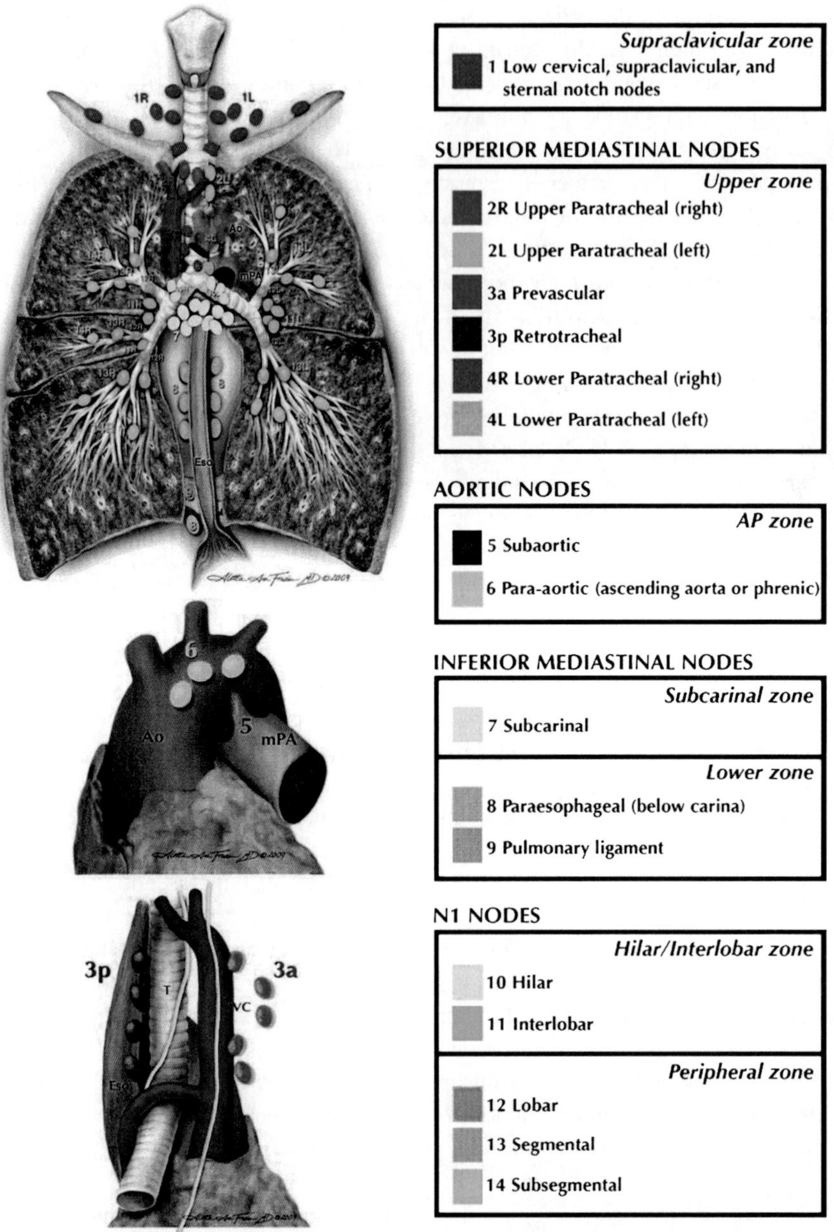

Fig. 5.1 The International Association for the Study of Lung Cancer (IASLC) lymph node map, including the proposed grouping of lymph node stations into "zones" for the purposes of prognostic analyses [reprinted courtesy of the International Association for the study of Lung Cancer and with permission of Aletta Frazier, MD. Copyright © 2009, 2010 Aletta Ann Frazier, MD]

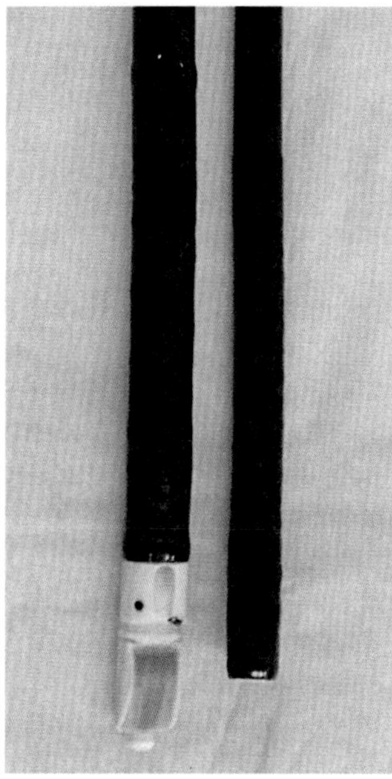

Fig. 5.2 Comparison of the EBUS-TBNA bronchoscope with a standard bronchoscope

as it emerges out of the distal tip. The channel angulation is needed to ensure real-time ultrasound visualization of the biopsy needle as it is advanced through the airway and into the lymph node (Fig. 5.5). One must only use a dedicated or proprietary TBNA needle with the EBUS scope. EBUS-TBNA needles are contained within a sheath similar to standard TBNA needles. However, EBUS-TBNA needles are longer (40 mm) than standard TBNA needles (13 mm) and are grooved at their distal end (Fig. 5.6) to make them hyperechoic that allows it to be seen more readily on ultrasound images. The EBUS-TBNA needle also has an inner stylet that prevents its contamination with bronchial cells during insertion into the lymph node. The EBUS scope is fitted with a balloon at the tip that can be filled with varying amounts of saline to achieve better contact between the ultrasound probe and the airway wall (Fig. 5.7). This may allow better visualization of structures outside the bronchial

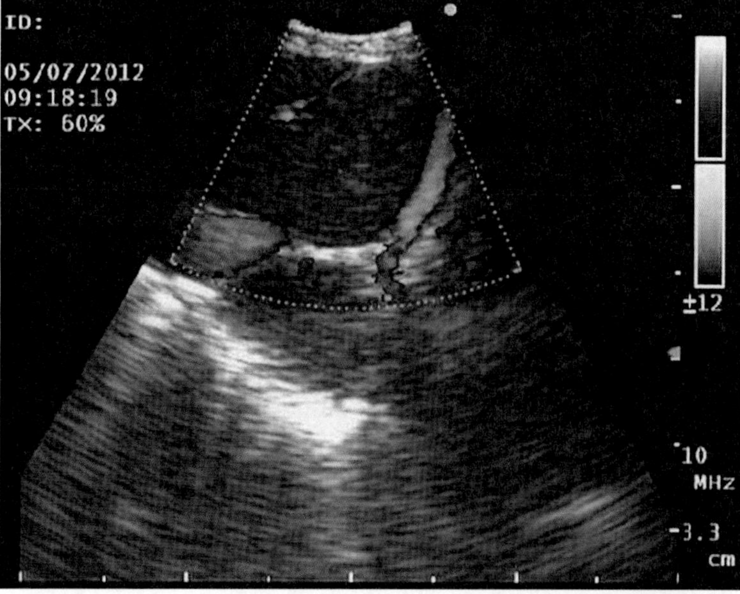

Fig. 5.3 Power Doppler flow within the lymph node

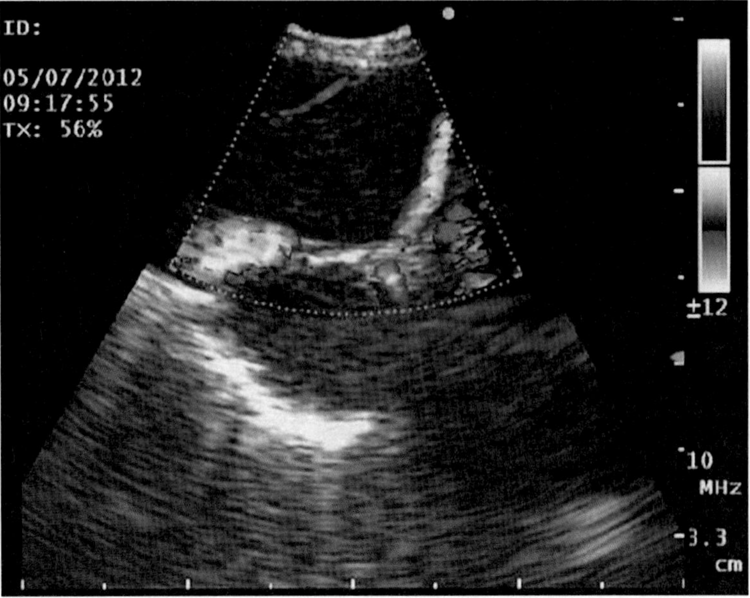

Fig. 5.4 Color Doppler flow within the lymph node

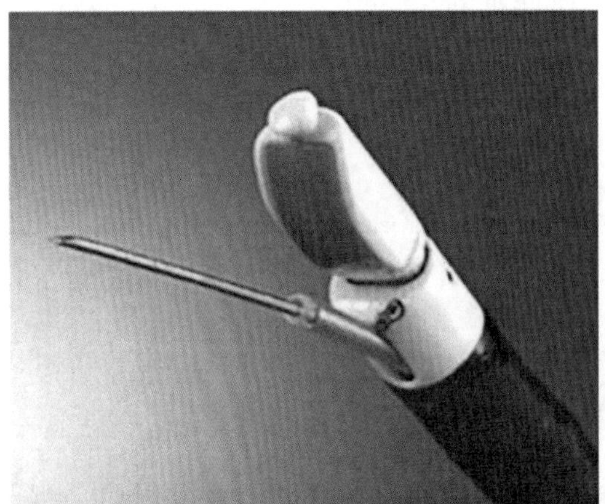

Fig. 5.5 The tip of the EBUS-TBNA scope and inserted TBNA needle

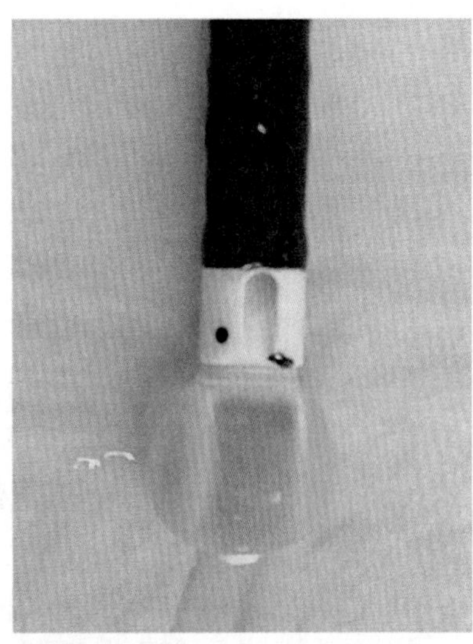

Fig. 5.7 EBUS-TBNA scope with inflated balloon filled with saline

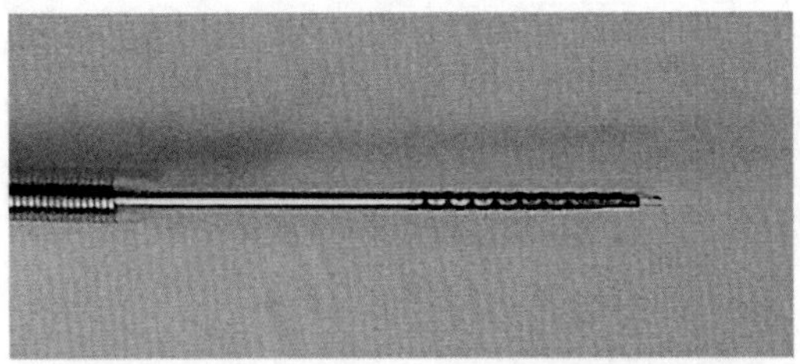

Fig. 5.6 Grooves on the EBUS-TBNA needle make it to be hyperechoic that allows it to be seen more readily on ultrasound images

lumen in some instances. The balloon is made up of latex material, and should not be used in patients known to have a latex allergy.

Procedure Technique

The scope can be introduced into the airway through the mouth, through a supraglottic airway (SGA) such as laryngeal mask airway (LMA), or through an endotracheal tube (ETT). Although some operators have placed the scope through the nose, the larger outer diameter of the EBUS scope makes the passage difficult and causes local trauma especially in subjects with narrow nasal passages. Therefore, it is best to use the oral passage for introduction of the EBUS scope in most circumstances.

Although optimal methodology for EBUS-TBNA has been suggested [32], there is no standardized technique, and approaches differ slightly across operators and institutions. In general, the following principles should be used. Identification of the node is made using the ultrasound image. Proper identification of the nodal station can be carried out through both direct visualization of where the tip of the scope lies as well as through the visualization of anatomic structures within the ultrasound image's field of view (Fig. 5.8). Once the node is identified, the EBUS needle catheter is advanced through the working channel and locked in position. To perform the procedure with proficiency, the operators must be thoroughly familiar with the operational aspects of the dedicated TBNA needle used during EBUS-guided TBNA (Fig. 5.9). Step-by-step approach to obtaining specimen from the target lymph nodes is summarized in Table 5.1. Advancement of the TBNA needle through the scope into its final position should be performed while the EBUS scope is held in neutral position. The distal part of the needle is relatively rigid and can cause damage to the EBUS scope if the operator inadvertently tries to force it through the distal end with the scope in flexed position. Once the needle is fully advanced and locked into place, the needle sheath is advanced until it can be seen protruding out of the distal end of the scope. Since the needle is somewhat rigid, the angulation from maximal flexing may be reduced compared to when the needle was not in the scope, thus changing the ultrasound view of the node compared to the prior view without the needle. Due to this reason, the EBUS scope often needs to be repositioned to visualize the lymph node to be biopsied. Once compensation has been accomplished and the node is ready for biopsy, the needle should be advanced through the airway wall into the lymph node (Fig. 5.10). The advancement of the needle into a lymph node is defined as an "excursion" in the cytology literature; a needle "pass" is a series of excursions starting from advancement into the node until withdrawal of the needle from the node. Once within the node, the inner stylet should be tapped or slightly withdrawn and advanced several times to eject any debris that may have collected during insertion through the bronchial wall. There is no general consensus regarding how many needle excursions should occur during each pass, how vigorous to make the needle excursions, where to make the needle excursions (cortical, medullary, or both parts of lymph node), or whether suction should be used during needle excursions in all cases. Once the biopsy is completed, the needle should be removed with the scope again in neutral position to avoid damage to the scope channel. Regardless of needle technique, the ideal result of a needle pass should be acquisition of lymphoid tissue and/or malignant cells that may have replaced the lymph node. The processing and interpretation of samples are discussed in the next section.

Specimen Handling

Each needle pass should provide sufficient material to make several slides with enough remaining to be placed into a preservative solution for cell block preparation. Depending on the preference of the cytopathologist, the slides can be air dried, fixed in alcohol, or both. After the needle is removed from the scope, the stylet is placed back into the TBNA needle, expressing the contents of the needle onto a slide for preparing smears. Smear(s) can be put into 95 % ethanol and/or air dried. At our institution, two smears are prepared from each pass; one slide is fixed in alcohol, and the other slide is air dried for rapid staining using a Diff-Quik stain. The remainder of the sample is placed in Cytolyt®. After the stylet is removed, the TBNA needle is first flushed with approximately 0.5 ml of normal saline and subsequently with air until all the saline has been flushed through the TBNA needle; this sample is also placed into Cytolyt® solution. The material collected in the Cytolyt® is used to make both a

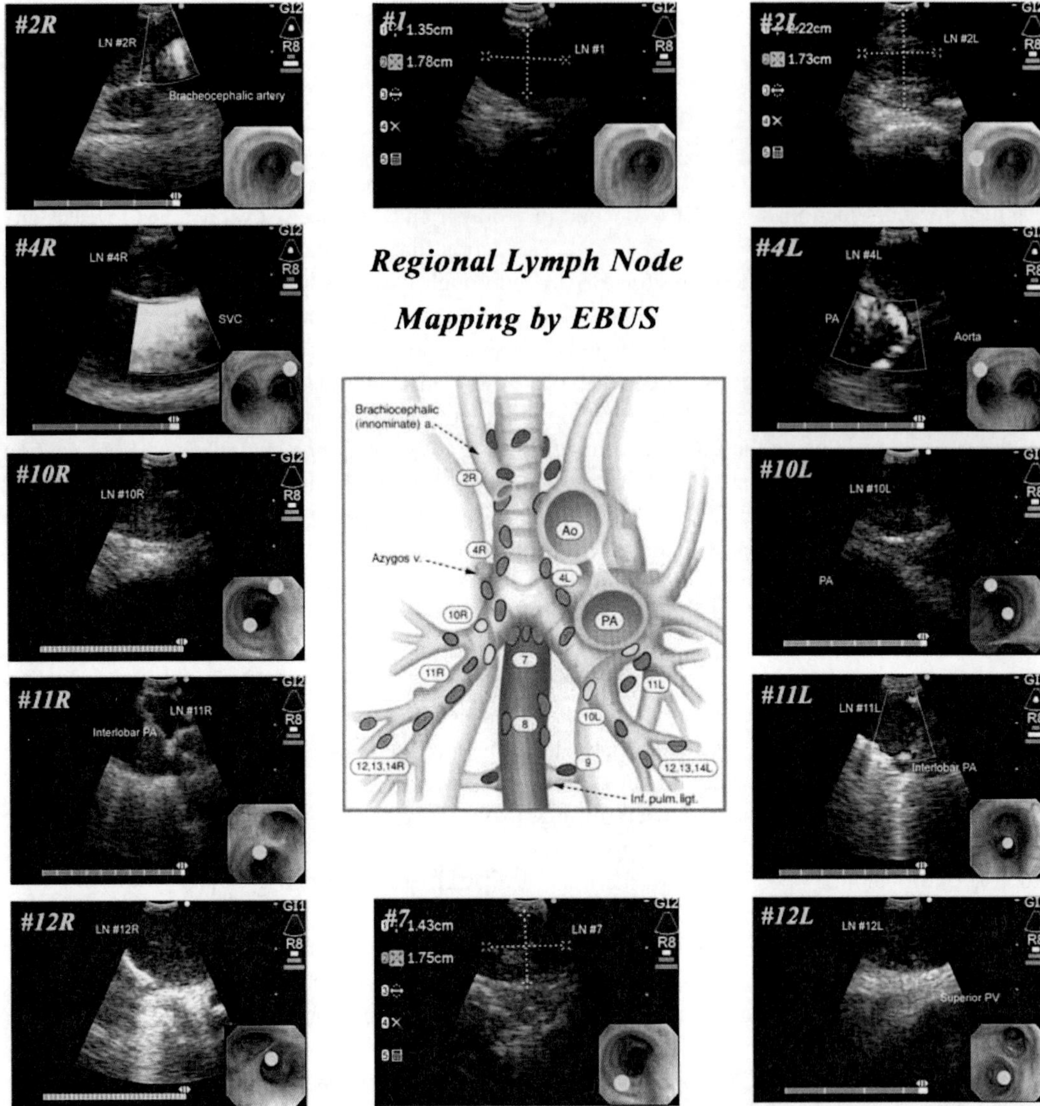

Fig. 5.8 EBUS images and corresponding bronchoscopic landmarks for different lymph node stations [reprinted from Yasufuku K. EBUS-TBNA Bronchoscopy. In: Ernst A, Herth FJX (eds.). Endobronchial Ultrasound: An Atlas and Practical Guide. New York: Springer Science+Business Media; 2009. With permission from Springer Science+Business Media]

ThinPrep slide and a cell block. There are some centers that prefer to place the initial sample into preservative solution, leaving the remainder for smear preparation. The goal of this approach is to minimize peripheral blood contamination on the smears. Once the specimen is obtained, the stylet is wiped with wet gauze (saline or ethanol) and placed back into the TBNA needle for the next biopsy pass.

If facility for on-site cytology review is available (also known as ROSE: rapid on-site evaluation), several staining methods can be used for immediate assessment of the adequacy and triage of the sample obtained with EBUS-TBNA. These include rapid H&E (≈4-min preparation time), rapid Papanicolaou (≈6–8-min preparation time), and Diff-Quik (≈1-min preparation time). Aspirated samples may be triaged for flow cytometry, microbiologic cultures, molecular testing,

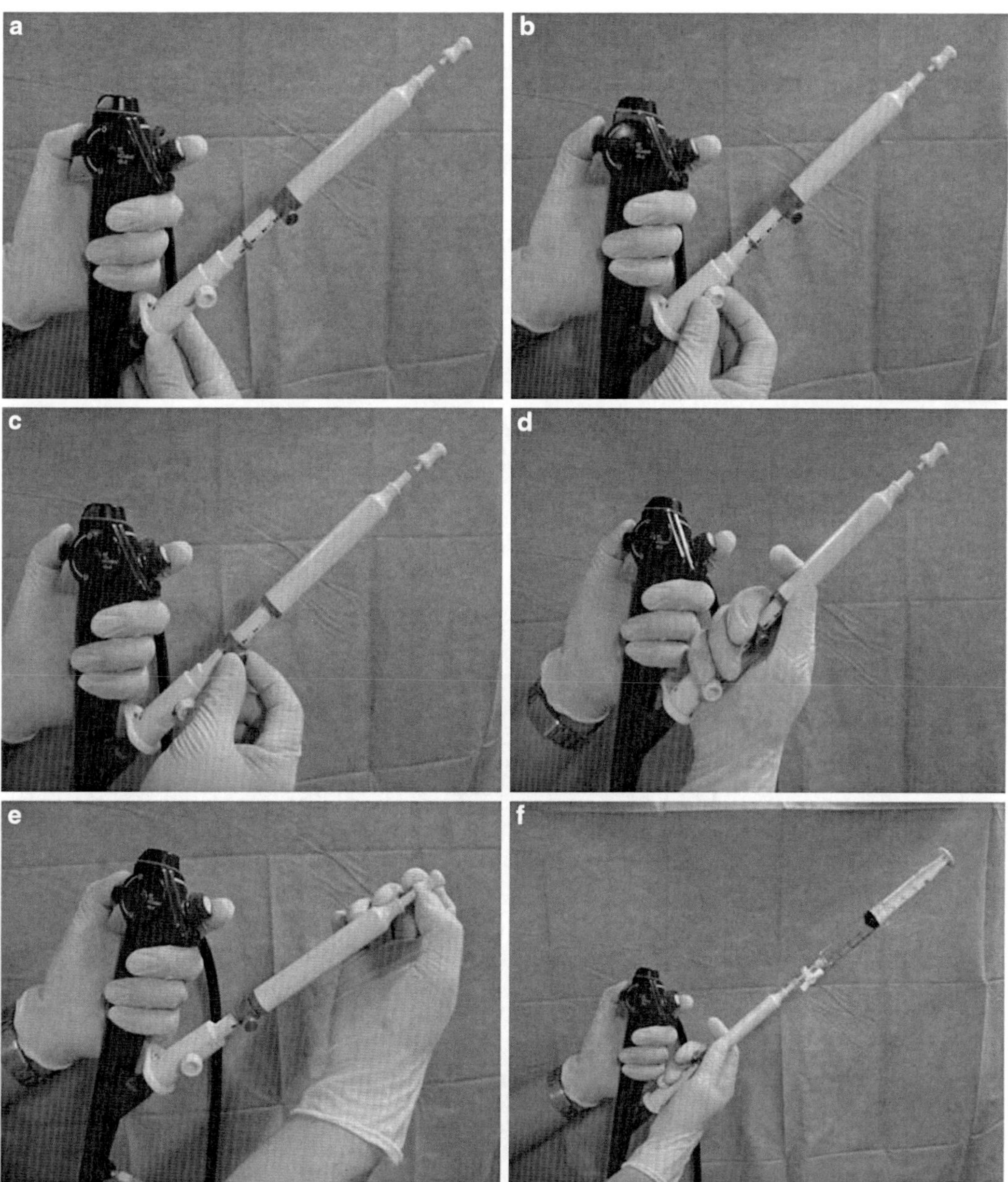

Fig. 5.9 Use of dedicated EBUS-TBNA needle for obtaining cytology specimen from lymph nodes. (**a**) The needle is attached to the working channel place by sliding the flange and locking it in place. (**b**) The sheath adjuster knob is unscrewed and the length is adjusted. (**c**) The needle adjuster knob is unscrewed. (**d**) Needle is advanced. (**e**) After lymph node puncture, the internal stylet is moved in and out a few times to remove the debris. (**f**) Suction is applied using Vaclok syringe [reprinted from Yasufuku K. EBUS-TBNA Bronchoscopy. In: Ernst A, Herth FJX (eds.). Endobronchial Ultrasound: An Atlas and Practical Guide. New York: Springer Science+Business Media; 2009. With permission from Springer Science+Business Media]

etc. ROSE results should serve to assess sample adequacy and for triage and not the final diagnosis. These results are analogous to a frozen section result on a surgical specimen. Although some studies have found ROSE to be beneficial when used in the setting of conventional TBNA [33–36], there is no evidence in the literature to date that ROSE improves yield in EBUS-TBNA. It would

Table 5.1 Steps to performing EBUS-TBNA

Step 1	Advance EBUS biopsy needle through the working channel in neutral position
Step 2	Secure the needle housing by sliding the flange and locking it in place
Step 3	Release the sheath screw
Step 4	Advance and lock the sheath when it is visualized at the top right corner of the monitor
Step 5	Release the needle guard
Step 6	Locate the target lymph node to be biopsied using ultrasound imaging
Step 7	Advance the needle using the quick "jab" technique
Step 8	Visualize needle entering target node
Step 9	Move the stylet in and out a few times to dislodge debris within the needle
Step 10	Withdraw the stylet
Step 11	Attach suction syringe to the biopsy needle
Step 12	Apply suction
Step 13	Pass the needle in and out of the node 10–15 times under ultrasound visualization
Step 14	Release suction
Step 15	Retract the needle into the sheath
Step 16	Unlock and remove the needle and sheath and prepare slide smears

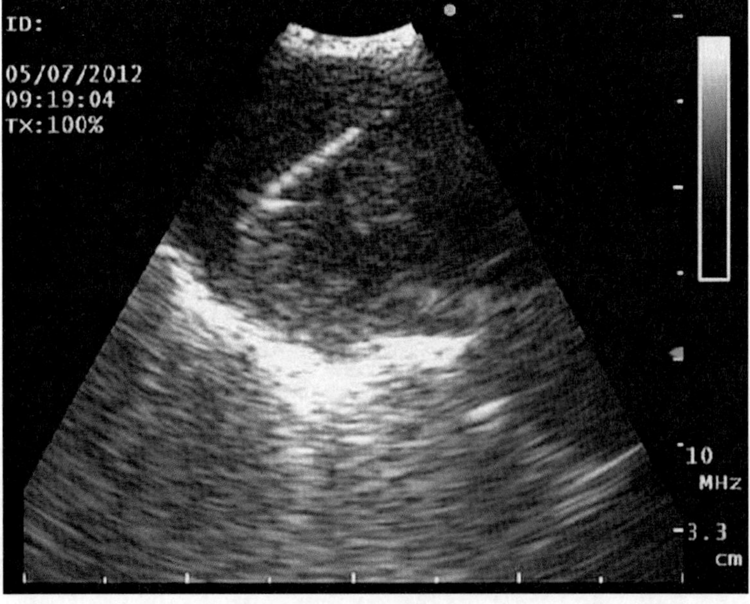

Fig. 5.10 EBUS-TBNA image showing an enlarged mediastinal lymph node with the biopsy needle clearly visible within it

seem intuitive to extrapolate from conventional TBNA data that ROSE can decrease the number of passes taken per lymph node station (due to sample adequacy analysis) and perhaps reduce procedure time when used in conjunction with EBUS-TBNA [37]. Furthermore, it would also seem that ROSE could decrease procedure cost by triaging specimens in a more targeted way, thus reducing unnecessary testing and potentially sparing the patient from additional procedures. Future studies need to address these issues.

In the absence of ROSE, there should be enough biopsy samples to ensure adequate specimen that is representative of the lymph node. In the setting of lung cancer staging, it has been suggested that three biopsy samples per lymph node should be adequate, and if tissue fragments have been acquired then only two passes are necessary [38]. Slides placed into ethanol can be processed with a Papanicolaou stain that allows for more robust evaluation of cell morphology. Specimen that is placed into preservative solution is concentrated for processing as a ThinPrep and cell block. The samples should be placed in the appropriate media for immunophenotyping and flow cytometry when a diagnosis other than lung cancer is suspected. For instance, if lymphoma is expected, Roswell Park Medical Institution (RPMI) media or its equivalent should be used. If infection is suspected, the aspirate should be submitted into sterile saline for cultures.

Anesthesia for EBUS-TBNA

There have been no studies addressing the optimal anesthesia for EBUS-TBNA. General anesthesia or deep sedation with short-acting agents such as propofol and fentanyl and/or short-acting paralytics (rocuronium) allows immobilization for better operating conditions, enhances patient comfort, and minimizes use of topical anesthetics. This form of anesthesia may shorten the procedure by optimizing scope placement and specimen procurement while the patient is immobilized. It may also shorten recovery time as most of the medications used for this purpose have a short half-life. However, general anesthesia is not available in most bronchoscopy suites, and if available, requires extra staffing and monitoring, and increases overall cost for the procedure. In many instances, EBUS-TBNA is performed in the operating rooms, which is associated with scheduling difficulties and cost issues. Conscious sedation is more readily available in a bronchoscopy suite, and can achieve levels of sedation that allow for EBUS-TBNA. There is no need for an artificial airway with conscious sedation, nor is there a need for dedicated anesthesia staff. It is unclear if EBUS-TBNA performed under conscious sedation has lower diagnostic yield than performed under deeper sedation, especially in experienced hands [39]. More studies are needed to assess if other procedure variables such as procedure time, patient comfort, number of passes needed to obtain a diagnosis, etc. are affected by the choice of anesthesia.

If general anesthesia is used, total intravenous anesthesia (TIVA) is preferred over the volatile anesthetics because frequent suctioning can lead to inconsistent delivery of volatile anesthetic gas levels to the patient [40]. Further, there is potential to contaminate the procedure room environment with volatile anesthetics, thus exposing operating room personnel to anesthetic vapors. To achieve TIVA, propofol is administered at a continuous rate between 75 and 250 mcg/kg/min [41], with or without intermittent administration of short-acting narcotics such as fentanyl or remifentanil. The doses of these agents should be titrated to maintain an adequate depth of anesthesia during the procedure. Muscle relaxation can be achieved through short-acting agents such as rocuronium or cisatracurium. Muscle relaxation during the procedure provides the advantage of mitigating patient movement and coughing, which if present can result in difficulty obtaining an adequate lymph node view and accurate insertion of the needle into the lymph node. Muscle relaxation also facilitates both SGA such as LMA and ETT insertion, and minimizes trauma to the vocal cords caused by frequent insertion and removal of the bronchoscope against contracted vocal cords. During muscle relaxation, the Bispectral index monitor (BIS Monitor®) (Covidien, Dublin, Ireland) can be used to help monitor the depth of anesthesia to minimize the chances of intraoperative recall [42]. The use of the BIS monitor can also help the anesthesiologist to titrate the doses of medication so as to avoid excessive anesthesia and hemodynamic compromise due to excessive doses and light anesthesia and possibly recall due to suboptimal doses.

If general anesthesia or deep sedation is used, it is advisable to use an LMA or an ETT. Consultation with the anesthesiologist to choose the ideal airway device prior to the procedure is recommended, as both airways have advantages and disadvantages that should be considered for each individual patient.

SGA is an ideal airway device for EBUS-TBNA procedures. The size 4 LMA has a large

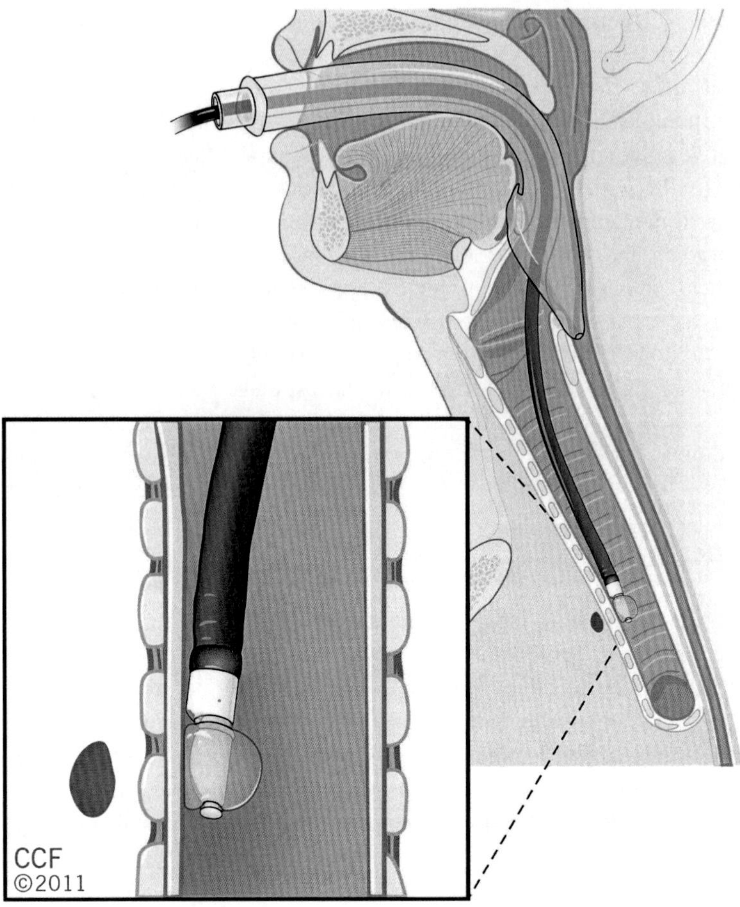

Fig. 5.11 Placement of the EBUS-TBNA scope within a laryngeal mask airway (LMA)

enough shaft diameter to allow for easy insertion of the relatively large EBUS bronchoscope and to ventilate around the bronchoscope (Fig. 5.11). Additionally, the SGA allows free mobility of the bronchoscope in the airway to bring the tip of the scope into close proximity of the bronchial wall, which is especially important in evaluating paratracheal lymph node stations. SGAs should be used with caution in patients who are at risk for aspiration of gastric contents, such as those with severe gastroesophageal reflux or hiatal hernias.

If an ETT is used, it must be large enough to accommodate the size of the EBUS scope (generally 8.5 and larger). The ETT should also be placed high in the trachea so that it does not interfere with paratracheal node evaluation (Fig. 5.12). As a general principle, ETT provides a more secure airway, which is helpful in patients with severe gastroesophageal reflux disease or hiatal hernia. Of note, the ETT will also provide protection to the vocal cords against repeated trauma and friction with the outer surface of the bronchoscope during long procedures that require multiple insertions and retractions of the instrument.

If conscious sedation is used, an adequate level of sedation should be attained to provide patient and operator comfort during the procedure. Sedation is typically achieved through the combination use of anxiolytics (i.e., midazolam) and narcotics (i.e., fentanyl). Randomized studies have reported better comfort, tolerance, and improved cough control with the combination of benzodiazepines and opiates over benzodiazepines alone [43]. Difficulties with this approach are commonly encountered due to the extended length of the procedure and lower tolerance of the large-diameter EBUS bronchoscope by the patient. As a result, larger doses of sedation than commonly used during routine bronchoscopy

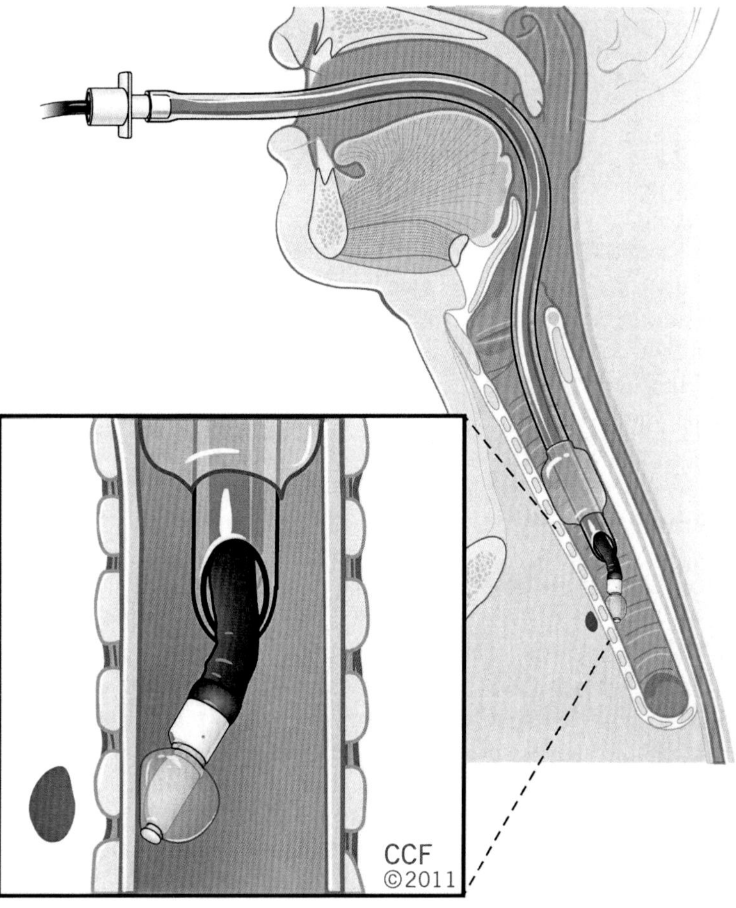

Fig. 5.12 Placement of the EBUS-TBNA scope within an endotracheal tube (ETT)

may need to be given to achieve better patient tolerance. The use of topical anesthetics should be used to adequately control cough during the procedure. The longer duration of the procedure and the need to mitigate cough may necessitate the use of larger total doses of topical anesthetics compared to a standard bronchoscopy, which increase the risk of toxicity to these agents [44]. One must be careful to limit the total lidocaine dose to under 7 mg/kg [45]. Lidocaine toxicity may result in involuntary movements, altered mental status, seizures, respiratory depression, unplanned intubation, hospital admission, and prolonged recovery time. Prolonged procedural time may especially be observed during procedures in which more than one lymph node station are being sampled, procedures in which smaller nodes are targeted, or procedures that are aimed at staging the mediastinum.

Indications of EBUS-TBNA

The main indications of EBUS-TBNA are the mediastinal and hilar staging of non-small-cell lung cancer (NSCLC), diagnosis of suspected cancer when no endobronchial lesion is present in patients with lymphadenopathy, and recurrence or restaging of NSCLC after chemotherapy or radiation. Other indications include any causes of mediastinal lymphadenopathy such as suspected sarcoidosis, infections such as tuberculosis, mediastinal lymphoma, thymoma, and mediastinal cysts. In addition, EBUS-TBNA can assist in guiding therapy by measuring the depth of tumor invasion into the airway wall, or for tissue banking and molecular testing. Future applications may include its utility in pulmonary vascular disease and assessing for airway remodeling.

Complications and Safety of EBUS-TBNA

EBUS-TBNA is well tolerated and is as safe as conventional TBNA [46, 47]. The procedure is less invasive and more safe than mediastinoscopy. Still, there have been few reports of pneumomediastinum, pneumothorax, hemomediastinum, mediastinitis, and bacteremia following EBUS-TBNA [48–50]. Similar to conventional TBNA procedure, bleeding complications are rare, even if major vessels are punctured inadvertantly.

Diagnostic Yield

Lung Cancer Staging

A full discussion of mediastinal staging of NSCLC is beyond the scope of this chapter. However, EBUS-TBNA has shown to be a powerful tool for the assessment of nodal metastases in the hilum and mediastinum in patients with NSCLC [47, 51]. Systematic mediastinal node sampling strategies have been proposed and validated for mediastinoscopy in patients with NSCLC. No such validated sampling strategy exists for EBUS-TBNA [14, 16, 52], although it would seem intuitive to extrapolate the mediastinoscopy strategies to EBUS-TBNA procedure when performed for the similar indication. Studies are needed to identify the most cost-effective strategy for EBUS-TBNA staging of lung cancer. Furthermore, it is unclear if N1 nodal data, which unlike mediastinoscopy can be sampled by EBUS-TBNA, should be incorporated into EBUS-TBNA staging strategies. Additionally, there seems to be no clear consensus on what lymph node size cutoff should be used for determination of biopsy; indeed there is a wide variation of size cutoffs used in the medical literature, with some using short axis diameters of 10 mm and others using 5 mm. The use of the 10 mm short axis cutoff is extrapolated from the CT scan literature [53–55]; however it has been shown that the biopsy of nodes using a short axis cutoff of 5 mm is not only feasible but also adds to the yield of EBUS-TBNA in staging of patients with NSCLC [37, 56, 57].

There has been some speculation that the appearance of the lymph node during EBUS imaging can be predictive of the involvement of lymph node with metastatic disease [58], although recent studies have cast doubt on this finding [37]. Some studies also suggest that Doppler imaging during EBUS-TBNA may have a role in predicting the spread of malignancy [31, 58, 59] by evaluating the vascular patterns within the mediastinal lymph nodes, as described in the endoscopic ultrasound (EUS) literature [60, 61].

EBUS as a staging modality was initially compared to radiographic staging, specifically positron emission tomography (PET) and computed tomography (CT) scanning. In the mediastinum, PET is more sensitive than conventional CT for assessing lymph nodes, although the negative predictive value of PET for mediastinal metastasis is determined by avidity for fluorodeoxy glucose (FDG) and tumor location [62]. Multiple studies [56, 63–68] have compared EBUS-TBNA with preoperative radiographic staging in patients with either a normal mediastinum or enlarged lymph nodes, which appear pathologic based on radiologic criteria [53–55] for both CT and PET-CT scans (Table 5.2). In these studies, EBUS-TBNA was shown to be superior to radiographic staging. EBUS-TBNA has also been shown to be superior to radiological staging for nodes between 5 and 20 mm, especially for adenocarcinoma, which is known to have a higher rate of mediastinal metastasis and lower PET activity [64]. In addition, combined EBUS-TBNA+EUS-FNA was superior to either EBUS-TBNA or EUS-FNA alone for sub-centimeter nodes on CT scans [68].

EBUS-TBNA Versus Conventional TBNA

The yield for TBNA for detection of mediastinal metastases varies widely in the literature (20–89 %) and appears to be related to the size and location of the lesion as well as operator experience [26, 69]. There have been a few trials comparing

Table 5.2 Studies comparing EBUS staging to computed tomography (CT) and positron emission tomography (PET) staging

Study	Year	No. of patients	Sensitivity			Specificity			NPV			Prevalance
			CT	PET	EBUS	CT	PET	EBUS	CT	PET	EBUS	
Yasufuku	2006	102	76.9 %	80 %	92.3 %	55.3 %	70.1 %	100 %	87.5 %	91.5 %	97.4 %	23.6 %
Herth	2008	97			89 %			100 %			98.9 %	8.2 %
Bauwens	2008	106		67 %	95 %			100 %		100 %	91 %	58 %
Wallace	2008	138	67 %	24 %	69 %			100 %			88 %	28 %
Hwangbo	2009	117		70 %	90 %		59.8 %	100 %		85.2 %	96.7 %	26 %
Rintoul	2009	109			91 %			100 %			60 %	71 %
Szlubowski	2010	120			68 % + EUS			98 % + EUS			91 % + EUS	22 %

conventional TBNA with EBUS-TBNA in the setting of lung cancer staging. In the large comparative prospective trial, EBUS-TBNA yield was superior to conventional TBNA (84 % vs. 58 %) at stations other than station 7 in 200 patients with suspected NSCLC. There was no statistically significant difference in the diagnostic yield from station 7, although a trend favoring EBUS-TBNA over conventional TBNA (86 % vs. 74 %) was pointed out by the authors [46] One must note, however, that in this study, the radial probe EBUS was used to locate the lymph nodes and the TBNA procedure was performed using the standard TBNA needle and conventional technique. In other words, this study was not a comparison between the convex probe EBUS-TBNA and the conventional TBNA. In fact, the use of radial probe EBUS for this purpose has more or less been abandoned in the recent times in favor of convex probe EBUS-TBNA. The second comparative prospective trial included 138 patients with known or suspected lung cancer based on lung or mediastinal abnormality on CT [67]. EBUS-TBNA and EUS-FNA were compared to conventional TBNA. EBUS and EUS revealed the same sensitivity (69 %) and NPV (88 %). However, conventional TBNA had lower values with regard to both sensitivity (36 %) and NPV (78 %). This study suggests that EBUS-TBNA has a higher sensitivity than conventional TBNA for the detection of metastatic disease in the mediastinal and hilar lymph nodes.

EBUS-TBNA Versus Mediastinoscopy

Several studies have established the usefulness of EBUS-TBNA in staging of lung cancer (Table 5.3). High success of EBUS-TBNA in cancer staging has started a debate over the ability of EBUS-TBNA to supplant mediastinoscopy as the procedure of choice for mediastinal staging [6, 70]. Numerous studies have shown robust sensitivity and negative predictive values [63, 71–73] which are comparable to mediastinoscopy [57, 74–76] (Table 5.4).

EBUS-TBNA as an initial procedure for mediastinal staging has been shown to reduce the need for subsequent mediastinoscopy [77]. The ACCP guidelines published in 2007 for mediastinal staging of lung cancer suggest EBUS-TBNA as one of the options for initial staging. If the EBUS-TBNA samples do not show metastasis it

Table 5.3 Studies evaluating the usefulness of EBUS-TBNA in staging of lung cancer

Study	Year	No. of patients	Study design	Sensitivity EBUS	Specificity EBUS	NPV EBUS	Disease prevalence
Szlubowski	2009	206	Prospective cohort	89 %	100 %	84 %	61 %
Rintoul	2009	109	Retrospective	91 %	100 %	60 %	71 %
Hwangbo	2010	150	Prospective	84 %	100 %	93 %	
Andrade	2010	98	Retrospective	88 %	97 %	84 %	

Table 5.4 Studies comparing EBUS-TBNA and mediastinoscopy (MED) for staging of lung cancer

Study	Year	No. of patients	Study design	Sensitivity EBUS	Sensitivity MED	Specificity	NPV EBUS	NPV MED	Disease prevalence
Ernst	2008	66	Prospective crossover	87 %	68 %	100 %	78 %	59 %	89 %
Annema	2010	241	Randomized controlled	94 % EBUS + EUS	79 %	100 %	93 % EBUS + EUS	86 %	49 %
Defranchi	2010	494	Retrospective			100 %	72 %	81 %	
Yasufuku	2011	153	Prospective crossover	87 %	68 %	100 %	91 %	90 %	35 %

is recommended that a confirmatory mediastinoscopy is performed as EBUS-TBNA does not have 100 % negative predictive value. For example, in one study from Mayo Clinic, 29 patients with suspected or confirmed lung cancer who had a negative EBUS-TBNA result underwent mediastinoscopy for suspected N2 disease [74]. Metastatic disease was found in 8 of 29 (28 %) patients. Based on these results, the authors concluded that mediastinoscopy should be performed in lung cancer patients with suspicion for N2 disease but a negative EBUS-TBNA. In contrast, other studies have suggested that a confirmatory mediastinoscopy may not be necessary in all of these cases [57, 77]. Clearly, EBUS-TBNA performance, specifically negative predictive value, is the determining factor if a confirmatory mediastinoscopy is routinely withheld after a negative EBUS-TBNA. The NPV of EBUS-TBNA is affected by several factors including operator skill, cytologist skill, pre-procedure probability of malignancy, and incidence of benign disease in the population (i.e., histoplasmosis). Therefore, until further data are available, confirmatory mediastinoscopy in an EBUS-TBNA-negative mediastinum is recommended in the proper clinical setting.

It should be stressed that EBUS-TBNA and mediastinoscopy should be seen as complementary procedures and not mutually exclusive of each other. As such, each individual institution should take into account all factors such as yield, operator experience, cytologist skill, and surgical expertise before setting up local standards of mediastinal staging.

EBUS-TBNA for Lymphoma

The diagnosis of lymphoma is based upon a multimodality approach as outlined by the WHO in 2008 [78]. This approach combines clinical, morphologic, immunophenotypic, and genotypic data to establish the diagnosis. Whereas historically the classification of lymphoma was based primarily on cytomorphologic analysis, recent advances in immunophenotyping (specifically flow cytometric analysis) and genotype analysis have led to less reliance upon cytomorphology for diagnosis and classification. While analysis of morphologic features generally requires more tissue than what can be obtained by FNA alone, it has been established that the amount of tissue obtained in FNA samples can be adequate for phenotypic and genotypic analyses [79–81]. Accordingly, several studies have shown that EBUS-TBNA is a viable option for the diagnosis of lymphoma [82–84]. The overall sensitivity of detecting lymphoma is approximately 76 %; however the sensitivity for detecting its subtype is lower, owing to the fact that certain lymphoma subtypes such as marginal cell, some follicular cell, and Hodgkin's lymphoma [85] are difficult to diagnose with small-volume specimens. Furthermore, despite advances in flow cytometry and genetic testing, several lymphoma subtypes such as diffuse large B-cell lymphoma, mantle cell lymphoma, Burkitt's lymphoma, several subtypes of follicular lymphoma, and Hodgkin's lymphoma remain difficult to diagnose using a cytology specimen [86]. In case of Hodgkin's lymphoma, the characteristic Reed–Sternberg cells are present in small numbers and lack cell markers that can be identified by flow cytometry [86]. Still, newer assays are in development that may make Hodgkin's lymphoma more readily detectable by flow cytometry [87].

EBUS-TBNA for Benign Diseases

Sarcoidosis

The diagnosis of sarcoidosis can be enigmatic since the hallmark pathology of the disease—the epithelioid non-necrotizing granulomata—is a nonspecific finding that can be seen in many other disease states. The diagnosis of sarcoidosis is based on clinical symptoms and radiographic findings, supported by pathologic findings on tissue biopsy. Bronchoscopy and transbronchial biopsy have high diagnostic yield for pulmonary sarcoidosis (Chap. 2). Similarly, several studies have shown feasibility of obtaining specimen from enlarged mediastinal lymph nodes with conventional TBNA to establish the diagnosis of sarcoidosis. Lymphocytosis and CD4/CD8 ratio of >3.5 on BAL fluid may provide for supportive evidence but are not considered diagnostic for sarcoidosis [88]. Variable yield of conventional TBNA to obtain diagnostic specimen for sarcoidosis from mediastinal nodes has been reported [89, 90], depending on the experience of the operator and whether or not a 19-G TBNA histology needle is used. EBUS-TBNA has been applied to the acquisition of nodal tissue for diagnosis of sarcoidosis with reported yields of up to 93 % [91] and pooled yields of approximately 80 % [92]. In some studies, EBUS-TBNA has seemingly outperformed conventional TBNA [93] and also transbronchial biopsy [94]. Based on these studies, it is reasonable to use EBUS-TBNA as an initial diagnostic test for Stage I and II sarcoidosis, especially when transbronchial biopsy cannot be performed or is non-diagnostic.

Infection

Several studies have shown EBUS-TBNA to be useful in the diagnosis of tuberculosis, specifically in smear-negative disease when combined with bronchoalveolar lavage culture and nucleic acid amplification testing [95, 96]. Additionally, EBUS-TBNA was shown to have a high sensitivity for diagnosis of isolated mediastinal tuberculous lymphadenitis, which may occur in up to 9 % of all cases [97].

Miscellaneous

Although the data is limited, EBUS-TBNA has been reported to have a high diagnostic yield in mediastinal masses of unknown origin [98], especially if the etiology is benign. EBUS-TBNA may also play a role in the diagnosis and treatment of bronchogenic cysts [99, 100].

Limitations of EBUS-TBNA

EBUS-TBNA is an exciting new technology, but it is still evolving. Many challenges and limitations need to be addressed to further enhance the clinical utility of this technique. The EBUS scope is larger than standard bronchoscope and it cannot be used for a thorough endobronchial examination or for obtaining bronchoscopic specimens other than TBNA sample. Therefore, standard bronchoscopy is needed along with the EBUS-TBNA procedure, which increases the cost and duration of the procedure. A sleeker design with the capability to perform standard bronchoscopy using the same scope will greatly enhance its clinical utility. Also, some operators routinely perform EBUS-TBNA under general anesthesia, which adds to the cost, scheduling conflicts, and risk of anesthesia. A better design of the bronchoscope may obviate the need for general anesthesia for this procedure. Another major issue is the current design of the dedicated TBNA needle, which is significantly more complicated and cumbersome to use than the TBNA needle used for the conventional procedure. Innovation in the TBNA needle design to make it more user friendly may help eliminate some of the steps needed during acquisition of TBNA specimen. Finally, the issue of cost must be mentioned. The initial capital needed for EBUS can be an important consideration in a resource-limited setting. Further, the need for general anesthesia, operating and recovery room time, and anesthesia charges may add significantly to the overall cost of the procedure. It must also be pointed out that the maintenance and repair cost of EBUS-TBNA scopes per procedure is significantly higher than the repair cost of standard flexible bronchoscopes per procedure [101]. Lastly, most pulmonologists are not trained in ultrasound imaging and there is a significant need for education and training before an operator can perform this procedure with sufficient proficiency.

Conclusions

In summary, EBUS-TBNA is an innovative procedure, which is increasingly used across the world in the diagnosis of both malignant and benign disorders. EBUS-TBNA offers a minimally invasive procedure which allows reliable access to lymph nodes within the hilum and mediastinum, and real-time sampling of lymph node tissue. As compared to conventional TBNA and mediastinoscopy, EBUS-TBNA may be more suitable to reach smaller and more distant nodes in the hilum and mediastinum. The yield of EBUS is robust in both the benign and malignant settings, and approaches that of mediastinoscopy. While mediastinoscopy still plays an important role in the diagnosis of mediastinal diseases, the use of EBUS-TBNA in these settings will continue to increase as expertise and availability of EBUS-TBNA increase.

References

1. Hurter T, Hanrath P. Endobronchial sonography in the diagnosis of pulmonary and mediastinal tumors. Dtsch Med Wochenschr. 1990;115:1899–905.
2. Shannon JJ, Bude RO, Orens JB, et al. Endobronchial ultrasound-guided needle aspiration of mediastinal adenopathy. Am J Respir Crit Care Med. 1996;153: 1424–30.
3. Kurimoto N, Murayama M, Yoshioka S, et al. Assessment of usefulness of endobronchial ultrasonography in determination of depth of tracheobronchial tumor invasion. Chest. 1999;115:1500–6.
4. Herth FJ, Ernst A, Becker HD. Endobronchial ultrasound-guided transbronchial lung biopsy in solitary pulmonary nodules and peripheral lesions. Eur Respir J. 2002;20:972–4.
5. Yasufuku K, Chiyo M, Sekine Y, et al. Real-time endobronchial ultrasound-guided transbronchial needle aspiration of mediastinal and hilar lymph nodes. Chest. 2004;126:122–8.
6. Rusch VW. Mediastinoscopy: an obsolete procedure? J Thorac Cardiovasc Surg. 2011;142:1400–2.
7. Disayabutr S, Tscheikuna J, Nana A. The endobronchial ultrasound-guided transbronchial lung biopsy in peripheral pulmonary lesions. J Med Assoc Thai. 2010;93 Suppl 1:S94–101.
8. Wang Memoli JS, Nietert PJ, Silvestri GA. Meta-analysis of guided bronchoscopy for the evaluation of the pulmonary nodule. Chest. 2012;142(2):385–93.
9. Kurimoto N, Miyazawa T, Okimasa S, et al. Endobronchial ultrasonography using a guide sheath increases the ability to diagnose peripheral pulmonary lesions endoscopically. Chest. 2004; 126:959–65.
10. Yoshikawa M, Sukoh N, Yamazaki K, et al. Diagnostic value of endobronchial ultrasonography with a guide sheath for peripheral pulmonary lesions without X-ray fluoroscopy. Chest. 2007;131: 1788–93.
11. Chao TY, Chien MT, Lie CH, et al. Endobronchial ultrasonography-guided transbronchial needle aspiration increases the diagnostic yield of peripheral pulmonary lesions: a randomized trial. Chest. 2009;136:229–36.
12. Cho JH, Kim J, Kim K, et al. A comparative analysis of video-assisted mediastinoscopy and conventional mediastinoscopy. Ann Thorac Surg. 2011;92:1007–11.
13. Zakkar M, Tan C, Hunt I. Is video mediastinoscopy a safer and more effective procedure than conventional mediastinoscopy? Interact Cardiovasc Thorac Surg. 2012;14:81–4.
14. Detterbeck F, Puchalski J, Rubinowitz A, et al. Classification of the thoroughness of mediastinal staging of lung cancer. Chest. 2010;137:436–42.
15. Ernst A, Gangadharan SP. A good case for a declining role for mediastinoscopy just got better. Am J Respir Crit Care Med. 2008;177:471–2.
16. Detterbeck FC, Jantz MA, Wallace M, et al. Invasive mediastinal staging of lung cancer: ACCP evidence-based clinical practice guidelines (2nd edition). Chest. 2007;132:202S–20.
17. Little AG, Rusch VW, Bonner JA, et al. Patterns of surgical care of lung cancer patients. Ann Thorac Surg. 2005;80:2051–6. discussion 2056.
18. Deneffe G, Lacquet LM, Gyselen A. Cervical mediastinoscopy and anterior mediastinotomy in patients with lung cancer and radiologically normal mediastinum. Eur J Respir Dis. 1983;64:613–9.
19. Hammoud ZT, Anderson RC, Meyers BF, et al. The current role of mediastinoscopy in the evaluation of thoracic disease. J Thorac Cardiovasc Surg. 1999; 118:894–9.
20. De Leyn P, Schoonooghe P, Deneffe G, et al. Surgery for non-small cell lung cancer with unsuspected metastasis to ipsilateral mediastinal or subcarinal nodes (N2 disease). Eur J Cardiothorac Surg. 1996;10:649–54. discussion 654–645.
21. Page A, Nakhle G, Mercier C, et al. Surgical treatment of bronchogenic carcinoma: the importance of staging in evaluating late survival. Can J Surg. 1987; 30:96–9.
22. Dillemans B, Deneffe G, Verschakelen J, et al. Value of computed tomography and mediastinoscopy in preoperative evaluation of mediastinal nodes in non-small cell lung cancer. A study of 569 patients. Eur J Cardiothorac Surg. 1994;8:37–42.
23. Leschber G, Sperling D, Klemm W, et al. Does video-mediastinoscopy improve the results of conventional mediastinoscopy? Eur J Cardiothorac Surg. 2008;33:289–93.
24. Schieppati E. Mediastinal puncture thru the tracheal carina. Rev Asoc Med Argent. 1949;63:497–9.
25. Schieppati E. Mediastinal lymph node puncture through the tracheal carina. Surg Gynecol Obstet. 1958;107:243–6.
26. Wang KP, Brower R, Haponik EF, et al. Flexible transbronchial needle aspiration for staging of bronchogenic carcinoma. Chest. 1983;84:571–6.
27. Holty JE, Kuschner WG, Gould MK. Accuracy of transbronchial needle aspiration for mediastinal staging of non-small cell lung cancer: a meta-analysis. Thorax. 2005;60:949–55.
28. Diacon AH, Schuurmans MM, Theron J, et al. Transbronchial needle aspirates: how many passes per target site? Eur Respir J. 2007;29:112–6.

29. Chin Jr R, McCain TW, Lucia MA, et al. Transbronchial needle aspiration in diagnosing and staging lung cancer: how many aspirates are needed? Am J Respir Crit Care Med. 2002;166:377–81.
30. Rusch VW, Asamura H, Watanabe H, et al. The IASLC lung cancer staging project: a proposal for a new international lymph node map in the forthcoming seventh edition of the TNM classification for lung cancer. J Thorac Oncol. 2009;4:568–77.
31. Nakajima T, Anayama T, Shingyoji M, et al. Vascular image patterns of lymph nodes for the prediction of metastatic disease during EBUS-TBNA for mediastinal staging of lung cancer. J Thorac Oncol. 2012;7:1009–14.
32. Nakajima T, Yasufuku K. How I do it–optimal methodology for multidirectional analysis of endobronchial ultrasound-guided transbronchial needle aspiration samples. J Thorac Oncol. 2011;6:203–6.
33. Trisolini R, Cancellieri A, Tinelli C, et al. Rapid onsite evaluation of transbronchial aspirates in the diagnosis of hilar and mediastinal adenopathy: a randomized trial. Chest. 2011;139:395–401.
34. Diette GB, White Jr P, Terry P, et al. Utility of on-site cytopathology assessment for bronchoscopic evaluation of lung masses and adenopathy. Chest. 2000; 117:1186–90.
35. Baram D, Garcia RB, Richman PS. Impact of rapid on-site cytologic evaluation during transbronchial needle aspiration. Chest. 2005;128:869–75.
36. Diacon AH, Schuurmans MM, Theron J, et al. Utility of rapid on-site evaluation of transbronchial needle aspirates. Respiration. 2005;72:182–8.
37. Memoli JS, El-Bayoumi E, Pastis NJ, et al. Using endobronchial ultrasound features to predict lymph node metastasis in patients with lung cancer. Chest. 2011;140:1550–6.
38. Lee HS, Lee GK, Kim MS, et al. Real-time endobronchial ultrasound-guided transbronchial needle aspiration in mediastinal staging of non-small cell lung cancer: how many aspirations per target lymph node station? Chest. 2008;134:368–74.
39. Ost DE, Ernst A, Lei X, et al. Diagnostic yield of endobronchial ultrasound-guided transbronchial needle aspiration: results of the AQuIRE Bronchoscopy Registry. Chest. 2011;140:1557–66.
40. Sarkiss M. Anesthesia for bronchoscopy and interventional pulmonology: from moderate sedation to jet ventilation. Curr Opin Pulm Med. 2011;17: 274–8.
41. Sarkiss M, Kennedy M, Riedel B, et al. Anesthesia technique for endobronchial ultrasound-guided fine needle aspiration of mediastinal lymph node. J Cardiothorac Vasc Anesth. 2007;21:892–6.
42. Avidan MS, Zhang L, Burnside BA, et al. Anesthesia awareness and the bispectral index. N Engl J Med. 2008;358:1097–108.
43. Stolz D, Chhajed PN, Leuppi JD, et al. Cough suppression during flexible bronchoscopy using combined sedation with midazolam and hydrocodone: a randomised, double blind, placebo controlled trial. Thorax. 2004;59:773–6.
44. Milman N, Laub M, Munch EP, et al. Serum concentrations of lignocaine and its metabolite monoethylglycinexylidide during fibre-optic bronchoscopy in local anaesthesia. Respir Med. 1998;92: 40–3.
45. Wahidi MM, Jain P, Jantz M, et al. American College of Chest Physicians consensus statement on the use of topical anesthesia, analgesia, and sedation during flexible bronchoscopy in adult patients. Chest. 2011;140:1342–50.
46. Herth F, Becker HD, Ernst A. Conventional vs endobronchial ultrasound-guided transbronchial needle aspiration: a randomized trial. Chest. 2004;125: 322–5.
47. Gu P, Zhao YZ, Jiang LY, et al. Endobronchial ultrasound-guided transbronchial needle aspiration for staging of lung cancer: a systematic review and meta-analysis. Eur J Cancer. 2009;45:1389–96.
48. Huang CT, Chen CY, Ho CC, et al. A rare constellation of empyema, lung abscess, and mediastinal abscess as a complication of endobronchial ultrasound-guided transbronchial needle aspiration. Eur J Cardiothorac Surg. 2011;40:264–5.
49. Moffatt-Bruce SD, Ross Jr P. Mediastinal abscess after endobronchial ultrasound with transbronchial needle aspiration: a case report. J Cardiothorac Surg. 2010;5:33.
50. Steinfort DP, Johnson DF, Irving LB. Incidence of bacteraemia following endobronchial ultrasound-guided transbronchial needle aspiration. Eur Respir J. 2010;36:28–32.
51. Khoo KL, Ho KY. Endoscopic mediastinal staging of lung cancer. Respir Med. 2011;105:515–8.
52. De Leyn P, Lardinois D, Van Schil PE, et al. ESTS guidelines for preoperative lymph node staging for non-small cell lung cancer. Eur J Cardiothorac Surg. 2007;32:1–8.
53. Staples CA, Muller NL, Miller RR, et al. Mediastinal nodes in bronchogenic carcinoma: comparison between CT and mediastinoscopy. Radiology. 1988; 167:367–72.
54. Silvestri GA, Gould MK, Margolis ML, et al. Noninvasive staging of non-small cell lung cancer: ACCP evidenced-based clinical practice guidelines (2nd edition). Chest. 2007;132:178S–201.
55. Dales RE, Stark RM, Raman S. Computed tomography to stage lung cancer. Approaching a controversy using meta-analysis. Am Rev Respir Dis. 1990;141: 1096–101.
56. Herth FJ, Eberhardt R, Krasnik M, et al. Endobronchial ultrasound-guided transbronchial needle aspiration of lymph nodes in the radiologically and positron emission tomography-normal mediastinum in patients with lung cancer. Chest. 2008;133:887–91.
57. Yasufuku K, Pierre A, Darling G, et al. A prospective controlled trial of endobronchial ultrasound-guided transbronchial needle aspiration compared with

mediastinoscopy for mediastinal lymph node staging of lung cancer. J Thorac Cardiovasc Surg. 2011; 142:1393–400. e1391.
58. Fujiwara T, Yasufuku K, Nakajima T, et al. The utility of sonographic features during endobronchial ultrasound-guided transbronchial needle aspiration for lymph node staging in patients with lung cancer: a standard endobronchial ultrasound image classification system. Chest. 2010;138:641–7.
59. Satterwhite LG, Berkowitz DM, Parks CS, et al. Central intranodal vessels to predict cytology during endobronchial ultrasound transbronchial needle aspiration. J Bronchol Intervent Pulmonol. 2011;18: 322–8.
60. Nakajima T, Shingyouji M, Nishimura H, et al. New endobronchial ultrasound imaging for differentiating metastatic site within a mediastinal lymph node. J Thorac Oncol. 2009;4:1289–90.
61. Sawhney MS, Debold SM, Kratzke RA, et al. Central intranodal blood vessel: a new EUS sign described in mediastinal lymph nodes. Gastrointest Endosc. 2007;65:602–8.
62. Currie GP, Kennedy AM, Denison AR. Tools used in the diagnosis and staging of lung cancer: what's old and what's new? QJM. 2009;102:443–8.
63. Rintoul RC, Tournoy KG, El Daly H, et al. EBUS-TBNA for the clarification of PET positive intra-thoracic lymph nodes-an international multi-centre experience. J Thorac Oncol. 2009;4:44–8.
64. Hwangbo B, Kim SK, Lee HS, et al. Application of endobronchial ultrasound-guided transbronchial needle aspiration following integrated PET/CT in mediastinal staging of potentially operable non-small cell lung cancer. Chest. 2009;135:1280–7.
65. Bauwens O, Dusart M, Pierard P, et al. Endobronchial ultrasound and value of PET for prediction of pathological results of mediastinal hot spots in lung cancer patients. Lung Cancer. 2008;61:356–61.
66. Yasufuku K, Nakajima T, Motoori K, et al. Comparison of endobronchial ultrasound, positron emission tomography, and CT for lymph node staging of lung cancer. Chest. 2006;130:710–8.
67. Wallace MB, Pascual JM, Raimondo M, et al. Minimally invasive endoscopic staging of suspected lung cancer. JAMA. 2008;299:540–6.
68. Szlubowski A, Zielinski M, Soja J, et al. A combined approach of endobronchial and endoscopic ultrasound-guided needle aspiration in the radiologically normal mediastinum in non-small-cell lung cancer staging–a prospective trial. Eur J Cardiothorac Surg. 2010;37:1175–9.
69. Gasparini S, Zuccatosta L, De Nictolis M. Transbronchial needle aspiration of mediastinal lesions. Monaldi Arch Chest Dis. 2000;55:29–32.
70. Shrager JB. Mediastinoscopy: still the gold standard. Ann Thorac Surg. 2010;89:S2084–9.
71. Hwangbo B, Lee GK, Lee HS, et al. Transbronchial and transesophageal fine-needle aspiration using an ultrasound bronchoscope in mediastinal staging of potentially operable lung cancer. Chest. 2010;138: 795–802.
72. Szlubowski A, Kuzdzal J, Kolodziej M, et al. Endobronchial ultrasound-guided needle aspiration in the non-small cell lung cancer staging. Eur J Cardiothorac Surg. 2009;35:332–5. discussion 335–336.
73. Andrade RS, Groth SS, Rueth NM, et al. Evaluation of mediastinal lymph nodes with endobronchial ultrasound: the thoracic surgeon's perspective. J Thorac Cardiovasc Surg. 2010;139:578–82. discussion 582–573.
74. Defranchi SA, Edell ES, Daniels CE, et al. Mediastinoscopy in patients with lung cancer and negative endobronchial ultrasound guided needle aspiration. Ann Thorac Surg. 2010;90:1753–7.
75. Ernst A, Anantham D, Eberhardt R, et al. Diagnosis of mediastinal adenopathy-real-time endobronchial ultrasound guided needle aspiration versus mediastinoscopy. J Thorac Oncol. 2008;3:577–82.
76. Annema JT, van Meerbeeck JP, Rintoul RC, et al. Mediastinoscopy vs endosonography for mediastinal nodal staging of lung cancer: a randomized trial. JAMA. 2010;304:2245–52.
77. Lee BE, Kletsman E, Rutledge JR, et al. Utility of endobronchial ultrasound-guided mediastinal lymph node biopsy in patients with non-small cell lung cancer. J Thorac Cardiovasc Surg. 2012;143:585–90.
78. Campo E, Swerdlow SH, Harris NL, et al. The 2008 WHO classification of lymphoid neoplasms and beyond: evolving concepts and practical applications. Blood. 2011;117(19):5019–32.
79. Young NA. Grading follicular lymphoma on fine-needle aspiration specimens–a practical approach. Cancer. 2006;108:1–9.
80. Young NA, Al-Saleem T. Diagnosis of lymphoma by fine-needle aspiration cytology using the revised European-American classification of lymphoid neoplasms. Cancer. 1999;87:325–45.
81. Caraway NP. Strategies to diagnose lymphoproliferative disorders by fine-needle aspiration by using ancillary studies. Cancer. 2005;105:432–42.
82. Steinfort DP, Conron M, Tsui A, et al. Endobronchial ultrasound-guided transbronchial needle aspiration for the evaluation of suspected lymphoma. J Thorac Oncol. 2010;5:804–9.
83. Marshall CB, Jacob B, Patel S, et al. The utility of endobronchial ultrasound-guided transbronchial needle aspiration biopsy in the diagnosis of mediastinal lymphoproliferative disorders. Cancer Cytopathol. 2011;119:118–26.
84. Kennedy MP, Jimenez CA, Bruzzi JF, et al. Endobronchial ultrasound-guided transbronchial needle aspiration in the diagnosis of lymphoma. Thorax. 2008;63:360–5.
85. Farmer PL, Bailey DJ, Burns BF, et al. The reliability of lymphoma diagnosis in small tissue samples is heavily influenced by lymphoma subtype. Am J Clin Pathol. 2007;128:474–80.

86. de Tute RM. Flow cytometry and its use in the diagnosis and management of mature lymphoid malignancies. Histopathology. 2011;58:90–105.
87. Fromm JR, Thomas A, Wood BL. Flow cytometry can diagnose classical Hodgkin lymphoma in lymph nodes with high sensitivity and specificity. Am J Clin Pathol. 2009;131:322–32.
88. Nagai S, Izumi T. Bronchoalveolar lavage. Still useful in diagnosing sarcoidosis? Clin Chest Med. 1997;18:787–97.
89. Gilman MJ, Wang KP. Transbronchial lung biopsy in sarcoidosis. An approach to determine the optimal number of biopsies. Am Rev Respir Dis. 1980;122: 721–4.
90. Koonitz CH, Joyner LR, Nelson RA. Transbronchial lung biopsy via the fiberoptic bronchoscope in sarcoidosis. Ann Intern Med. 1976;85:64–6.
91. Oki M, Saka H, Kitagawa C, et al. Real-time endobronchial ultrasound-guided transbronchial needle aspiration is useful for diagnosing sarcoidosis. Respirology. 2007;12:863–8.
92. Agarwal R, Srinivasan A, Aggarwal AN, et al. Efficacy and safety of convex probe EBUS-TBNA in sarcoidosis: a systematic review and meta-analysis. Respir Med. 2012;106:883–92.
93. Tremblay A, Stather DR, Maceachern P, et al. A randomized controlled trial of standard vs endobronchial ultrasonography-guided transbronchial needle aspiration in patients with suspected sarcoidosis. Chest. 2009;136:340–6.
94. Nakajima T, Yasufuku K, Kurosu K, et al. The role of EBUS-TBNA for the diagnosis of sarcoidosis–comparisons with other bronchoscopic diagnostic modalities. Respir Med. 2009;103:1796–800.
95. Lin SM, Chung FT, Huang CD, et al. Diagnostic value of endobronchial ultrasonography for pulmonary tuberculosis. J Thorac Cardiovasc Surg. 2009;138:179–84.
96. Lin SM, Ni YL, Kuo CH, et al. Endobronchial ultrasound increases the diagnostic yields of polymerase chain reaction and smear for pulmonary tuberculosis. J Thorac Cardiovasc Surg. 2010;139:1554–60.
97. Navani N, Molyneaux PL, Breen RA, et al. Utility of endobronchial ultrasound-guided transbronchial needle aspiration in patients with tuberculous intrathoracic lymphadenopathy: a multicentre study. Thorax. 2011;66:889–93.
98. Yasufuku K, Nakajima T, Fujiwara T, et al. Utility of endobronchial ultrasound-guided transbronchial needle aspiration in the diagnosis of mediastinal masses of unknown etiology. Ann Thorac Surg. 2011;91:831–6.
99. Galluccio G, Lucantoni G. Mediastinal bronchogenic cyst's recurrence treated with EBUS-FNA with a long-term follow-up. Eur J Cardiothorac Surg. 2006;29:627–9. discussion 629.
100. Anantham D, Phua GC, Low SY, et al. Role of endobronchial ultrasound in the diagnosis of bronchogenic cysts. Diagn Ther Endosc. 2011;2011: 468237.
101. Hergott CA, MacEachern P, Stather DR, Tremblay A. Repair cost for endobronchial ultrasound bronchoscopes. J Bronchol Intervent Pulmonol. 2010;17: 223–7.

Electromagnetic Navigation Bronchoscopy

6

Thomas R. Gildea and Joseph Cicenia

Abstract

Electromagnetic navigation bronchoscopy (ENB) has been in continuous evolution since its introduction in 2004. The basic components of this global positioning system-like technology include a magnetic field generator, a sensor and computer integration, and a computed tomography scan used as a three-dimensional map. Its value has been documented for individuals with small peripheral pulmonary nodules and clearly represents a significant improvement over standard non-guided bronchoscopy. Variances and worldwide practice have shown how ENB fits into regional work flows and opens several important questions about the values of adjunct technology such as fluoroscopy, peripheral ultrasound, biopsy technique, and anesthesia technique, etc. This chapter reviews the literature on ENB and discusses the evolution as well as the technical aspects of the procedure. Also described is the ideal patient population based on the literature and our own expertise.

Keywords

Solitary pulmonary nodule • Electromagnetic navigation bronchoscopy • Bronchoscopy

Introduction

Solitary pulmonary nodules (SPNs) are common incidental findings, and their incidence is rising, which is likely due to the increased use of chest CT, which is more sensitive at discovering a SPN than traditional plain chest radiography [1]. The detection of SPNs is likely to increase since the advent of the National Lung Screening Trial (NLST) [2]. The majority of SPNs is not malignant; even in high-risk patients only 1 % of SPNs are malignant [2].

T.R. Gildea, M.D., M.S. (✉)
Bronschoscopy, Cleveland Clinic, Respiratory Institute, 9500 Euclid Ave/A90, Cleveland, OH 44195, USA
e-mail: gildeat@ccf.org

J. Cicenia, M.D.
Respiratory Institute - Department of Interventional Pulmonary, Cleveland Clinic, Cleveland, OH, USA

A.C. Mehta and P. Jain (eds.), *Interventional Bronchoscopy: A Clinical Guide*, Respiratory Medicine 10,
DOI 10.1007/978-1-62703-395-4_6, © Springer Science+Business Media New York 2013

Therefore, minimizing invasiveness while maximizing accuracy can impact the diagnosis-related morbidity in profound ways. In broad terms, the approach to the SPN can be broken down into three strategies: (1) serial imaging to detect interval changes in the nodule ("watchful waiting"), (2) minimally invasive diagnostic procedures (bronchoscopy and transthoracic needle biopsy), and (3) surgical excision. The pretest probability of the malignant potential of the SPN in addition to the patient's ability to withstand morbidity should impact which strategy to be followed [3].

Computed tomography-guided fine needle aspiration (CT-FNA) is a common strategy of tissue procurement, with a pooled sensitivity for malignancy of approximately 90 % [4, 5]. However, the procedure is complicated by pneumothorax in up to 30 %, with the need for a chest tube in up to 6 % [5]. Risk factors for pneumothorax include older age, the presence of underlying COPD or emphysema, distance from the pleura, and smaller lesion size [5]. Of SPNs that result in surgical resection, up to 20 % are subsequently found to be benign [6]. This high rate of nontherapeutic thoracotomy may expose patients to unnecessary morbidity and mortality.

The diagnostic yield of conventional bronchoscopy has historically been disappointing, with sensitivities for malignancy ranging from 14 to 63 % [7, 8], with multiple factors affecting yield. These factors include nodule size (> or < 2 cm), biopsy method, number of biopsies taken, and the presence of an air bronchus sign [9].

The addition of radial-probe ultrasound [10, 11] has improved yield of conventional bronchoscopic biopsy to about 70 % [12]. However broad application of this technology is highly dependent on operator skill and availability of the technology. Additionally, its yield drops significantly as the size of the nodule decreases [11]. The ability of the probe to articulate with an accessible airway is likely related to the nodule size, and as such, smaller nodules may be difficult to reach with ultrasound guidance alone if a steerable catheter is not used.

Electromagnetic navigation bronchoscopy (ENB) was cleared for use in the United States via FDA 510 K in 2004. The basic principles of the technology are the use of the CT scan as a three-dimensional map and the use of sensors in a low-power electromagnetic field to give positional information. The addition of catheter steering capacity and computer feedback of relative position functions similarly to global positioning system (GPS)-like technology. The locatable guide sensor can be removed from the extended working channel (EWC) leaving a direct pathway to the target through which standard biopsy instruments can be passed. There have been several studies over time and multiple software and hardware evolutions. Studies have been done in a number of different clinical environments using different biopsy techniques, anesthesia techniques, adjunctive imaging techniques, and different thresholds for error. Despite all these differences there is a surprising consistency of yield around 70 %. This chapter addresses the basics of ENB and the latest version of the technique as well as a description of the method we use at the Cleveland Clinic.

System Components

The superDimension system is composed of both hardware and software components, collectively known as the iLogic® system. The system is composed of both planning and procedure stations. The planning station consists of a laptop computer. The laptop allows for portability and obviates the need to perform planning functions on the procedural tower. CT data, in the form of DICOM files, can be loaded into the laptop either through a CD-ROM or networked directly into the computer via an Ethernet (or similar) connection. The procedure station consists of a central processing unit (CPU), video screen, location amplifier, location board, locatable guide, and patient sensor triplets. The software used for the procedure is composed of planning and procedural/navigation components. The planning component of the software is placed on both the laptop computer and procedure CPU. The procedural tower CPU contains both planning and navigation software elements. Additionally it contains a location amplifier that serves to integrate the peripheral system components used during the procedure, processing, and sending of navigation data to the CPU. The location board generates a low-frequency electromagnetic field known as the "sensing volume" through which the navigational procedure takes place and is positioned under the patient, typically between the mattress and stretcher, and should extend generally from the thoracic inlet to the diaphragm (Fig. 6.1). The sensing volume created by the location board is approximately 40 cm × 40 cm in the x- and y-axes, and 23 cm in the z-axis, with the z-axis beginning 5 cm above the board. The patient's thoracic space must fit in this volume for the procedure to occur which can present challenges for morbidly obese patients. Patient sensor triplets are connected to the patient to assess for patient movement and to correct for this during the procedure. Typically these are placed near the sternal notch and along the lower rib cage in a triangular fashion. The locatable guide (LG) is a miniaturized sensor that feeds positional data to the CPU. Positional data includes x-, y-, and z-coordinates in addition to roll, pitch, and yaw; data is delivered to the CPU 166 times per second. During navigation, the LG fits into a catheter known as the extended working channel (EWC) (Fig. 6.2a); the EWC allows for steerability. There are two iterations of the EWC: the classic EWC with manual 8-direction steerability (achieved through struts within the LG device), and the more recent Edge catheters that have inherent distal curvatures of 45°, 90°, and 180° (Fig. 6.2b).

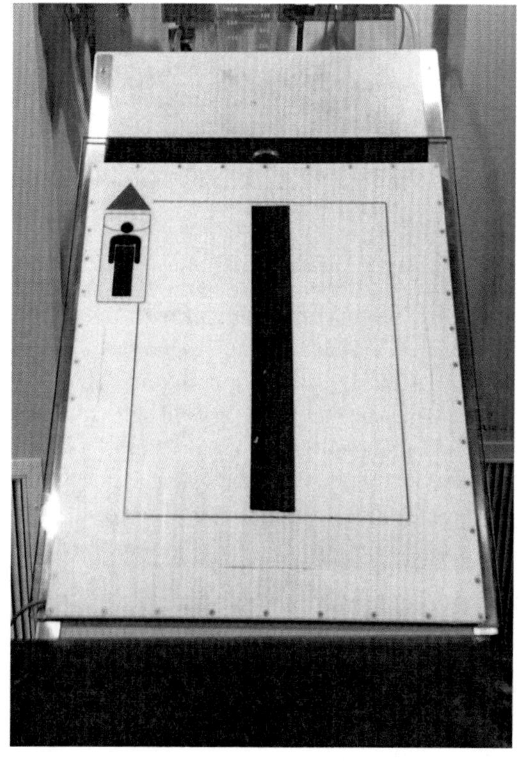

Fig. 6.1 Electromagnetic location board, placed at the head end of the table

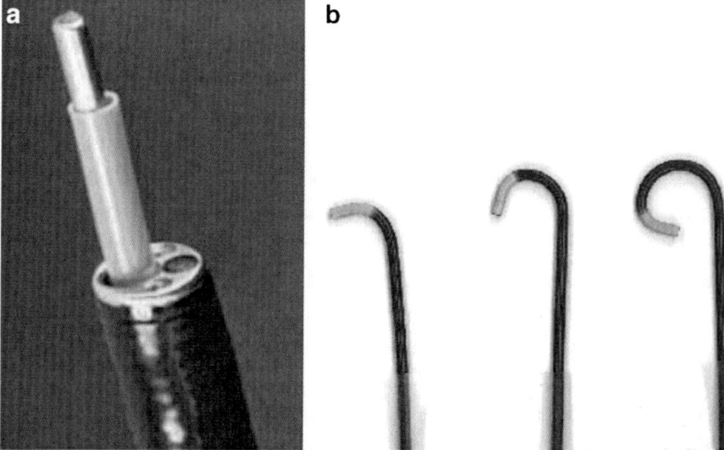

Fig. 6.2 (**a**) Extended working channel (EWC) (*blue*) through which locatable guide (LG) has been placed. Both EWC and LG are navigated to the lesion after the tip of the bronchoscope is wedged into the chosen bronchus. (**b**) The edge catheter comes in 45, 90 and 180 degree angulations

These Edge catheters are designed similar to vascular catheters that use torquability properties to facilitate smoother steerability. The distal curves of the Edge catheters may also allow for directional biopsies if the lesion does not articulate directly with the airway.

CT Scan Formats

The CT scan is the basic map from which all ENB can occur. It requires some specific configuration that has changed over time. Initially a CT with 3 mm cuts at 1.5 intervals was the ideal used for optimal virtual airway rendering. However, since the migration to the new version, higher resolution scans are now preferable. The interval and slice thickness should have 25–50 % overlap and the soft tissue kernel is best to reduce CT artifact. We have noted some initial issues with some of the dose reduction protocols for losing some of the small airways, but for the initial planning and target acquisition these have been adequate. Ideal CT acquisition and reconstruction specifications vary across manufacturers. These specifications have been validated by superDimension, and are available from them upon request.

Procedure Planning

For the purposes of this chapter, we will be describing planning on the most current software version, which according to most estimates have approximately 90 % market penetration. In the past, registration was done manually using registration points selected during the planning process; currently registration is performed automatically in the most current software iteration. It is still recommended, however, to prepare for a manual registration in case the automatic registration cannot be achieved. We discuss each registration technique below; however it will be discussed from the standpoint of the most current software version at the time of this writing. Procedure planning occurs most commonly on a freestanding laptop computer with the dedicated planning software. The planning process begins with the patient's CT data being uploaded from DICOM files to the laptop via a CD-ROM or directly off a *picture archiving and communication system* (PACS). If the CT scan is appropriately configured and in the proper format, each image series with its corresponding parameters will show up on the import page. The image series that conform to the ideal recommended parameters will be identified by the software; image series with acceptable but not ideal parameters will also be listed; however there will be a warning message stating that these images may result in suboptimal reconstructions for the procedure. The operator will then select the image series to be processed. As the images are processed, the software will construct a virtual 3D tracheobronchial tree for the operator to approve. Ideally this tree should include a minimum of four generations of bronchi. Once the 3D tree is approved, the screen will generally show three panels of multiplanar CT reconstructions (axial, coronal, and sagittal planes) and a fourth panel with a virtual airway reconstruction with standard tool bars for interacting with the software and CT data (Fig. 6.3).

Typically we then next identify registration points in case a manual registration needs to be performed during the procedure. This is accomplished by identifying points on the virtual bronchoscopy that can be easily identified during bronchoscopy procedure. Typically these points include the main carina, the upper, middle, and one lower lobe segmental carina on the right; the carina separating the left upper and left lower lobe; and one segmental left lower lobe bifurcation. These registration points should be spatially separated, and should extend into the lower lobes. After registration points are selected and marked, the target is then identified, marked, and sized. Once the target has been identified the software will generate a tentative pathway to the closest central airway to the lesion (Fig. 6.4). This will be represented as a gray dot on the screen, which represents a proposed exit point of the airway to the lesion. At this stage we examine this pathway, and if validated, we save the pathway. The pathway may not be able to be validated for several

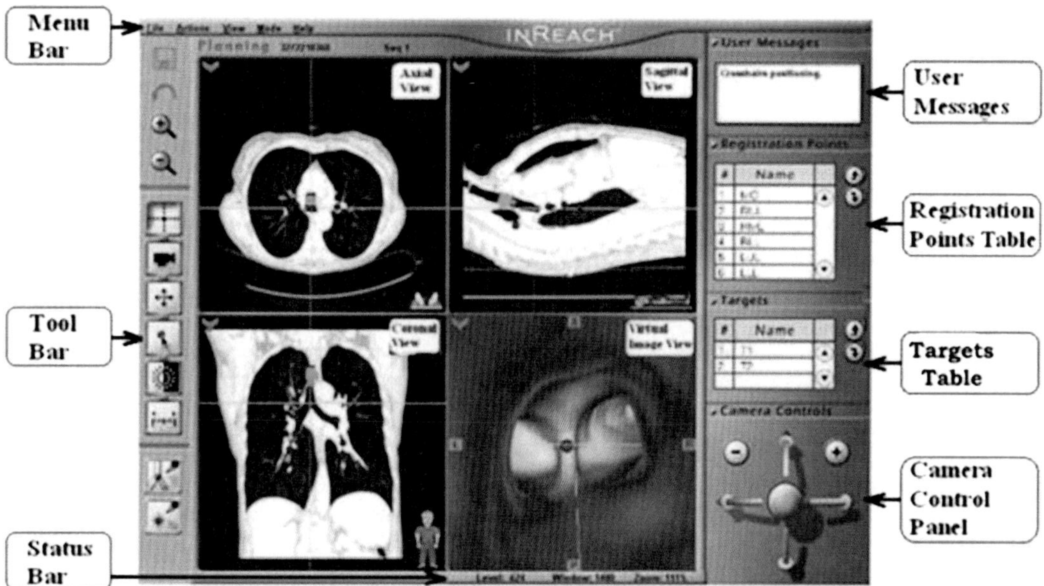

Fig. 6.3 Computer interphase showing the coronal, axial, and sagittal views of chest computed tomography and the virtual bronchoscopy image

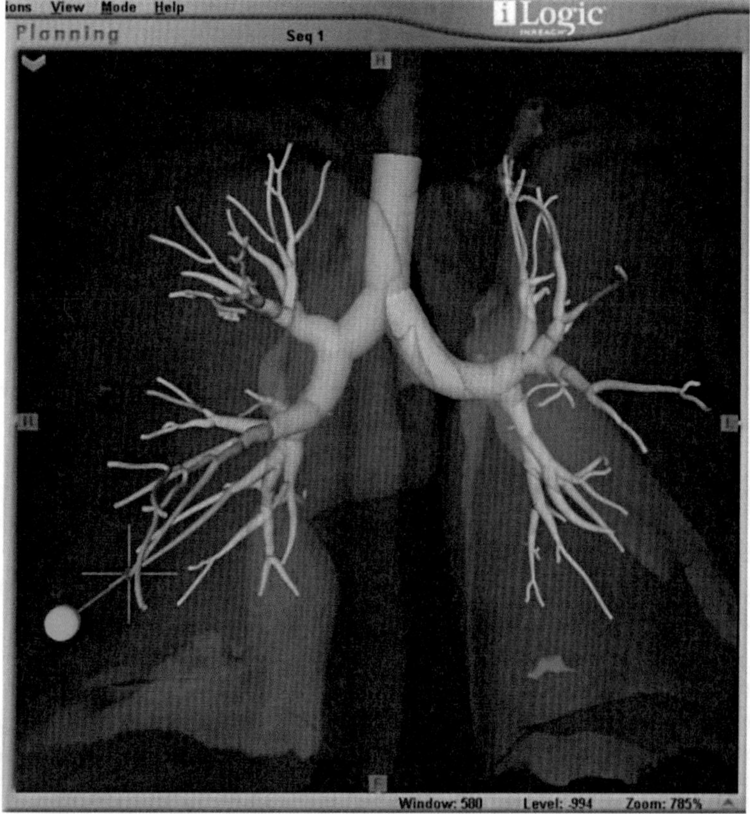

Fig. 6.4 Automatic pathway to the lesion (*shown as green dot*)

reasons: the software may not identify distal airways to the lesion; there may be a closer or different airway path to the lesion, among other things. If a closer airway or a completely different airway is identified, we can manually place intermediate points within this airway, sometimes called "bread crumbs," and confirm the new exit point by clicking on the gray dot. Once the exit point is confirmed the pathway then turns purple and we can review the pathway in a virtual bronchoscopic "fly through." At this point additional targets may be chosen in a similar fashion. Although more than one target can be selected given the clinical circumstance, we do not approach targets in contralateral lung due to the risk of potentially causing bilateral pneumothoraces. Once planning is completed, the data is saved first on the laptop, and then can be exported to a flash drive for the procedure.

Also, there is the potential for planning mediastinal biopsies. In this work flow it is important to place the virtual camera facing the general direction of the mediastinal lymph node we wish to biopsy and after target selection, where the size of the target center actually is important, we can make the airway translucent by changing the slide bar to the right of the image. During the procedure, this image will be available on the navigation screen for directing the approach of the needle biopsy.

Procedure Registration

Once planning is accomplished and the data saved, the procedure can be commenced. The procedure begins by laying the patient on the procedure table (or stretcher) which has the location board attached to it. The patient should be positioned so that they are aligned properly with the location board, and that their thorax will be contained within the sensing volume. At our institution, we have a preset position for the board to be attached to the stretcher, and the stretcher is also marked to allow for proper patient positioning, so that patient repositioning during the procedure is minimized. Once the patient is positioned, patient sensors are placed on the patient to ensure placement within the sensing volume, and to detect and correct for patient movement during the procedure. Typically these sensors are placed on the cephalad sternum, and in the midaxillary lines bilaterally. For the procedure to commence, all connections to the procedure CPU must first be verified by the software; once this is accomplished the operator will move forward with the registration procedure.

Automatic Registration

When the registration component is begun, the locatable guide is placed through the working channel of the bronchoscope until its tip can be seen protruding out of the distal end of the scope. The bronchoscope is then advanced through the airways starting in the mid-trachea; as the bronchoscope is advanced through the airways, it is placed into each lobar bronchus (to ensure best accuracy, the bronchoscope should be advanced an equal distance into each lobar bronchus). During this process, the LG passively makes several hundred position ascertainments as it moves through the central airways and matches this to the volume of the virtual 3D tracheobronchial tree. Once the software has enough data points to create an accurate registration, a virtual bronchoscopic image (with its panel outlined in a green border) will appear on the screen. At this point the scope should be withdrawn and placed at the main carina, and the virtual bronchoscopic image should be manually rotated on the screen to match the orientation of the real-time bronchoscopic image. Once this is performed, the operator presses "registration complete" manually on the screen and navigation procedure can be commenced.

Manual Registration

There are instances where automatic registration cannot be completed, or there is concern regarding accuracy of the registration process. If this occurs, then a manual registration can be performed. This process is similar to the original registration process required in prior software versions. In this technique, the LG is placed serially upon preset registration points identified and saved during the planning process (see above). Each point's coordinate within the sensing volume will be correlated with the preset point in the CT volume. This process should include at least five registration points, with one of the points being the main carina, and two of the points being in each lower lobe bronchi. The effect should be to create a triangle that extends out from the main carina. Because this is not a dynamic process, the registration algorithm will incur variable CT to body error also known as average fiducial target registration error (AFTRE), and will be reported by the software once registration is completed. If the AFTRE score is acceptable (<5 mm), the operator will accept the registration and move on to the navigation phase of the procedure. If the AFTRE score is not acceptable, the manual registration process can be restarted.

The AFTRE is the average of the sum of all the variances between the observed and expected distances between each of the registration points in the virtual patient compared to those measured in the actual patient. The end result is a value in millimeters that represents a sphere of uncertainty about the location of tip of the probe in the actual patient and the location in the virtual patient. Beyond that sphere there is potential of two other kinds of error. Translational error is the possibility that all the registration points are systematically moved in the same direction so that the error and its correction may be a matter of a linear adjustment. There is also the potential for rotational error where there may be asymmetric error: anteriorly on one side and posteriorly on the other. In this case there is a magnifying effect and the error increases as one moves away from the mediastinum and the central airways. The last kind of error is the inability to account for the complexity of lung movement. Although there is a tracking mechanism for anterior and subtle other movements of the thorax, these do not account for diaphragm excursion. This is particularly troubling in individuals with normal lung function where a breath hold CT and a CT at functional residual capacity (FRC) may vary with as much as 5 cm of diaphragm movement in the cephalad direction but also may slide forward or backward as the lesion slides in the lung over the diaphragm. Adjusting and recognizing error are relatively simple when there is a significant translational error that one can check at the end of registration making sure that the probe is not significantly different in location in the virtual and actual endobronchial images. The impact of error on yield was noted by Makris and colleagues where a CT–body error of <4 mm was associated with higher diagnostic yield [13].

Difference in Registration Processes

The release of iLogic® introduced the automatic registration process, which has several advantages over manual registration. The automatic registration process is dependent on the availability of a good virtual bronchoscopic image and the balance of the airway survey. Unlike manual registration, automatic registration does not require the manual planning and acquisition of predefined anatomical landmarks in the tracheobronchial tree. In automatic registration, instead of individually registering each point the LG passively makes several hundred-position ascertainments as it moves through the central airways and matches this to the volume of the virtual 3D tracheobronchial tree. In automatic registration an actual measure of error is not reported but according to the manufacturer, it is in between 3 and 4 mm or it will not register, thus ensuring that a procedure will not commence without an accurate registration.

Anesthesia Techniques

Anesthesia for ENB is not uniform in any published data. The earliest trials in Europe were performed under general anesthesia with rigid bronchoscopy as is typical of those clinics [14, 15]. In the first US trial and our center, all procedures were done under conscious sedation using morphine and midazolam and lidocaine sedation and analgesia [16]. Other centers have tried alternative techniques including nitrous oxide [17]. Although not specifically compared, there is no significant difference in yields or complications in centers that use one particular type of anesthesia versus another, with potential benefits and risks on both sides. It is theoretically possible to have an increased risk of pneumothorax while on positive pressure ventilation during transbronchial biopsies; conversely, the patient is likely to cough unexpectedly during transbronchial biopsies if only under moderate sedation. Also, there is a potential for change in the severity of the planned versus actual lung of individuals under sedation. The CT scan obtained for procedure planning is typically performed with a deep inspiratory breath hold where as under sedation the patients breathe close to functional residual capacity with small tidal volumes. In patients with normal lung function there may be significant difference in thoracic volume and movement of the diaphragms such that lower lung lesions may be much more mobile than upper lobe lesions. In individuals with severe obstructive lung disease and emphysema this movement is minimized. During general anesthesia it is possible to instill a large breath and to mimic the CT scan. It may be difficult to reproduce this mechanism with the patient under moderate sedation. Overall, choice of anesthesia still depends on the center as it has not been shown that differences in anesthesia techniques are associated with different outcomes or complications.

Fluoroscopy Versus No Fluoroscopy

In the user's manuals, the use of biplane fluoroscopy is recommended during the performance of ENB. We have found single-plane fluoroscopy to be useful in our center. Most European centers published data specifically not using fluoroscopy, and these show very similar yields and complications. It is our experience that using fluoroscopy is helpful identifying how and if the EWC becomes displaced during biopsy procedures because the instrument passing through the working channel has varying characteristics of stiffness and trackability, which may increase the possibility of a non-diagnostic biopsy. If fluoroscopy is going to be used, it is important to know that the fluoroscope cannot be in position during registration and navigation since the c-arm itself may represent a form of ferromagnetic interference with the location board. Only after navigation is completed should the fluoroscopy unit be brought into the field to localize the lesion relative to the working channel and probe.

Adjunctive Imaging

There has been a good deal of interest in using radial probe endobronchial ultrasound (R-EBUS) as a real-time imaging technique that can confirm accurate navigation. R-EBUS has an advantage over fluoroscopy in that it does not depend on planar images, and that it can detect small lesions that cannot be seen on fluoroscopy. In a prospective randomized trial there was a benefit of using both R-EBUS and EMB together with 88 % yield [18] but in subsequent trials by the same group the combined yield was 75 % [19]. Furthermore, it is estimated that fewer than 5 % of centers with superDimension systems in the United States have R-EBUS availability. Despite this, R-EBUS is used routinely at our institution to assess for navigational success. Additionally, with the use of the curved Edge catheters, R-EBUS can aid in obtaining the ideal catheter orientation for biopsy (by torquing the catheter until the image shows the lesion in greatest dimension), especially in those lesions which do not articulate directly with the airway (i.e., those lesions without an air bronchus sign).

Navigation and Tissue Acquisition

The bronchoscope is wedged into the subsegment leading to the target lesion. The EWC and LG are then slowly advanced toward the lesion. The objective during navigation is to steer and advance the LG along the pathway (purple line in Fig 6.5) generated on virtual bronchoscopy images to the target. The LG can either be steered with the directional instrument in the old system or now directed with rotation of the Edge catheter

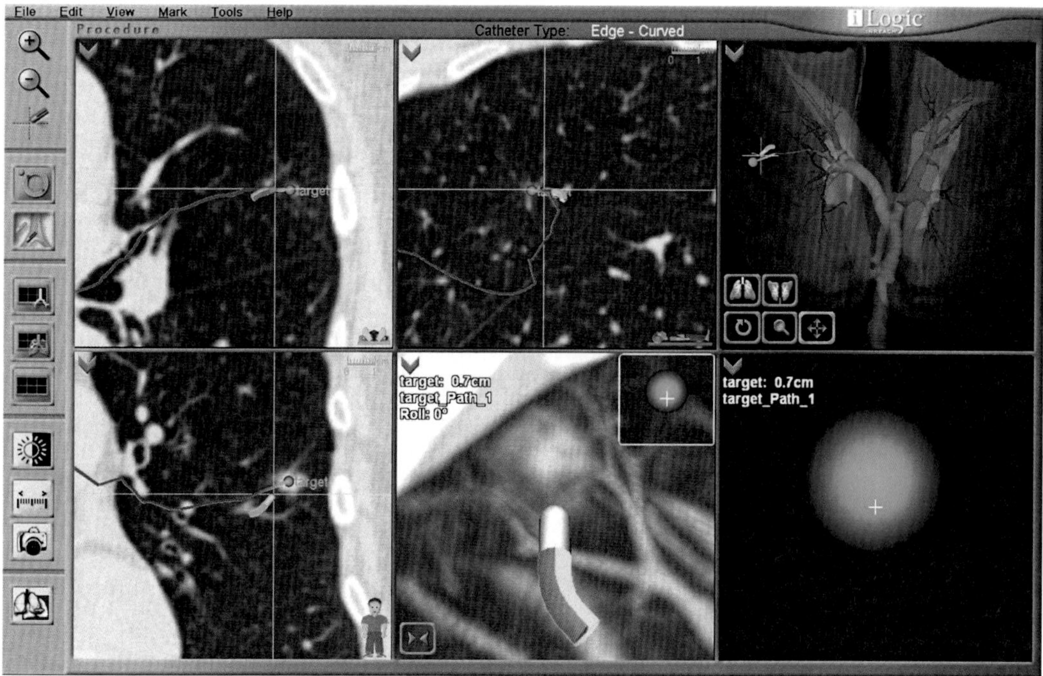

Fig. 6.5 The 6 panel navigation view using the edge catheter has the multiplanar CT views but also options for maximum intensive projection MIP (bottom center) and a dynamic airway view top right as well and the standard target window noting distance to lesion center with a graphic view of lesion relation to probe tip

along the pathway. The lesion is represented as a green sphere. The lesion is represented as a green sphere on all of the system viewports (Fig. 6.5). As the distal LG gets closer to the lesion, the green dot continues to get larger in a relative fashion. Once the LG reaches the desired location close to the target, the EWC or edge catheter is fixed at the proximal end of the biopsy channel of the bronchoscope by a locking mechanism and the LG is withdrawn. Fluoroscopy can be performed to view the LG in the desired location before its removal. Bronchoscopic accessories such as a biopsy forceps, transbronchial aspiration needle, and endobronchial brush can be inserted via the EWC to obtain a tissue specimen. An endobronchial ultrasound probe can also be inserted for additional location confirmation. The EWC can accommodate all standard bronchoscopic biopsy tools. There is some difficulty advancing standard Wang needles if the bend in the EWC is toward the upper lobes or in the superior segment of the lower lobes due to the angulation. Several centers have reported yields based on TBBx alone while others have used a variety of tools such as cytology brushes, cytology needles, transbronchial biopsy forceps, needle-brush, and cytology aspirates. There is clearly no best instrument but they are complementary in that in some cases one instrument yields a diagnosis while others are negative and a different combination in different cases. It has been our protocol to obtain as many types of specimens as possible. There has been one paper looking at the yield of a catheter aspiration vs. transbronchial biopsy. There is a clear benefit to the catheter aspiration even in cases where there is a 50 % yield even in the absence of identifiable EBUS images [19].

Diagnostic Yield. There is a very large amount of variation in several factors of the technique that may have an effect on yield and yet there is a surprising similarity across centers. A recent meta-analysis pooled yield prior to 2010 was 70 % [12]. There is a trend toward higher yields in more recent literature that may have to do with the various technical upgrades, changes in biopsy tools, and better patient selection with a positive bronchus sign [9]. Table 6.1 summarizes the

Table 6.1 Diagnostic yield of electromagnetic navigation bronchoscopy

Reference	Technique	*N*	Size (mm) range or mean	Diagnostic yield	RE/NE	Duration of bronchoscopy (min)	Anesthesia	PNX (%)
Becker (2005) [15]	ENB + fluoro	29	12–106	69 %	RE: 6.1 ± 1.7	N/A	GA	3.3
Hautmann (2005) [20]	ENB + fluoro	16	22 ± 6	Not given	4.2	N/A	CS	0
Schwarz (2006) [21]	ENB + fluoro	13	15–50	69 %	NE: 5.7	46 min	CS	0
Gildea (2006) [16]	ENB + fluoro	58	PPL: 22.8 LN: 28.1	PPL: 74 % LN: 100 %	RE: 6.6 ± 2.1 NE: 9 ± 5	51 ± 6 min	CS	3.4
Wilson (2007) [22]	ENB + fluoro + ROSE	248	PPL: 2.1 LN: 1.8	70–86 %	RE: 0.5 ± 0.02	N/A	CS	1.2
Makris (2007) [13]	ENB	40	23.5	62.5 %	RE :4 ± 0.15 NE: 8.7 ± 0.8	N/A	GA	7.5
Eberhardt (2007) [14]	ENB	89	24	67 %	RE: 4.6 ± 1.8 NE: 9 ± 6	29.9 ± 6.5 min	GA or CS	2.2
Eberhardt (2007) [18]	ENB	39	26	88 %	N/A	N/A	GA or CS	6
Lamprecht (2009) [23]	ENB + PET-CT + ROSE	13	30	76.9 %	N/A	60 min	–	0
McLemore (2007) [24]	ENB + EBUS	48	23 (6–60)	90 %	N/A	N/A	–	2.1
Bertoletti (2009) [17]	ENB	53	31.2	77.3 %	RE: 4.7 ± 1.3 NE: 10 ± 5.9	29.5 min	Nitrous oxide	4
Seijo (2010) [9]	ENB + ROSE	51	25 (15–35)	67 %	RE: 4	N/A	–	0
Eberhardt (2010) [19]	ENB + EBUS	53	23.3 (11–29)	75.5 %	RE: 3.6 (1.8–5.7)	25.7 (16–45) min	–	1.9
Mahajan (2011) [25]	ENB + fluoro	48	20 ± 13	77 %	N/A	N/A	CS	10
Lamprecht (2012) [26]	ENB + PET-CT + ROSE	112	27.1 ± 1.3	83.9 %	N/A	45 min	GA	1.8
Pearlstein (2012) [27]	ENB + ROSE	104	28	85 %	RE: 4.0 (2.4–7)	70 min (25–157)	GA	5.8

CS conscious sedation, *ENB* electromagnetic navigation bronchoscopy, *EBUS* endobronchial ultrasound, *GA* general anesthesia, *LN* lymph nodes, *PPL* peripheral pulmonary lesions, *PNX* pneumothorax, *ROSE* rapid on-site examination, *RE* registration error, *NE* navigation error, *N/A* not available results of studies addressing the diagnostic role of ENB in patients with peripheral pulmonary nodules.

Use of ENB in Therapeutic Interventions

ENB is becoming increasingly popular in bronchoscopic placement of fiducial markers prior to stereotactic radiosurgery or cyberknife treatment. This treatment option is generally reserved for patients who have a localized lung cancer but are medically unfit to undergo lung tumor resection [28]. With this technology, the tumor is exposed to a more concentrated doses of radiation while sparing the surrounding structures, thereby reducing the risk of collateral radiation-induced damage. For an exact tumor ablation, cyberknife requires fiducial marker placement in and close to the tumor. Traditional method of placing fiducials via transthoracic route under CT guidance is associated with high risks of pneumothorax. For example, in one series 47 % of patients developed pneumothorax and required chest tube drainage after transthoracic placement of fiducial markers [29]. The risk of pneumothorax is significantly lower when fiducials are placed via bronchoscopic route. However, bronchoscopic placement of fiducials requires a navigation tool for accurate localization of peripheral tumors [30]. Several studies have attested to the feasibility of using ENB to facilitate accurate placement of fiducials. In one study, a total of 39 fiducial markers were deployed in 8 of 9 patients using ENB guidance without any significant complications [31, 32]. In another study, fiducials were placed in 15 patients via transthoracic route and in 8 patients via transbronchial route with ENB guidance. Pneumothorax developed in 8 of 15 patients who had fiducials placed via transthoracic route, 6 of which required chest tube drainage. No pneumothorax developed in patients who had fiducial markers placed via ENB-guided bronchoscopy [33].

There is a potential for bronchoscopically deployed fiducials to dislodge from their original location. Linear gold fiducial markers have a smooth surface and have been reported to dislodge in 10–30 % of cases when placed using ENB guidance [32, 34]. Better results have been reported with the use of coil-spring fiducial markers in nonoperative lung cancer patients undergoing cyberknife treatment [35]. In one study, a total of 52 consecutive patients underwent fiducial marker placement using ENB. Of these, 4 patients received 17 linear fiducial markers and 49 patients with 56 tumors received 217 coil-spring fiducial markers. At cyberknife planning, 215 (99 %) of 217 coil-spring fiducial markers were still in place whereas only 8 (47 %) of 17 linear fiducial markers remained in their original location ($P=0.0001$). Two of the four patients who had initially received linear fiducial markers required additional fiducial placements while none of the patients with coil fiducial markers required additional procedures. Pneumothorax developed in 3 (5.8 %) study patients. These results suggest that coil-spring markers may be more suitable for bronchoscopic placement under ENB guidance than the linear gold fiducial markers.

ENB has also been used to place fiducial markers in sub-pleural location in vicinity of small pulmonary nodules, which can be helpful in locating non-visible and non-palpable lesions during video-assisted thoracoscopic surgery [36].

In recent years, interstitial brachytherapy has been explored as one of the therapeutic options for localized but inoperable lung cancer. In one study, use of ENB was described to facilitate brachytherapy for treatment of a medically inoperable peripheral non-small-cell lung cancer patient [37]. The investigators first localized the right upper lobe tumor using ENB guidance. After successful localization of the lesion, EBUS was performed and a brachytherapy catheter was placed directly within the tumor. A repeat EBUS and CT after the application of high-dose-rate brachytherapy demonstrated a partial while histology showed a complete remission of the tumor. Similarly, with the ENB and EBUS guidance, Becker and associates treated 18 inoperable peripheral lung cancer patients with interstitial brachytherapy. A complete remission was achieved in 9 of 18 patients (50 %), and the majority of the remaining patients achieved a partial remission [38].

Complications

Pneumothorax is the most common complication of ENB with an incidence of 0–10 % in different studies (Table 6.1). No study has specifically addressed the factors associated with increased risk of pneumothorax after ENB procedure. In theory, the rate of pneumothorax could be affected by AFTRE because an error of even a few millimeters could be crucial in the small peripherally located or sub-pleural lesions. This is especially true if the fluoroscopic guidance is not employed during the procedure.

Self-limiting bleeding may be encountered in some cases [15, 22]. Possibly, the presence of EWC is helpful in controlling the bleeding by allowing the scope to remain wedged at the subsegmental bronchus throughout the process [16, 18]. In a single case, repeated insertion and removal of biopsy forceps perforated the EWC [14].

Limitations

Despite an elegant navigational software and locatable guide system, the diagnostic yield of this technique has remained in the range of 70 %. There are several explanations for inability to achieve a higher diagnostic yield. First, there is always some difference in CT-based virtual and actual patient anatomy. Second, the biopsy in this technique is not performed under a real-time guidance. This is especially true when fluoroscopy is not used. Third, the respiratory movements tend to hinder the biopsy procedure, especially from lower lobes. Four, some areas of lung are simply difficult to reach with the flexible bronchoscope and the navigational catheter. Finally, there is always a possibility that EWC is dislodged from its primary site during the sampling of the tissue. The bronchoscopist must be vigilant for this possibility and if suspected, repeat the navigational stage of the procedure.

Another important issue relates to the learning curve of the technique. Successful application of this technique requires a well-trained team of bronchoscopist and bronchoscopy assistants. The procedure is relatively complicated and requires a careful pre-procedural planning. Still, some studies have reported a very steep learning curve [13]. It is unclear as to how many procedures are needed before a bronchoscopist can be considered proficient in the technique. In this regard, it is encouraging to note that this technique has been used successfully in community hospital setting with minimal formal training [22, 27]. Clearly, it is important to have training and mastery in basic bronchoscopy skills before ENB is adopted in bronchoscopy practice. As a matter of common sense, the diagnostic yield is likely to improve as the bronchoscopists gain more experience in the technique.

Another issue relates to the total duration of procedure when ENB is used for obtaining specimen from peripheral pulmonary nodule. As shown in Table 6.1, the average duration of bronchoscopy has varied from 25 to 70 min. Most studies do not explicitly report additional time required during the planning phase, but with experience, it can be achieved in less than 10 min.

The presence of pacemakers and automatic implanted cardiac defibrillators (AICD) is considered a relative contraindication to the use of ENB due to potential risk of malfunction under the magnetic field that is used during the procedure. In a recent study, ENB was performed in 24 subjects with a pacemaker and AICD, with cardiac electrophysiologist in attendance during the procedure [38]. None of the patients experienced cardiac arrhythmia or pacemaker dysfunction during the procedure. The authors concluded that ENB is safe when performed in patients with pacemakers and AICDs. Notwithstanding, extreme caution is warranted in these cases, and we believe that further studies are needed to independently validate these results.

Finally, and most importantly, EBN is an expensive technique. The initial setup requires a substantial investment. The locatable guide and EWC are disposable and add very significantly to the cost of an individual procedure. As such, the procedure is not adequately reimbursed by the third-party payers. The cost is further increased if the procedure is performed under general anesthesia, and if multi-modality approach using radial probe EBUS in addition to ENB is used to optimize the diagnostic yield. Routine addition of ROSE comes with its own price tag. Clearly, the cost of the procedure is prohibitive for resource-limited areas.

Conclusion

ENB is one more modality of the new class of advanced diagnostic bronchoscopy techniques designed for improving accuracy in diagnosing peripheral lung lesions. This and the other procedures are now considered standard of care in our institution for individuals with high risk for CT-FNA or those for whom a biopsy is desirable for those inoperable patients. Over time the yield of ENB in the published literature continues to increase in part due to patient selection (i.e., presence of a bronchus sign) and possibly related to availability of the newer generation of software and the better design of the locatable guide. Exciting new developments are also taking place in the application of ENB to facilitate advanced nonsurgical therapies for patients with localized lung cancers who cannot undergo curative resection. We believe that innovation in this area will continue to advance the diagnostic and therapeutic uses of ENB.

References

1. Henschke CI, McCauley DI, Yankelevitz DF, Naidich DP, McGuinness G, Miettinen OS, et al. Early lung cancer action project: overall design and findings from baseline screening. Lancet. 1999;354:99–105.
2. Aberle DR, Adams AM, Berg CD, Black WC, Clapp JD, Fagerstrom RM, et al. Reduced lung-cancer mortality with low-dose computed tomographic screening. N Engl J Med. 2011;365:395–409.
3. Ost D, Fein AM, Feinsilver SH. Clinical practice. The solitary pulmonary nodule. N Engl J Med. 2003;348: 2535–42.
4. Gould MK, Ananth L, Barnett PG. A clinical model to estimate the pretest probability of lung cancer in patients with solitary pulmonary nodules. Chest. 2007;131:383–8.
5. Wiener RS, Schwartz LM, Woloshin S, Welch HG. Population-based risk for complications after transthoracic needle lung biopsy of a pulmonary nodule: an analysis of discharge records. Ann Intern Med. 2011; 155:137–44.
6. Davies B, Ghosh S, Hopkinson D, Vaughan R, Rocco G. Solitary pulmonary nodules: pathological outcome of 150 consecutively resected lesions. Interact Cardiovasc Thorac Surg. 2005;4:18–20.
7. Popovich Jr J, Kvale PA, Eichenhorn MS, Radke JR, Ohorodnik JM, Fine G. Diagnostic accuracy of multiple biopsies from flexible fiberoptic bronchoscopy. A comparison of central versus peripheral carcinoma. Am Rev Respir Dis. 1982;125:521–3.
8. Rivera MP, Mehta AC. Initial diagnosis of lung cancer: Accp evidence-based clinical practice guidelines (2nd edition). Chest. 2007;132:131S–48.
9. Seijo LM, de Torres JP, Lozano MD, Bastarrika G, Alcaide AB, Lacunza MM, et al. Diagnostic yield of electromagnetic navigation bronchoscopy is highly dependent on the presence of a bronchus sign on CT imaging: results from a prospective study. Chest. 2010;138:1316–21.
10. Kikuchi E, Yamazaki K, Sukoh N, Kikuchi J, Asahina H, Imura M, et al. Endobronchial ultrasonography with guide-sheath for peripheral pulmonary lesions. Eur Respir J. 2004;24:533–7.
11. Paone G, Nicastri E, Lucantoni G, Dello Iacono R, Battistoni P, D'Angeli AL, et al. Endobronchial ultrasound-driven biopsy in the diagnosis of peripheral lung lesions. Chest. 2005;128:3551–7.
12. Memoli JS, El-Bayoumi E, Pastis NJ, Tanner NT, Gomez M, Huggins JT, et al. Using endobronchial ultrasound features to predict lymph node metastasis in patients with lung cancer. Chest. 2011;140:1550–6.
13. Makris D, Scherpereel A, Leroy S, Bouchindhomme B, Faivre JB, Remy J, et al. Electromagnetic navigation diagnostic bronchoscopy for small peripheral lung lesions. Eur Respir J. 2007;29:1187–92.
14. Eberhardt R, Anantham D, Herth F, Feller-Kopman D, Ernst A. Electromagnetic navigation diagnostic bronchoscopy in peripheral lung lesions. Chest. 2007; 131:1800–5.
15. Becker HD, Herth F, Ernst A, Schwarz Y. Bronchoscopic biopsy of peripheral lung lesions under electromagnetic guidance: a pilot study. J Bronchol Intervent Pulmonol. 2005;12:9–13.
16. Gildea TR, Mazzone PJ, Karnak D, Meziane M, Mehta AC. Electromagnetic navigation diagnostic bronchoscopy: a prospective study. Am J Respir Crit Care Med. 2006;174:982–9.
17. Bertoletti L, Robert A, Cottier M, Chambonniere ML, Vergnon JM. Accuracy and feasibility of electromagnetic navigated bronchoscopy under nitrous oxide sedation for pulmonary peripheral opacities: an outpatient study. Respiration. 2009;78:293–300.
18. Eberhardt R, Anantham D, Ernst A, Feller-Kopman D, Herth F. Multimodality bronchoscopic diagnosis of peripheral lung lesions: a randomized controlled trial. Am J Respir Crit Care Med. 2007;176:36–41.
19. Eberhardt R, Morgan RK, Ernst A, Beyer T, Herth FJ. Comparison of suction catheter versus forceps biopsy

for sampling of solitary pulmonary nodules guided by electromagnetic navigational bronchoscopy. Respiration. 2010;79:54–60.
20. Hautmann H, Schneider A, Pinkau T, et al. Electromagnetic catheter navigation during bronchoscopy: validation of a novel method by conventional fluoroscopy. Chest. 2005;128:382–7.
21. Schwarz Y, Greif J, Becker HD, et al. Real-time electromagnetic navigation bronchoscopy to peripheral lung lesions using overlaid CT images: the first human study. Chest. 2006;129:988–94.
22. Wilson DS, Barlett RJ. Improved diagnostic yield of bronchoscopy in a community practice: a combination of electromagnetic navigation system and rapid on-site evaluation. J Bronchol. 2007;14:227–32.
23. Lamprecht B, Porsch P, Pirich C, Studnicka M. Electromagnetic navigation bronchoscopy in combination with PET-CT and rapid on-site cytopathologic examination for diagnosis of peripheral lung lesions. Lung. 2009;187:55–9.
24. McLemore TL, Bedekar AR. Accurate diagnosis of peripheral lung lesions in a private community hospital employing electromagnetic guidance bronchoscopy (EMB) coupled with radial endobronchial ultrasound (REBUS). Chest. 2007;132:452S.
25. Mahajan AK, Patel S, Hogarth DK, Wightman R. Electromagnetic navigational bronchoscopy. An effective and safe approach to diagnose peripheral lung lesions unreachable by conventional bronchoscopy in high-risk patients. J Bronchol Intervent Pulmonol. 2011;18:133–7.
26. Lamprecht B, Porsch P, Wegleitner B, Strasser G, Kaiser B, Studnicka M. Electromagnetic navigation bronchoscopy (ENB): increasing diagnostic yield. Respir Med. 2012;106:710–5.
27. Pearlstein D, Quinn CC, Burtis CC, Ahn KW, Katch AJ. Electromagnetic navigation bronchoscopy performed by thoracic surgeons: one center's early success. Ann Thorac Surg. 2012;93:944–50.
28. Sherwood JT, Brock MV. Lung cancer: new surgical approaches. Respirology. 2007;12:326–32.
29. Pennathur A, Luketich JD, Heron DE, et al. Stereotactic radiosurgery for the treatment of stage I non-small cell lung cancer in high-risk patients. J Thorac Cardiovasc Surg. 2009;137:597–604.
30. Linden PA. Use of navigation bronchoscopy for biopsy and endobronchial fiducial placement. Innovations (Phila). 2011;6:271–5.
31. Anantham D, Feller-Kopman D, Shanmugham LN, et al. Electromagnetic navigation bronchoscopy-guided fiducial placement for robotic stereotactic radiosurgery of lung tumors: a feasibility study. Chest. 2007;132:930–5.
32. Kupelian PA, Forbes A, Willoughby TR, et al. Implantation and stability of metallic fiducials within pulmonary lesions. Int J Radiat Oncol Biol Phys. 2007;69:777–85.
33. Harley DP, Krimsky WS, Sarkar S, et al. Fiducial marker placement using endobronchial ultrasound and navigational bronchoscopy for stereotactic radiosurgery: an alternative strategy. Ann Thorac Surg. 2010;89:368–74.
34. Schroeder C, Hejal R, Linden PA. Coil spring fiducial markers placed safely using navigation bronchoscopy in inoperable patients allows accurate delivery of cyberknife stereotactic radiosurgery. J Thorac Cardiovasc Surg. 2010;140:1137–42.
35. Andrade RS. Electromagnetic navigation bronchoscopy-guided thoracoscopic wedge resection of small pulmonary nodules. Semin Thorac Cardiovasc Surg. 2010;22:262–5.
36. Harms W, Krempien R, Grehn C, et al. Electromagnetically navigated brachytherapy as a new treatment option for peripheral pulmonary tumors. Strahlenther Onkol. 2006;182(2):108–11.
37. Becker HD, McLemore T, Harms W. Electromagnetic navigation and endobronchial ultrasound for brachytherapy of inoperable peripheral lung cancer. Chest. 2008;134:S396.
38. Khan AY, Berkowitz D, Krimsky WS, et al. Safety of pacemakers and defibrillators in electromagnetic navigation bronchoscopy. Chest 2013;143:75–81.

Practical Application of Virtual Bronchoscopic Navigation

7

Fumihiro Asano

Abstract

Transbronchial biopsy (TBBx) for peripheral pulmonary lesions (PPLs) is associated with fewer complications than percutaneous biopsy. However, the diagnostic yield using TBBx can be inadequate, and depends on the operator's skill. Virtual bronchoscopic navigation (VBN) is a method in which a bronchoscope is guided using virtual bronchoscopy (VB) images on the bronchial route to a peripheral lesion. A system that allows automatic search for the route to the target, production of VB images, and matched display with real images has been developed. This system is used for diagnosis of peripheral lesions, marker placement for surgery or radiotherapy, and education and training. VBN is used in combination with CT-guided ultrathin bronchoscopy, endobronchial ultrasonography with a guide-sheath (EBUS-GS), and bronchoscopy with or without X-ray fluoroscopy. Based on prospective studies, the diagnostic yield is 74 % for all PPLs and 68 % for lesions ≤2 cm. In a recent randomized study, use of VBN in association with EBUS-GS increased the diagnostic yield for ≤3 cm lesions from 67 to 80 %, and shortened the total examination time. A meta-analysis has also revealed the usefulness of VBN. There are many advantages of VBN. Even beginners can readily use this technique for peripheral lesions, and a high diagnostic rate can be obtained. To increase the diagnostic yield using VBN, it is important to clarify the relationship between the lesion and extracted bronchi, select appropriate bronchoscopic techniques, and combine them with VBN. CT should be performed under appropriate conditions. VBN is a useful method to support bronchoscopy; wider use and further development of this system are expected.

F. Asano, M.D., F.C.C.P. (✉)
Department of Pulmonary Medicine,
Gifu Prefectural General Medical Center,
4-6-1 Noishiki, Gifu 5008717, Japan
e-mail: asano-fm@ceres.ocn.ne.jp

A.C. Mehta and P. Jain (eds.), *Interventional Bronchoscopy: A Clinical Guide*, Respiratory Medicine 10,
DOI 10.1007/978-1-62703-395-4_7,

Keywords
CT-guided ultrathin bronchoscopy • Endobronchial ultrasonography • Navigation system • Peripheral pulmonary lesions • Transbronchial biopsy • Ultrathin bronchoscope • Virtual bronchoscopy • Virtual bronchoscopic navigation

Abbreviations

EBUS	Endobronchial ultrasonography
EBUS-GS	Endobronchial ultrasonography with a guide-sheath
EMN	Electromagnetic navigation
PPL	Peripheral pulmonary lesion
TBBx	Transbronchial biopsy
VB	Virtual bronchoscopy
VBN	Virtual bronchoscopic navigation

Introduction

Peripheral pulmonary lesion (PPL) is a common finding on chest computed tomography (CT). Due to the widespread use of CT in clinical practice, it is common to encounter small PPL as an incidental finding [1]. Based on the results of the National Lung Screening Trial (NLST), many physicians are expected to adopt lung cancer screening using CT in their clinical practice [2]. The majority of lung nodules detected on CT have a benign etiology. The challenge is to detect lung cancer at an early stage among these small peripheral lesions. This is a difficult task. Pathological confirmation is essential for diagnosis of lung cancer. The options for collecting specimen from the lung nodules include surgical biopsy, percutaneous needle biopsy, and transbronchial biopsy (TBBx) [3]. Although surgical biopsy is most accurate, it is also the most invasive method. Since most of PPLs detected incidentally or on screening are benign and do not require resection, it is unacceptable to subject all of these patients to a major thoracic surgery with its attendant cost and complications. The American College of Chest Physicians (ACCP) guidelines recommend percutaneous needle biopsy as a preferred diagnostic method for small lesions, which has a sensitivity of 90 % and a specificity of 97 % [4]. However, the diagnostic sensitivity of percutaneous needle biopsy differs according to whether CT is used, the lesion size, and whether the lesion is malignant or benign [4]. In addition, the incidence of complications is high; pneumothorax develops in 21 %, and hemoptysis in 5 % [5]. In Japan, Tomiyama et al. investigated 9,783 CT-guided needle biopsy cases in 124 institutions, and reported a mortality rate of 0.07 %, severe complication (tension pneumothorax, hemopneumothorax, air embolism, and dissemination) rate of 0.75 %, and pneumothorax rate of 35 % [6]. TBBx has a better safety profile. According to a survey by the Japanese Society for Respiratory Endoscopy that included 37,485 cases, TBBx was associated with a mortality rate of 0.003 % and an overall complication rate of 1.79 % (bleeding, 0.73 %; pneumothorax, 0.63 %) [7]. Even though these investigations are not directly comparable, these studies were performed under similar conditions and on similar patient population in Japan and their results suggest that TBBx has a better safety profile than CT-guided percutaneous biopsy. However, the diagnostic yield of standard bronchoscopy for peripheral lesions is inadequate. According to the evidence-based review published by ACCP, the diagnostic yield of TBBx was 78 % for all lesions and 34 % for lesions ≤2 cm [4]. Therefore, the ACCP guidelines do not recommend bronchoscopic examination for these lesions. In bronchoscopic diagnosis of peripheral solitary lesions, the major lesion-associated factors that affect the diagnostic yield are size [8, 9], location [8], presence or absence of involved bronchi [10], and whether the disease is benign or malignant [9]. The major operator-associated factors that affect the yield are the operator's skills and experience [11]. At present,

PPLs are approached using a bronchoscope with an external diameter of about 5–6 mm under X-ray fluoroscopy guidance. A major problem that limits the usefulness of TBBx in these patients is the difficulty in guiding the bronchoscope and biopsy instruments toward the lesion. To reach peripheral lesions, correct guidance of the bronchoscope and biopsy instruments through the bronchi is needed as the instruments must pass through many bronchial branching sites. For this, bronchoscopists generally select the bronchial path toward the lesion during the examination by mentally reconstructing the bronchial arrangement in three dimensions using two-dimensional (2D) planar axial CT data obtained before procedure. Unfortunately, as expected, this method often proves inaccurate [12] and is not applicable to more peripheral bronchi that cannot be traced on CT and can only be observed directly using a thin or an ultrathin bronchoscope. Therefore, there is a need for an accurate navigation method that can be used to approach peripheral lesions with a greater degree of accuracy.

Virtual bronchoscopy (VB) is a method that can produce images from three-dimensional (3D) helical CT data that simulate real bronchoscopic images [13]. This method is noninvasive, and has been used for evaluation and treatment planning of central airway stenosis [14, 15], but not for PPLs. Virtual bronchoscopic navigation (VBN) is a technique that is designed to guide the bronchoscopist to peripheral lesions on the basis of VB images of the bronchial tree [16]. Under direct visualization of the bronchial path to the lesion displayed on the VB images, this technique allows the bronchoscope to be readily guided to the target in a short time, irrespective of the bronchoscopist's skill level. In addition, the systems that automatically searches for the bronchial route to the target when the target is set, produces VB images on the route, and displays VB images matched with real images, have been developed and clinically applied [17, 18]. VBN has been used in conjunction with CT-guided ultrathin bronchoscopy and endobronchial ultrasonography with a guide-sheath (EBUS-GS), and excellent results have been reported [17–22]. A randomized study has shown improvement in the diagnostic yield and decreases in the bronchoscope guidance time and total examination time using VBN with EBUS-GS [23]. Likewise, a meta-analysis of previous studies has also shown the usefulness of VBN [24]. In this chapter, the scientific basis, clinical applications, clinical results, procedures, measures that can be taken to improve diagnostic yield, and limitations of VBN are discussed.

Scientific Basis

Virtual Bronchoscopy

Helical CT provides continuous 3D volumetric data. There are various 3D display methods for these data. VB is a method for 3D display of images of the bronchi and bronchial lumen, and simulates the live view of an actual bronchoscopy [13].

VB images reflect real anatomical findings [25], and may provide useful information for bronchoscope guidance such as the branching patterns as observed from the bronchial lumen. This information includes the shapes of the bronchial orifices, sizes of bronchi at the branching sites, branching angles, and the bronchial arrangement after branching.

VB has several advantages. (1) Unlike actual bronchoscopy, VB is noninvasive. (2) Since observation from any viewpoint or direction is possible, thin bronchi and bronchi distal to stenosis that cannot be evaluated with a real bronchoscope can be observed on virtual bronchoscopy. (3) Semitransparent display of bronchial wall allows visualization of structures beyond the bronchial wall. (4) The length, area, and volume of the bronchi can be accurately measured. The disadvantages of VB are as follows. (1) The resolution of VB images depends on the CT images. (2) Subtle changes in mucosal lining cannot be detected with VB images. (3) Specimen for tissue diagnosis cannot be collected.

VB has been used for evaluation of airway stenosis [14, 15], and for planning of interventional procedures such as stent insertion [26], detection of foreign matters in the airway [27], and bronchoscopy training [28, 29]. However,

VB had not previously been used for peripheral lesions because of difficulty in producing VB images of peripheral bronchi. This limitation was not only due to the performance of CT but also due to nonavailability of thin or ultrathin bronchoscopes that could be advanced into peripheral areas. Recently, multi-detector CT has allowed high-speed detailed scanning of the chest region during a single breath-hold, removing the artifacts due to respiration and cardiac motion and improving temporal and spatial resolution. Using data from multi-detector CT, it is now feasible to construct bronchial path to the peripheral lesion in majority of cases.

Ultrathin Bronchoscope

In recent years, bronchoscopes have become thinner. In particular, ultrathin bronchoscopes can be advanced into more distal bronchi under direct observation [30]. An ultrathin bronchoscope with an external diameter of 2.8 mm and forceps channel of 1.2 mm that allows biopsy procedure is also commercially available [31]. Ultrathin bronchoscopes are useful for diagnosis of PPLs because they can be advanced to close to the lesion, thereby facilitating guidance of biopsy instruments with greater accuracy [32]. Lesions such as those on the mediastinal side of the lung apex that are difficult to reach using conventional bronchoscopes can also be reached using the ultrathin bronchoscopes [33]. A survey in 2010 reported the use of ultrathin bronchoscopes in 44 % of board-certificated institutions of the Japanese Society for Respiratory Endoscopy.

Virtual Bronchoscopy Navigation

Virtual bronchoscopy navigation is a more advanced clinical application of VB for peripheral lesions. In this technique, VB images of the bronchial path to the lesion are produced and displayed simultaneously with the corresponding real bronchoscopic images, helping the operator to navigate the bronchoscope to the chosen target. We reported our initial experience in 2002 [16]. In this report, VB images were produced to the tenth-generation bronchi delineating the bronchial path to the target. VB images were displayed simultaneously with real images, and an ultrathin bronchoscope was advanced to sites close to the lesion according to the path [16]. In the studies from Japan, including this study, the Japanese nomenclature of bronchial branches has been used. According to this system, all subsegmental bronchi are regarded as third-generation bronchi, and the bronchial generation is calculated by adding a number for each subsequent branch [34]. Therefore, caution is necessary when studies from Japan are compared with those from western countries.

VB can be performed using software provided with the CT system in each institution, but there are some cautionary items when it is clinically used as VBN. There are surface rendering and volume rendering VB methods. In the production of VB images, determination of the threshold is important. The border between the air within the bronchus and the bronchial wall is determined by selecting the threshold. This is important because the VB images are altered with change in the threshold. As a result, sometimes the operator may receive inaccurate information because some branches are missed, while holes that resemble opening of a branch in the absence of an actual branch may form on some VB images, particularly those from peripheral airways [15, 35]. Whenever there is a difference in the number of branches on the route between the VB and real images, the bronchoscope might be guided to an incorrect site. When a virtual bronchoscope is advanced toward a lesion using fly-through display, it is important to produce the correct VB images that reflect each branching. It is also prudent that the presence or the absence of branching is confirmed on axial, sagittal, or coronal images. The other cautionary item is related to rotation of images at the time of bronchoscopy. Unlike VB that can be manipulated in several different ways, the bronchoscope tip can only be moved up and down, and therefore, appropriate rotation is always necessary at the time of advancement. When the bronchoscope is rotated, real images shift from previously produced VB images. Since bifurcation into two bronchi is frequently observed in the peripheral area, rotation of ≥90° causes considerable difficulty in determining the bronchus into which the bronchoscope should be advanced to reach target. This bifurcation pattern is repeatedly observed on the route. Therefore, correction of VB image is frequently necessary to achieve consistency between VB and real images at each branching site in order to avoid taking an incorrect bronchial route.

VBN System

VBN using conventional VB software has two serious problems. First, the production of VB images on the route while a virtual bronchoscope is advanced to the target using flight-through display is time-consuming, and requires skill to select the threshold. Second, rotation cannot be accommodated, which introduces inaccuracies as discussed above. To overcome these problems, we developed a navigation system that allows automatic production of VB images in the bronchial path (called automatic VB image production function) [18] and displays VB images in comparison with real images (called navigation function) [17]. This system became commercially available as Bf-NAVI® (Cybernet systems, Tokyo, Japan) in Japan in 2008, and was used in 12 % of board-certified and -related institutions in Japan in 2010. In the United States, LungPoint® (Bronchus Technologies, Inc., CA, USA) has been commercially available since 2009, and subsequently began to be covered by health insurance as a type of navigational bronchoscopy [36].

The navigation system has two important functions. First is VB image production and provision of information, called the editor or planning function. Both Bf-NAVI® and LungPoint® systems automatically select the route and produce VB images, but LungPoint® searches for the route only after setting the target at the lesion, and therefore, can be more readily used. Composite display of three cross-sectional CT images (axial, sagittal, and coronal images) and the bronchial tree is also possible [37]. Using Bf-NAVI, the end point other than the target should be set. When the end point is set, the bronchial lumens that are automatically extracted are displayed in blue on the three cross-sectional CT images, and extraction of the bronchi can be confirmed. Since bronchi that have not yet been extracted are not visualized on VB images and their branches are also not displayed, accurate navigation cannot be performed. Therefore, confirmation of extracted bronchi is a very important prerequisite for increasing navigation accuracy. In addition, using Bf-NAVI, when there are bronchi that are not automatically extracted (such as peripheral bronchi near the lesion or bronchi peripheral to stenosis), the bronchi can be manually extracted. In this way, the end point can be established as a pinpoint in the extracted bronchus near the lesion. Such establishment of the end point seems to be complicated, but using this procedure, the route to a site near the lesion can be accurately displayed. If the end point is established in a range that overlaps with the target, but has a longer radius than the target, Bf-NAVI (as with LungPoint) automatically searches for extracted bronchi in the end of the range. This is done in the order of increasing distance to the lesion, and displays multiple routes. Although VB images are produced prior to bronchoscopy, image production time depends on the quantity of CT data and the specification of the processing computer.

The other important function of VBN systems is the navigation function, also called the viewer or procedure function. The navigation function can be manual or automatic. Manual navigation systems display VB images at each branching site, and show the appropriate bronchus for bronchoscope advancement on the route to the lesion as reference images. The operator advances the bronchoscope by manually matching VB images with real images. When VB images matched with real bronchoscopic images are displayed, the bronchoscope tip is displayed in the bronchial tree and corresponding CT images. Bf-NAVI is a representative manual navigation system. Automatic navigation systems automatically acquire information on the position of the bronchoscope tip, and display the real-time position of the bronchoscope on CT images. For automatic tracking of the bronchoscope, tracking of position information on the bronchoscope tip needs to be performed by a reliable method. At present, there are two position information tracking methods: image registration [38–41] and magnetic position sensors [42]. The image registration method predicts bronchoscope motion based on similarity between real and virtual images. A VB image that is the most similar to the real image is automatically selected by pattern recognition. Based on information on the viewpoint and view direction of the VB image, bronchoscope motion is predicted and the bronchoscope is tracked. LungPoint has this function. Information on VB images such as the route and distance to the target lesion, bronchial names, and major blood vessels outside the bronchi can be superimposed on the live bronchoscopic view captured in the system. This method is more straightforward and accurate than the magnetic sensor method described below. However, matching of VB images with the real images requires time due to the computer processing, and the bronchoscope needs to be manipulated considerably slowly. In addition, when the bronchial lumen becomes invisible due to conditions such as coughing, tracking is interrupted, and there are still many other problems that require improvement. An option of manual navigation is also available in these systems. The magnetic sensors provide position information using a magnetic sensor incorporated into the bronchoscope tip or a specially designed bronchoscopic accessory. Concretely, multiple landmarks established on VB images are directly touched during actual bronchoscopy using a magnetic sensor, information is acquired, and the position information from the magnetic sensor is superimposed on the CT information. This enables real-time display of the position of the bronchoscope tip on CT images. This method is called electromagnetic navigation (EMN) which was approved by the FDA in 2004 [43, 44]. This method differs from VBN because in EMN system, the VB images of the central bronchi are used only for calibration, not for navigation, and guidance is performed using a magnetic position sensor. Errors during calibration and those due to respiratory motion are problems. In recent years, for calibration, EMN has used information on the centerline of the bronchi obtained from CT images, not VB images. Assuming that the bronchoscope is advanced on the bronchial centerline, the position information on the magnetic sensor obtained during actual bronchoscopy is concretely matched with CT images. Presently, iLogic™ (SuperDimension, Herzliya, Israel) and Spin Drive™ (Veran Medical Technologies, St. Louis, USA) are commercially available as EMN systems.

Clinical Applications

The clinical applications of VBN include diagnosis of peripheral lesions, marker placement for surgery and radiotherapy, and educational training.

Diagnosis of Peripheral Lesions

Since VBN does not allow confirmation of arrival of the biopsy instruments at the lesion, it is often used in combination with CT, X-ray fluoroscopy, or endobronchial ultrasonography (EBUS). The results of each combination in previous studies on the diagnosis of PPLs using VBN and its system are summarized in Table 7.1 and are discussed briefly in the following section.

CT-Guided Ultrathin Bronchoscopy

Real-time CT imaging during bronchoscopy can confirm the arrival of biopsy instruments at the lesion even if it cannot be observed using fluoroscopy. In some studies, it is found useful for the diagnosis of PPLs [45, 46]. Since VBN is performed on the basis of CT data, CT during examination can also accurately confirm the accuracy of VBN. The diagnostic yield using VBN in combination with CT-guided ultrathin bronchoscopy has been reported to be 65–86 % for all lesions and 65–81 % for lesions ≤2 cm in diameter [17, 19, 20, 22]. A retrospective comparison also showed shortening of the time until arrival at the lesion using a VBN system [22].

Table 7.1 Results of VBN

Author	VBN system	Confirmation of arrival	No. of lesions examined	Diagnostic yield (%)	No. of lesions <2 cm	Diagnostic yield for lesions <2 cm	Examination time
Asano et al. [19]	Not used	CT and X-ray fluoroscopy	36	86.1	26	80.8 %	n/a
Shinagawa et al. [20]	Not used	CT fluoroscopy	26	65.4	26	65.4 %	29.3 min
Asahina et al. [21]	Not used	EBUS	30	63.3	18	44.4 %	25.7 min
Asano et al. [17]	Bf-NAVI	CT and X-ray fluoroscopy	38	81.6	26	80.8 %	24.9 min
Shinagawa et al. [22]	Bf-NAVI	CT fluoroscopy	71	70.4	71	70.4 %	24.5 min
Tachihara et.al. [52]	Bf-NAVI	X-ray fluoroscopy	96	62.5	77	54.5 %	24.1 min
Asano et al. [18]	Bf-NAVI	EBUS	32	84.4	15	73.3 %	22.3 min
Eberhardt et al. [37]	LungPoint	Without fluoroscopy	25	80.0	n/a	n/a	15 min
Ishida et al. [23]	Bf-NAVI	EBUS	99	80.8	58	75.9 %	24 min
Summary			453	74.0	317	67.5 %	

Ground glass opacities (GGO) are difficult to visualize on fluoroscopy or EBUS-GS. In comparison, GGO is readily identified on CT images. Therefore, VBN with CT-guided ultrathin bronchoscopy may be the most suitable technique to obtain biopsy specimens from lesions that show predominantly ground glass changes on the CT. However, because of radiation exposure issues and extra cost associated with the occupation of the CT room, this combination of diagnostic strategy should be limited to a few highly selected cases. The factors contributing to diagnosis have been reported to be the presence or the absence of the involved bronchi and the advancement range of the ultrathin bronchoscope [47]. In addition, the amount of specimen collected with an ultrathin bronchoscope is limited and may only be sufficient for cytodiagnosis [48].

EBUS with a Guide Sheath

In recent years, studies have shown the usefulness of radial type EBUS for identification of the location of the lesion during bronchoscopy for PPLs [49]. With EBUS-GS, the arrival at the lesion is confirmed using an ultrasonic probe, and biopsy of the lesion is performed through a guide sheath placed in the lesion [50]. The diagnostic yield of VBN in combination with EBUS-GS has been reported to be 63–84 % for all lesions and 44–73 % for lesions ≤2 cm in diameter [18, 21, 23]. To objectively confirm the usefulness of the VBN system with EBUS-GS, we performed a multicenter joint randomized study (NINJA Study) [23]. Biopsy was performed using EBUS-GS after randomizing 200 patients with PPLs ≤3 cm in diameter into VBN-assisted (VBNA) and non-VBN-assisted (NVBNA) groups. A thin bronchoscope was guided using a VBN system in the VBNA group and guided using previously obtained axial CT images as a reference in the NVBNA group. In the VBNA group, VB images to the fourth- through the twelfth (median, sixth)-generation bronchi could be acquired, and the rate of consistency between the VB and real images was 98 %. The diagnostic yield in the VBNA group (80 %) was significantly higher than that in the NVBNA group (67 %). In addition, the time until the initiation of biopsy and the total duration of bronchoscopy were significantly shorter in the VBNA group (median, 8.1 and 24.0 min, respectively) than in the NVBNA group (9.8 and 26.2 min, respectively).

An EBUS system is necessary for this method. However, the system is not expensive to purchase, and the procedure is straightforward. In addition, lesions that cannot be observed using fluoroscopy can be identified, and specimens can be collected through the guide sheath accurately and repeatedly. The results of the above randomized study and the high diagnostic yield suggest that the combination of the VBN system, a thin bronchoscope, and EBUS-GS has a potential to become a routine approach to PPLs. Recently, use of EBUS-GS without fluoroscopy was also reported [51]. Since accurate bronchoscope guidance without X-ray fluoroscopy is possible using a VBN system, a high diagnostic rate may be obtained even without X-ray fluoroscopy.

X-Ray Fluoroscopy

Tachihara et al. [52] used a navigation system in 96 lesions with PPLs ≤3 cm, and reported a diagnostic yield of 63 % for all lesions and 55 % for lesions ≤2 cm and an examination time of 24.1 min. Their study is the only study on VBN under X-ray fluoroscopy. However, since fluoroscopy-guided bronchoscopy is a straightforward and a widely used method for TBBx, further studies on its usefulness in conjunction with VBN are necessary.

No Fluoroscopic Assistance

Eberhardt et al. [37] used ultrathin bronchoscope with VBN guidance without X-ray fluoroscopy to obtain biopsy specimens from 25 PPLs with a median size of 28 mm. The investigators reported a high diagnostic rate of 80 % with this technique.

Diagnostic Yield Using VBN for Peripheral Lesions

Based on the above prospective studies on VBN, the diagnostic yield is 74 % for all PPLs and 68 % for lesions that are ≤2 cm in size [53]. Since the diagnostic yield is affected by not only the lesion size but also the underlying disease process, the location of the lesion, and the presence/absence of the involved bronchi, comparison with traditional methods is generally difficult. Still, these diagnostic yields are significantly higher compared with 34 % diagnostic yield according to the ACCP guidelines [4]. Memoli and her colleagues undertook a meta-analysis to determine the overall diagnostic yield of guided bronchoscopy for pulmonary nodules using one or a combination of electromagnetic navigation bronchoscopy (ENB), VB, radial endobronchial ultrasound (R-EBUS), ultrathin bronchoscope, and guide sheath [24]. A total of 3,004 patients with 3,052 lesions from the 39 studies were included. The yield for VB was 72 % (95 % confidence interval, 66–79 %), although one study for mediastinal and hilar lesions (not for peripheral lesions) and a retrospective study were included.

Marker Placement for Peripheral Lesions

VBN can be applied not only to diagnosis but also to treatment [54]. We performed CT-guided transbronchial marker placement to show the location of the lesion and resection range during thoracoscopic surgery for 31 lesions (≤1 cm) with a pure GGO pattern that could not be visualized on X-ray fluoroscopy [55]. After an ultrathin bronchoscope was guided to a median of a sixth-generation bronchus using VBN, barium markings were placed near the lesion using a special catheter under CT guidance. The median distance between the marker and lesion was 4 mm, and the marker could be placed within 1 mm for 27 lesions. No complications developed in any patient. In thoracoscopic partial resection, all lesions could be resected along with the barium markers. As this method does not cause pneumothorax or bleeding, it can be used for multiple lesions. Since the procedure is straightforward, multiple markers can be placed for one lesion to show the resection range in 3D. VBN is also applicable to fiducial marker placement for stereotactic radiotherapy.

Education and Training

Display of the bronchial tree and naming of bronchi can increase anatomical knowledge of the airway, and is useful for education. VBN can also be used in the education of patients to help them understand the outline of bronchoscopy. For operators, VBN improves the understanding of the relationship between the lesion and airways with a 3D target view, allowing bronchoscopy simulation.

Comparison with Other Methods

As discussed above, EMN is another navigation method [43, 44, 56]. (See Chap. 6.) With EMN system, arrival at the lesion can be confirmed since a magnetic sensor is incorporated into a biopsy instrument and not the bronchoscope. However, there are errors between information on the position of the EM sensor and CT images. In addition, arrival is confirmed using CT images obtained prior to examination. Therefore, the diagnostic sensitivity was reported to increase using EMN combined with methods allowing real-time confirmation of the lesion such as EBUS [57]. A meta-analysis has shown a diagnostic yield of 67 % (range 46–88 %) using EMN, which appears to be similar to that using VBN [24]. Since EMN requires a disposable EM sensor, the cost per patient is high. In addition, unlike conventional bronchoscopy, guidance using an EM sensor requires certain training. In comparison, VBN requires only the cost of the VBN system, and its technique can be more readily mastered. Even beginners can readily perform bronchoscopy for peripheral lesions, and a high diagnostic rate can be obtained.

Procedure

Selection of Patients: VBN is indicated in patients with peripheral lesions requiring TBBx. Most suitable lesions are those that clearly show an involved bronchus on CT images. VBN is also indicated in patients with peripheral lesions requiring marker placement for thoracoscopic surgery or radiotherapy.

Instruments: Bronchoscopy under VBN guidance requires DICOM data of helical CT, a VBN system (LungPoint or Bf-NAVI), a bronchoscope (preferably a thin bronchoscope), and a set of standard bronchoscopy accessories. When necessary, a radial type EBUS probe and EBUS system can also be used alongside VBN system to obtain biopsy from PPL.

Procedure:

(a) *Preparation of CT DICOM data*: CT is performed under the conditions recommended by each VBN system, and images are reconstructed. A recommended slice thickness (as well as reconstruction interval) is ≤1 mm. In general, with thinner slices, VB images of more peripheral areas can be produced. When images are poor due to respiratory artifacts, the accuracy of VB images cannot be expected.

(b) *Production of VB images on the route to the lesion:*

For LungPoint

1. Import a CT scan: DICOM data of thin-section CT is imported into the system, with which bronchi are automatically extracted.
2. Define any object or area as the target: The lesion is defined as the target, and is semiautomatically traced (Fig. 7.1).
3. Review the interactive VB animation and airway paths to the target: A maximum of three routes to the lesion are displayed. Each branching on the route is automatically registered. 3D-CT cross-sectional images (axial, sagittal, and coronal images), a 3D-bronchial tree, and a VB image corresponding to the position of the virtual bronchoscope are simultaneously displayed, and the screen can be changed by switching (Fig. 7.2). While observing these images, the route that is the closest to the lesion is selected. Markedly bent routes on the bronchial tree or VB images are avoided due to difficulty in the guidance of the bronchoscope and biopsy instruments. When the lesion is away from the end point of the route, navigation cannot be performed in this interval, resulting in a decrease in the diagnosis rate (Fig. 7.3). Version 3 of LungPoint is

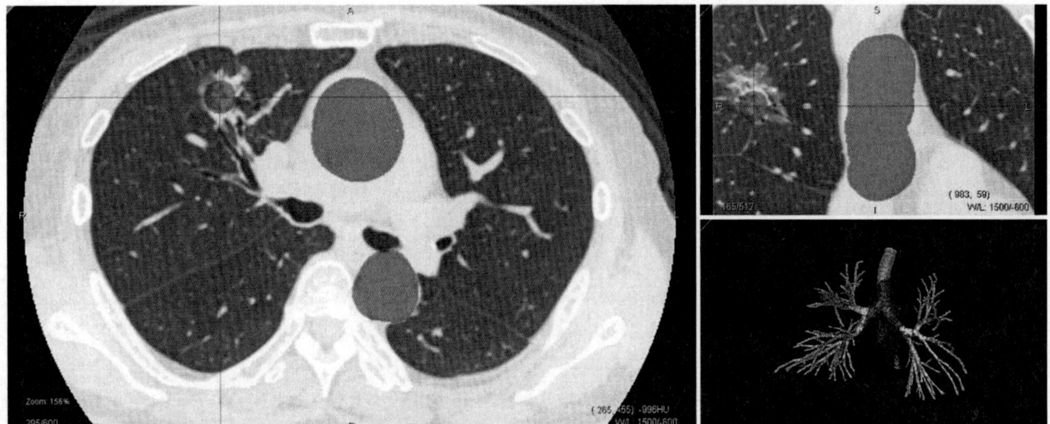

Fig. 7.1 LungPoint target setting. There is a lesion (2.5 cm) in the right S3. In this area, a *purple circle* is set as the target. The right lower image shows the extracted bronchial tree. The aorta is shown in *red*

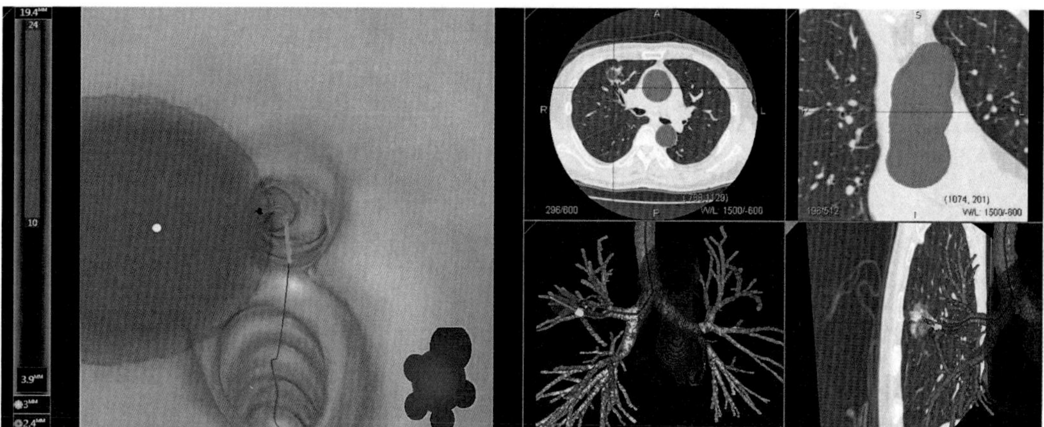

Fig. 7.2 Route display. The left image is a VB image. The bronchial centerline to the target lesion is shown in *light blue* and the target as a *pink circle*. The lower image at the center shows the bronchial tree on which the route to the target is indicated in *blue*. The right lower image is a composite image of a sagittal CT slice of the lesion area, the bronchial tree, and the location of the virtual bronchoscope, allowing the understanding of the relationship between the lesion and bronchial tree

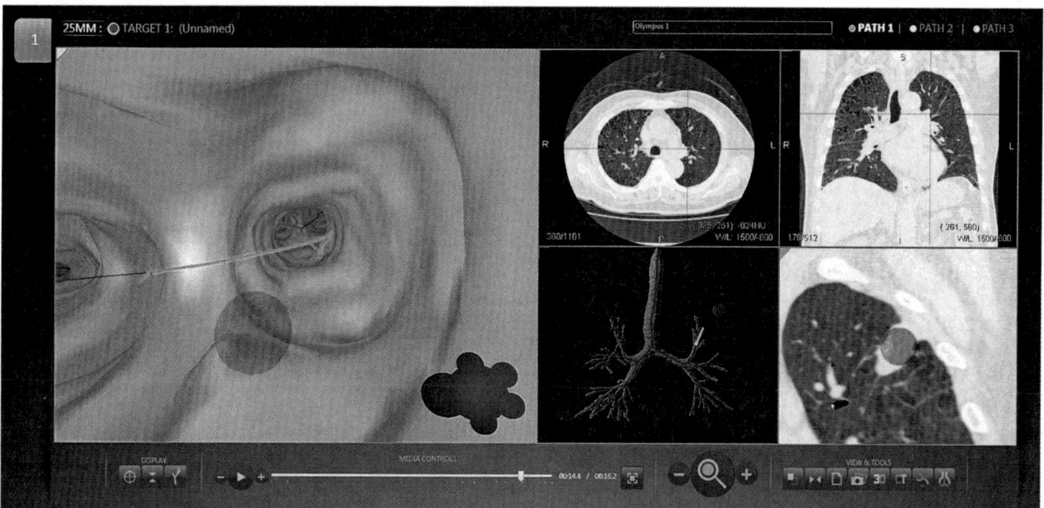

Fig. 7.3 Interval between the lesion and the end point of the route. When the lesion is apart from the end point of the route as shown in the lower image at the center, navigation of this interval is impossible, and the diagnostic yield decreases

applicable to fiducial marker placement for stereotactic body radiation therapy. With fluoroscopic rendering, the target and route can be displayed on a fluoroscopic type image (virtual fluoroscopy view) (Fig. 7.4).

For Bf-NAVI

1. CT DICOM data are imported into the system.
2. Target is set: The target is set so that it can surround the lesion on each cross section. When the target is set, bronchi automatically extracted are shown in blue.
3. End point is set (Fig. 7.5): An end point is placed in the extracted bronchus that is the closest to the lesion. When an involved bronchus reaching the lesion is present, but is not automatically

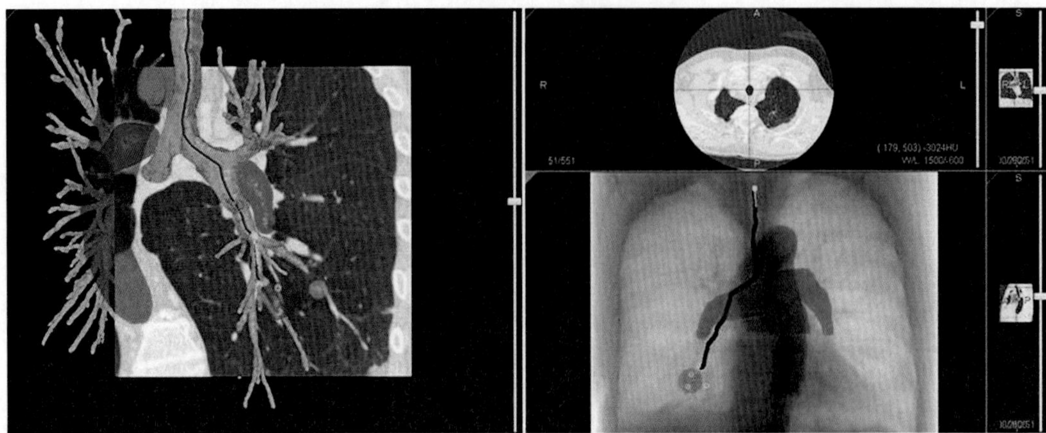

Fig. 7.4 Fiducial marker placement. The *purple circle* indicates the lesion, and the four small *yellow circles* around it indicate the recommended sites for fiducial marker placement. A virtual fluoroscopy view is shown on the right side

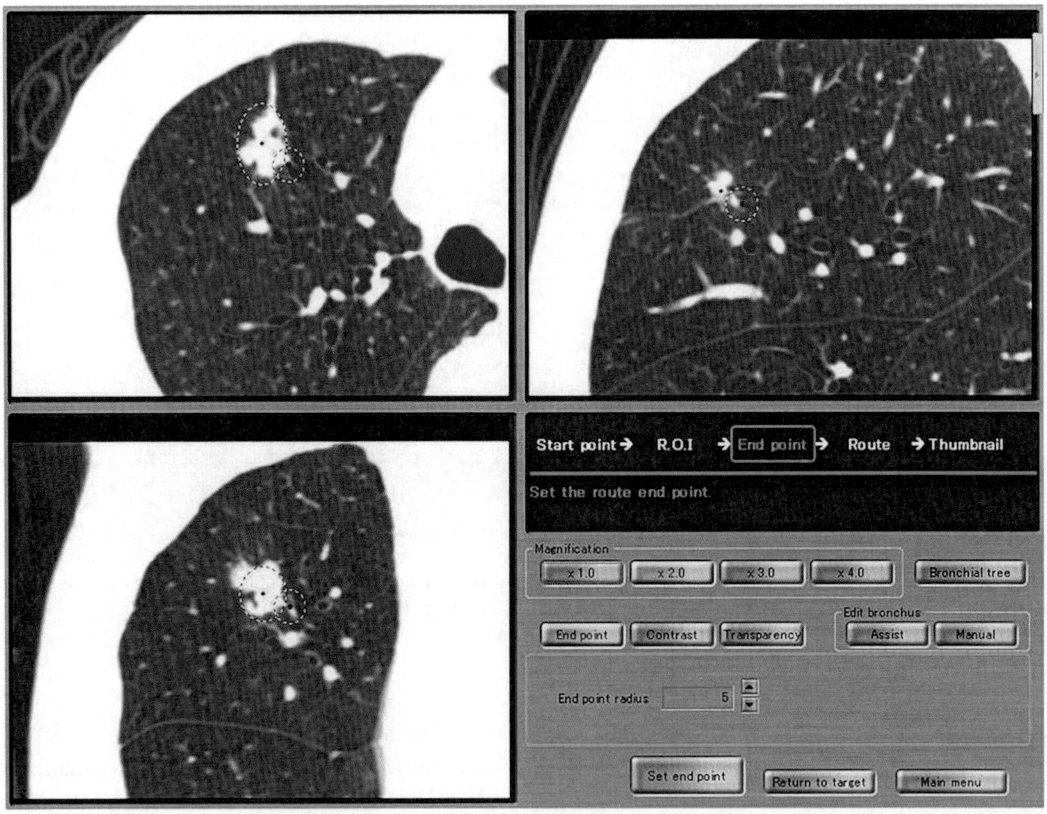

Fig. 7.5 Bf-NAVI setting of the end point. The larger *red broken line* indicates the target. The smaller *red broken line* represents the end point. The extracted bronchi are shown in *blue*

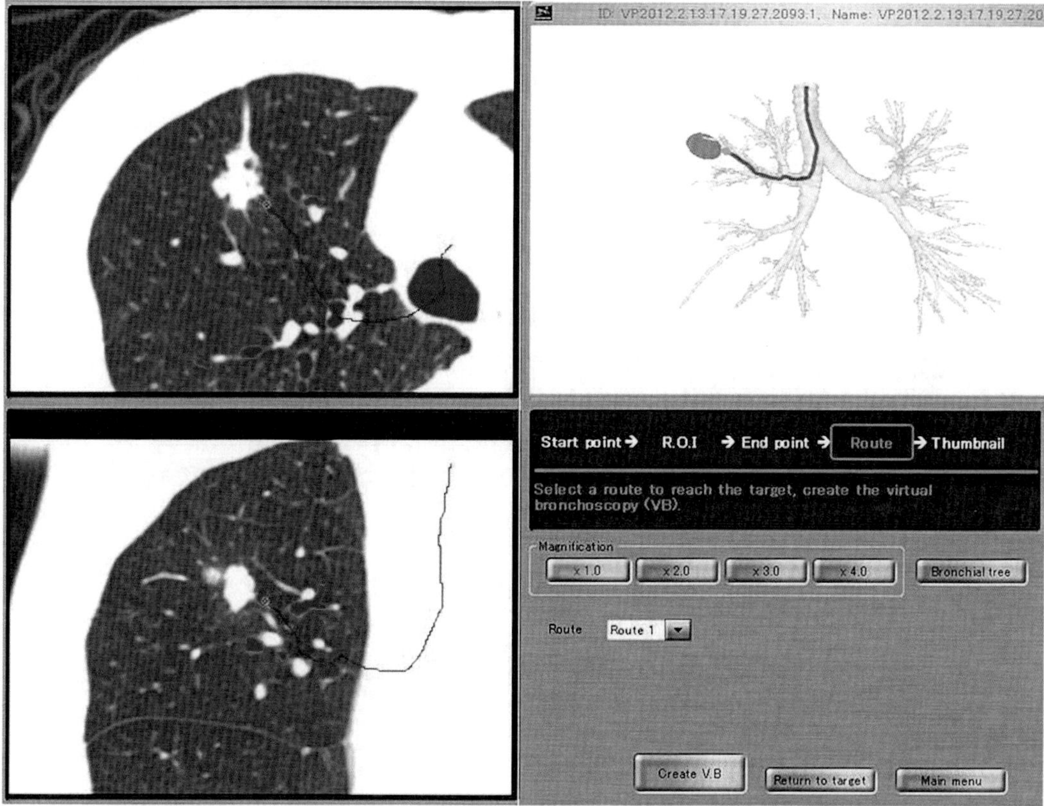

Fig. 7.6 Confirmation of the route. The *red line* indicates the route to the end point. The *green point* is the position of the virtual bronchoscope, and corresponding cross-sectional images are shown

extracted, additional extraction is possible. The screen is scrolled, and the involved bronchus is tracked centrally from the end point to confirm whether all bronchi branching from the involved bronchial route have been extracted. When they have not been extracted, their branching sites are not recognized on VB images, and therefore, additional extraction using the below-described method is always necessary.

4. The route is confirmed (Fig. 7.6): When the end point is set, the route to the end point is instantly displayed on each cross section. The route can also be confirmed on the bronchial tree.
5. Thumbnails are registered (Fig. 7.7): While VB images on the route are moved from the start point to end point, each branching site is registered as a thumbnail. During VBN, when VB images are advanced, the advancement stops at each thumbnail. According to the operator's preference, each branching site is registered. When multiple branching sites can be observed, marking/registration of only the innermost bronchus for advancement is performed.
6. Additional extraction of bronchi is processed (Figs. 7.8 and 7.9): When the distance between the terminal end of the extracted bronchus and the lesion is long, VB image information in this interval is absent, and the diagnostic yield decreases. Using Bf-NAVI, VB images close to the lesion can be generated by additional extraction. Automatic additional extraction is performed from the end of the extracted bronchus. Manual additional

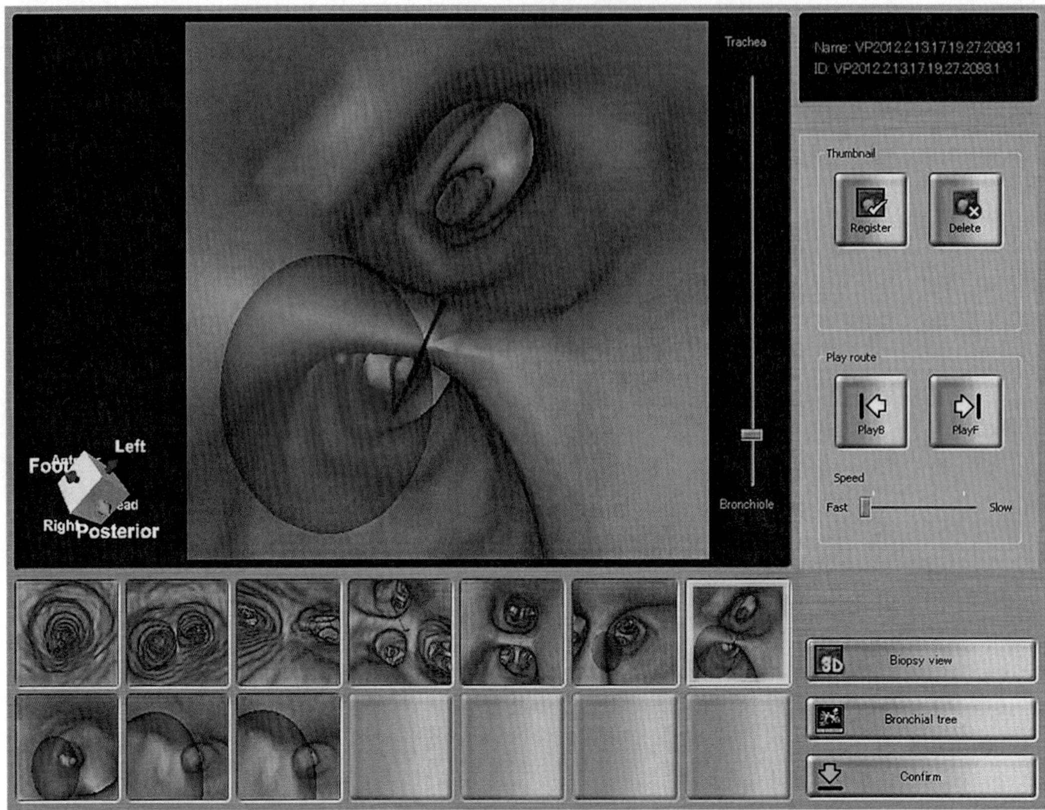

Fig. 7.7 VB images and thumbnail registration. The lower column shows registered thumbnails

extraction is forced extraction and is used for stenotic or bent areas. For example, when there is a bronchus branching from the route reaching the lesion, information that there is branching is indispensable. If this information is absent, this branching is not displayed on VB images, resulting in inconsistency between VB images and real bronchial branching. However, information on the periphery of the branching bronchus is not necessary for navigation. Therefore, only the bronchus immediately after branching is forcefully extracted using manual additional extraction. VB images added by manual extraction are shown in yellow.

(c) *Bronchoscope guidance (Navigation)*

For LungPoint

Using the procedure (VBN), the bronchoscope is advanced based on the route information superimposed on virtual or real images (Fig. 7.10). For manual navigation, see the procedure for Bf-NAVI.

For Bf-NAVI

In the examination room, the Bf-NAVI viewer is placed as close as possible to the bronchoscope monitor. VB data produced using the editor are imputed into the viewer, and the assistant (navi operator) controls VB images using the forward, backward, and rotation buttons. It is important to advance VB images forward and rotate them to match them with real images at each branching site. When becoming familiar with the procedure, the operator should keep the assistant informed about the rotation direction, and the location of the bronchoscope so that VB images can be matched with real images. When the operator and assistant begin to work together smoothly, VB and real images can be displayed as if they were synchronized.

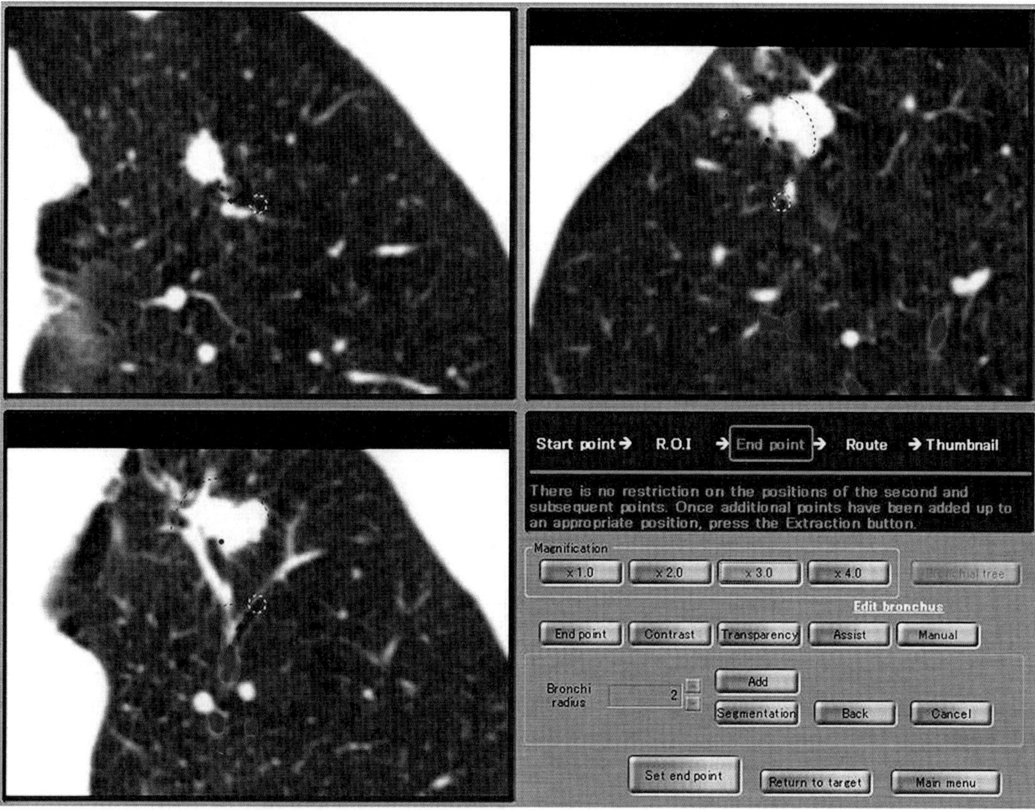

Fig. 7.8 Manual extraction. The point (*red point*) is placed at the end of the extracted bronchus, and continuously placed in the bronchus requiring further extraction

(d) *TBBx*

Biopsy (such as forceps biopsy, needle aspiration biopsy, brush cytology, and lavage cytology) is performed from the target area. See Chap. 4 for EBUS-GS procedure.

Tips for Increasing Diagnostic Yield

A higher diagnostic yield is expected for lesions that show type I or type II tumor–bronchus relationship [58, 59]. It is important to evaluate the relationship between the lesion and involved bronchus on the CT, and confirm the correct production of VB images to a site near the lesion. In particular, extraction of bronchial branching from the route should be confirmed on each cross-sectional image. Using Bf-NAVI, when extraction is inadequate, additional extraction should be performed, and the end point should be placed as close to the lesion as possible. When VB images are generated, techniques for combined use are selected, and the difficulty level is estimated based on the presence/absence of the involved bronchi, the number of bronchial branches approaching the target, and the degree of their bending. For VBN, a bronchoscope as thin as possible is desirable, but the amount of collected specimens becomes smaller as the bronchoscope becomes thinner due to the small forceps channel. In our hospital, a thin bronchoscope with an external diameter of 4.0 mm (P260, Olympus, Tokyo, Japan) and a working channel of 2 mm that can accommodate a guide sheath with an external diameter of 2.0 mm for EBUS-GS is now used for routine examination. When there are only a few branches beyond the bronchoscopic view, and the degree of bronchial bending is slight, the lesion

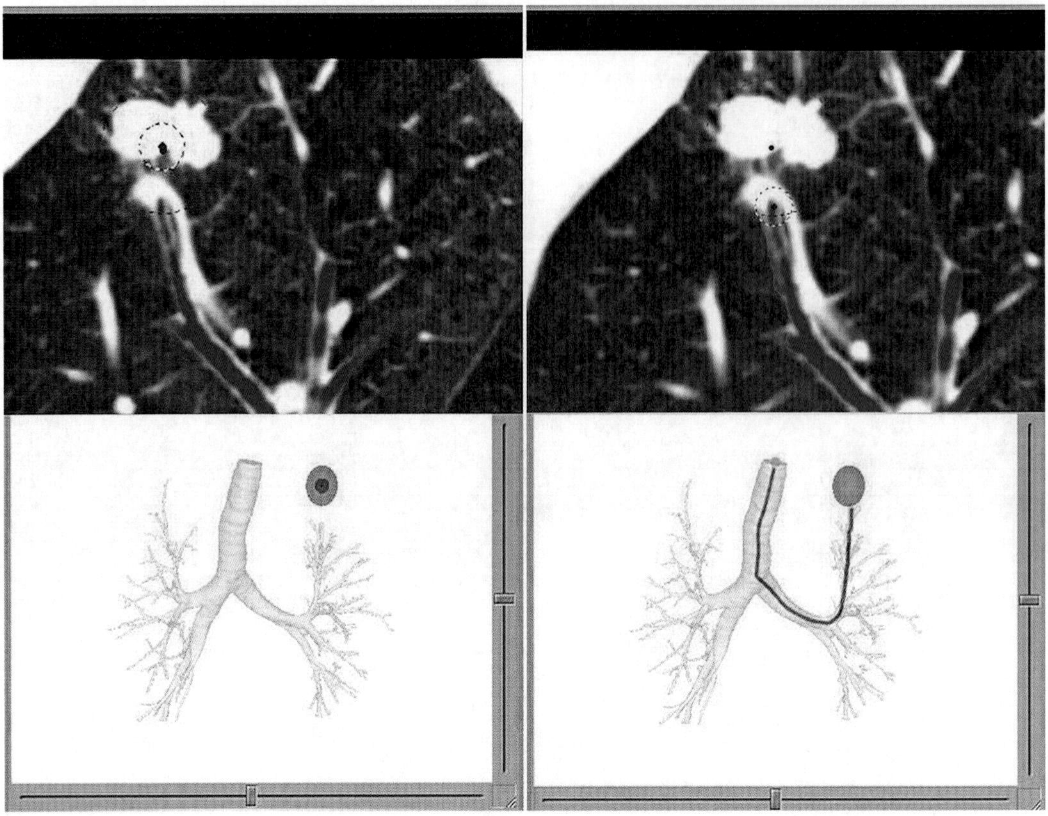

Fig. 7.9 Additional extraction. The left image is before additional extraction, and the right image is after additional extraction. Additional extraction allows extraction of the bronchi to a site immediately before the lesion, and the end point of the bronchial tree comes into contact with the lesion

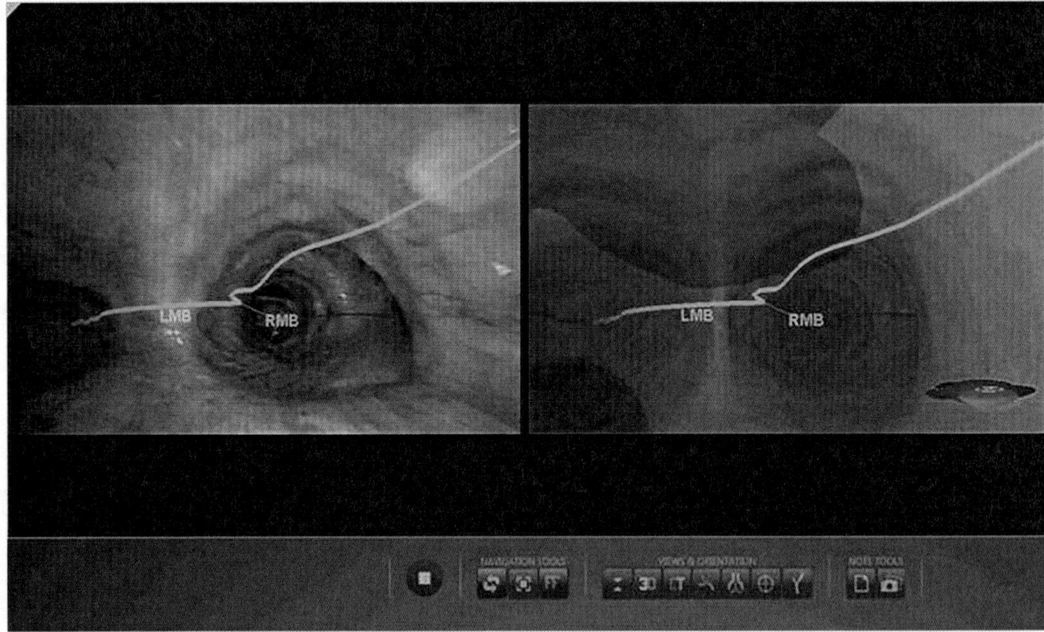

Fig. 7.10 Navigation. The right and left images show VB and real images, respectively. Both images are synchronized, and a VB image matched with the real image is displayed. On the real image, the bronchial *centerline* and route are superimposed

can be frequently visualized only by inserting an EBUS probe, thus allowing biopsy. In the randomized study mentioned above, [23] we were able to visualize the target lesions in 92 % of cases using EBUS in the VBNA group. In some of these cases, guidance from EBUS probe may not be necessary when a correct bronchial path is chosen with VBN and thin bronchoscope is employed to navigate toward the lesion. However, for sixth-generation and higher bronchi and in markedly bent bronchi (such as B6), bronchoscopy should be performed using an ultrathin bronchoscope under X-ray fluoroscopy.

Complications

Pneumothorax was observed in 2 (0.4 %) of 453 previously reported cases. This complication rate is similar to that for conventional TBBx. There are no special complications due to the VBN itself.

Limitations

CT conditions: The level of anatomical details visualized by VB depends on the volume data obtained with chest CT. Therefore, CT needs to be performed under conditions appropriate for individual VBN system. CT parameters for acquisition of volume data differ among scanners, but generally, minimizing collimation and overlapping the image reconstruction by at least 50 % will be suitable for use with VBN systems.

Cost: The necessary recurring cost is only that of CT examination. Due to the patient's exposure to radiation, CT examination is performed only once whenever possible.

Procedure time: The time required for bronchoscopy clearly decreases with the use of VBN guidance [23]. However, production of VB images requires 10–15 min of extra time prior to bronchoscopy.

Learning curve: Since only a bronchoscope is guided according to VB images, no special training is necessary. Familiarity with VB image production and procedure in a few cases is necessary.

Contraindication: There are no contraindications to VBN in patients in whom bronchoscopy and TBBx are otherwise indicated.

Indications for other measures: Even when there is no involved bronchus on CT images, the bronchoscope can be guided to the bronchus that is the closest to the lesion using VBN. However, in some patients, the subsequent guidance of forceps to the lesion is difficult and the diagnostic yield is low. In such patients, transbronchial needle aspiration biopsy might be useful, but there are no data. Alternatively, in patients in whom neither the bronchus nor pulmonary arteries involved in the lesion are confirmed, CT-guided percutaneous biopsy or surgical biopsy should be considered.

Future Directions

Randomized studies and meta-analysis have shown that VBN improves diagnostic yield and reduces examination time. Since its cost is also low, VBN may be widely used in the future. Bronchoscopy is associated with a lower complication rate than percutaneous biopsy. However, further studies are necessary to determine whether the diagnostic yield using VBN is comparable to that using percutaneous biopsy, and to identify the lesions for which VBN is most useful. More work is also needed to improve the accuracy of the automatic tracking and image registration with VBN.

Conclusions and Summary

TBBx for PPLs is associated with fewer complications than percutaneous biopsy. However, the diagnostic yield using TBB can be inadequate, and depends on the operator's skill. VBN is a method in which a bronchoscope is guided using VB images on the bronchial route to a peripheral lesion. A system that allows automatic search for the route to the target, production of VB images, and matched display with real images has been developed. This system is used for diagnosis of peripheral lesions, marker placement for surgery or radiotherapy, and education and training. VBN is used in combination with CT-guided ultrathin bronchoscopy, EBUS-GS, and bronchoscopy with or without X-ray fluoroscopy. Based on prospective studies, the diagnostic yield is 74 % for all PPLs and 68 % for lesions ≤2 cm. In a recent randomized study, use of VBN in association with EBUS-GS increased the diagnostic yield for ≤3 cm lesions from 67 to 80 %, and shortened the total examination time. A meta-analysis has also revealed the usefulness of VBN. There are many advantages of VBN. Even beginners can readily use this technique for peripheral lesions, and a high diagnostic rate can be obtained. To increase the diagnostic yield using VBN, it is important to clarify the relationship between the lesion and extracted bronchi, select appropriate bronchoscopic techniques, and combine them with VBN. CT should be performed under appropriate conditions. VBN is a useful method to support bronchoscopy; wider use and further development of this system are expected.

References

1. Kaneko M, Eguchi K, Ohmatsu H, Kakinuma R, Naruke T, Suemasu K, et al. Peripheral lung cancer: screening and detection with low-dose spiral CT versus radiography. Radiology. 1996;201:798–802.
2. Aberle DR, Adams AM, Berg CD, Black WC, Clapp JD, Fagerstrom RM, et al. Reduced lung-cancer mortality with low-dose computed tomographic screening. N Engl J Med. 2011; 365:395–409.
3. Yung RC. Tissue diagnosis of suspected lung cancer: selecting between bronchoscopy, transthoracic needle aspiration, and resectional biopsy. Respir Care Clin N Am. 2003;9:51–76.
4. Rivera MP, Mehta AC. Initial diagnosis of lung cancer: ACCP evidence-based clinical practice guidelines (2nd edition). Chest. 2007;132:131S–48S.
5. Manhire A, Charig M, Clelland C, Gleeson F, Miller R, Moss H, et al. Guidelines for radiologically guided lung biopsy. Thorax. 2003;58:920–36.
6. Tomiyama N, Yasuhara Y, Nakajima Y, Adachi S, Arai Y, Kusumoto M, et al. CT-guided needle biopsy of lung lesions: a survey of severe complication based on 9783 biopsies in Japan. Eur J Radiol. 2006;59:60–4.
7. Asano F, Aoe M, Ohsaki Y, Okada Y, Sasada S, Sato S, et al. Deaths and complications associated with respiratory endoscopy: a survey by the Japan society for respiratory endoscopy in 2010. Respirology. 2012;17:478–85.
8. Chechani V. Bronchoscopic diagnosis of solitary pulmonary nodules and lung masses in the absence of endobronchial abnormality. Chest. 1996;109:620–5.
9. Baaklini WA, Reinoso MA, Gorin AB, Sharafkaneh A, Manian P. Diagnostic yield of fiberoptic bronchoscopy in evaluating solitary pulmonary nodules. Chest. 2000;117:1049–54.
10. Naidich DP, Sussman R, Kutcher WL, Aranda CP, Garay SM, Ettenger NA. Solitary pulmonary nodules. CT-bronchoscopic correlation. Chest. 1988;93:595–8.
11. Minami H, Ando Y, Nomura F, Sakai S, Shimokata K. Interbronchoscopist variability in the diagnosis of lung cancer by flexible bronchoscopy. Chest. 1994;105:1658–62.
12. Dolina MY, Cornish DC, Merritt SA, Rai L, Mahraj R, Higgins WE, et al. Interbronchoscopist variability in endobronchial path selection: a simulation study. Chest. 2008;133:897–905.
13. Vining DJ, Liu K, Choplin RH, Haponik EF. Virtual bronchoscopy. Relationships of virtual reality endobronchial simulations to actual bronchoscopic findings. Chest. 1996;109:549–53.
14. Hoppe H, Dinkel HP, Walder B, von Allmen G, Gugger M, Vock P. Grading airway stenosis down to the segmental level using virtual bronchoscopy. Chest. 2004;125:704–11.
15. De Wever W, Vandecaveye V, Lanciotti S, Verschakelen JA. Multidetector CT-generated virtual bronchoscopy: an illustrated review of the potential clinical indications. Eur Respir J. 2004;23:776–82.
16. Asano F, Matsuno Y, Matsushita T, Seko A. Transbronchial diagnosis of a pulmonary peripheral small lesion using an ultrathin bronchoscope with virtual bronchoscopic navigation. J Bronchol. 2002; 9:108–11.
17. Asano F, Matsuno Y, Shinagawa N, Yamazaki K, Suzuki T, Ishida T, et al. A virtual bronchoscopic navigation system for pulmonary peripheral lesions. Chest. 2006;130:559–66.
18. Asano F, Matsuno Y, Tsuzuku A, Anzai M, Shinagawa N, Yamazaki K, et al. Diagnosis of peripheral pulmonary lesions using a bronchoscope insertion guidance system combined with endobronchial ultrasonography with a guide sheath. Lung Cancer. 2008;60:366–73.
19. Asano F, Matsuno Y, Takeichi N, Matsusita T, Ohoya H. Virtual bronchoscopy in navigation of an ultrathin bronchoscope. J Jpn Soc Bronchol. 2002; 24:433–8.
20. Shinagawa N, Yamazaki K, Onodera Y, Miyasaka K, Kikuchi E, Dosaka-Akita H, et al. CT-guided transbronchial biopsy using an ultrathin bronchoscope with virtual bronchoscopic navigation. Chest. 2004;125:1138–43.
21. Asahina H, Yamazaki K, Onodera Y, Kikuchi E, Shinagawa N, Asano F, et al. Transbronchial biopsy

using endobronchial ultrasonography with a guide sheath and virtual bronchoscopic navigation. Chest. 2005;128:1761–5.
22. Shinagawa N, Yamazaki K, Onodera Y, Asano F, Ishida T, Moriya H, et al. Virtual bronchoscopic navigation system shortens the examination time—feasibility study of virtual bronchoscopic navigation system. Lung Cancer. 2007;56:201–6.
23. Ishida T, Asano F, Yamazaki K, Shinagawa N, Oizumi S, Moriya H, et al. Virtual bronchoscopic navigation combined with endobronchial ultrasound to diagnose small peripheral pulmonary lesions: a randomised trial. Thorax. 2011;66:1072–7.
24. Wang Memoli JS, Nietert PJ, Silvestri GA. Meta-analysis of guided bronchoscopy for the evaluation of the pulmonary nodule. Chest. 2012;142(2):385–93.
25. Rodenwaldt J, Kopka L, Roedel R, Margas A, Grabbe E. 3D virtual endoscopy of the upper airway: optimization of the scan parameters in a cadaver phantom and clinical assessment. J Comput Assist Tomogr. 1997;21:405–11.
26. Ferretti GR, Thony F, Bosson JL, Pison C, Arbib F, Coulomb M. Benign abnormalities and carcinoid tumors of the central airways: diagnostic impact of CT bronchography. AJR Am J Roentgenol. 2000;174: 1307–13.
27. Adaletli I, Kurugoglu S, Ulus S, Ozer H, Elicevik M, Kantarci F, et al. Utilization of low-dose multidetector CT and virtual bronchoscopy in children with suspected foreign body aspiration. Pediatr Radiol. 2007;37:33–40.
28. Colt HG, Crawford SW, Galbraith 3rd O. Virtual reality bronchoscopy simulation: a revolution in procedural training. Chest. 2001;120:1333–9.
29. Ost D, DeRosiers A, Britt EJ, Fein AM, Lesser ML, Mehta AC. Assessment of a bronchoscopy simulator. Am J Respir Crit Care Med. 2001;164:2248–55.
30. Tanaka M, Takizawa H, Satoh M, Okada Y, Yamasawa F, Umeda A. Assessment of an ultrathin bronchoscope that allows cytodiagnosis of small airways. Chest. 1994;106:1443–7.
31. Saka H. Ultra-fine bronchoscopy: biopsy for peripheral lesions. Nippon Rinsho. 2002;60 Suppl 5:188–90.
32. Asano F, Matsuno Y, Komaki C, Kato T, Ito M, Kimura T, et al. CT-guided transbronchial diagnosis using ultrathin bronchoscope for small peripheral pulmonary lesions. Nihon Kokyuki Gakkai Zasshi. 2002;40:11–6.
33. Asano F, Kimura T, Shindou J, Matsuno Y, Mizutani H, Horiba M. Usefulness of CT-guided ultrathin bronchoscopy in the diagnosis of peripheral pulmonary lesions that could not be diagnosed by standard transbronchial biopsy. J Jpn Soc Bronchol. 2002;24:80–5.
34. Fujisawa T, Tanaka M, Saka H. Report by the Bronchus Nomenclature Working Group. J Jpn Soc Bronchol. 2000;22:330–1.
35. Seemann MD, Seemann O, Luboldt W, et al. Hybrid rendering of the chest and virtual bronchoscopy [corrected]. Eur J Med Res. 2000;5:431–7.
36. Edell E, Krier-Morrow D. Navigational bronchoscopy: overview of technology and practical considerations—new current procedural terminology codes effective 2010. Chest. 2010;137:450–4.
37. Eberhardt R, Kahn N, Gompelmann D, Schumann M, Heussel CP, Herth FJ. LungPoint—a new approach to peripheral lesions. J Thorac Oncol. 2010;5:1559–63.
38. Mori K, Deguchi D, Sugiyama J, Suenaga Y, Toriwaki J, Maurer CR, Jr., et al. Tracking of a bronchoscope using epipolar geometry analysis and intensity-based image registration of real and virtual endoscopic images. Med Image Anal. 2002;6:321–36.
39. Higgins WE, Helferty JP, Lu K, Merritt SA, Rai L, Yu KC. 3D CT-video fusion for image-guided bronchoscopy. Comput Med Imaging Graph. 2008;32: 159–73.
40. McLennan G, Ferguson JS, Thomas K, Delsing AS, Cook-Granroth J, Hoffman EA. The use of MDCT-based computer-aided pathway finding for mediastinal and perihilar lymph node biopsy: a randomized controlled prospective trial. Respiration. 2007;74:423–31.
41. Merritt SA, Gibbs JD, Yu KC, Patel V, Rai L, Cornish DC et al. Image-guided bronchoscopy for peripheral lung lesions: a phantom study. Chest. 2008;134: 1017–26.
42. Mori K, Deguchi D, Kitasaka T, Suenaga Y, Hasegawa Y, Imaizumi K, et al. Improvement of accuracy of marker-free bronchoscope tracking using electromagnetic tracker based on bronchial branch information. Med Image Comput Comput Assist Interv. 2008;11:535–42.
43. Schwarz Y, Mehta AC, Ernst A, Herth F, Engel A, Besser D, et al. Electromagnetic navigation during flexible bronchoscopy. Respiration. 2003;70:516–22.
44. Schwarz Y, Greif J, Becker HD, Ernst A, Mehta A. Real-time electromagnetic navigation bronchoscopy to peripheral lung lesions using overlaid CT images: the first human study. Chest. 2006;129:988–94.
45. Wagner U, Walthers EM, Gelmetti W, Klose KJ, von Wichert P. Computer-tomographically guided fiberbronchoscopic transbronchial biopsy of small pulmonary lesions: a feasibility study. Respiration. 1996;63:181–6.
46. Kobayashi T, Shimamura K, Hanai K. Computed tomography- guided bronchoscopy with an ultrathin fiberscope. Diagn Ther Endosc. 1996;2:229–32.
47. Shinagawa N, Yamazaki K, Onodera Y, Asahina H, Kikuchi E, Asano F, et al. Factors related to diagnostic sensitivity using an ultrathin bronchoscope under CT guidance. Chest. 2007;131:549–53.
48. Matsuno Y, Asano F, Shindoh J, Abe T, Shiraki A, Ando M, et al. CT-guided ultrathin bronchoscopy: bioptic approach and factors in predicting diagnosis. Intern Med. 2011;50:2143–8.
49. Herth FJ, Ernst A, Becker HD. Endobronchial ultrasound-guided transbronchial lung biopsy in solitary pulmonary nodules and peripheral lesions. Eur Respir J. 2002;20:972–4.
50. Kurimoto N, Miyazawa T, Okimasa S, Maeda A, Oiwa H, Miyazu Y, et al. Endobronchial ultrasonography using a guide sheath increases the ability to diagnose peripheral pulmonary lesions endoscopically. Chest. 2004;126:959–65.

51. Yoshikawa M, Sukoh N, Yamazaki K, Kanazawa K, Fukumoto S, Harada M, et al. Diagnostic value of endobronchial ultrasonography with a guide sheath for peripheral pulmonary lesions without X-ray fluoroscopy. Chest. 2007;131:1788–93.
52. Tachihara M, Ishida T, Kanazawa K, Sugawara A, Watanabe K, Uekita K, et al. A virtual bronchoscopic navigation system under X-ray fluoroscopy for transbronchial diagnosis of small peripheral pulmonary lesions. Lung Cancer. 2007;57:322–7.
53. Asano F. Virtual bronchoscopic navigation. Clin Chest Med. 2010;31:75–85.
54. Asano F, Matsuno Y, Ibuka T, Takeichi N, Oya H. A barium marking method using an ultrathin bronchoscope with virtual bronchoscopic navigation. Respirology. 2004;9:409–13.
55. Asano F, Shindoh J, Shigemitsu K, Miya K, Abe T, Horiba M, et al. Ultrathin bronchoscopic barium marking with virtual bronchoscopic navigation for fluoroscopy-assisted thoracoscopic surgery. Chest. 2004;126:1687–93.
56. Gildea TR, Mazzone PJ, Karnak D, Meziane M, Mehta AC. Electromagnetic navigation diagnostic bronchoscopy: a prospective study. Am J Respir Crit Care Med. 2006;174:982–9.
57. Eberhardt R, Anantham D, Ernst A, Feller-Kopman D, Herth F. Multimodality bronchoscopic diagnosis of peripheral lung lesions: a randomized controlled trial. Am J Respir Crit Care Med. 2007;176:36–41.
58. Tsuboi E, Ikeda S, Tajima M, Shimosato Y, Ishikawa S. Transbronchial biopsy smear for diagnosis of peripheral pulmonary carcinomas. Cancer. 1967;20:687–98.
59. Gaeta M, Pandolfo I, Volta S, Russi EG, Bartiromo G, Girone G, et al. Bronchus sign on CT in peripheral carcinoma of the lung: value in predicting results of transbronchial biopsy. AJR Am J Roentgenol. 1991;157:1181–5.

Part III

Therapeutic Interventional Bronchoscopy

Therapeutic Bronchoscopy for Central Airway Obstruction

8

Sarah Hadique, Prasoon Jain, and Atul C. Mehta

There are in fact two things, science and opinion; the former begets knowledge, the latter ignorance.

Hippocrates

Abstract

Central airway obstruction (CAO) results from a variety of malignant and nonmalignant causes. Advanced lung cancer is the most common etiology. The clinical presentation varies from slowly progressive cough and dyspnea to rapidly developing respiratory distress and asphyxia. A close collaboration among interventional pulmonologists, radiologists, anesthesiologists, and thoracic surgeons is essential for optimal outcome in these challenging situations. Immediate goals of the therapy are to secure the airway and to restore the patency of airway lumen. Several therapeutic bronchoscopy techniques are available using flexible or rigid bronchoscope to achieve these goals. The choice of technique depends on the underlying cause, type of obstruction, severity of CAO and availability of the instruments and expertise. Immediate relief in symptoms can be achieved with mechanical debridement, laser photoresection, electrocautery, argon plasma coagulation, cryorecanalization, and balloon dilation (Balloon bronchoplasty). Brachytherapy, photodynamic therapy, and cryotherapy have delayed effects and therefore are not suitable when immediate relief in symptoms is needed.Airway stents are helpful in patients with extrinsic central airway compression. A combination of these procedures is usually successful in rapid palliation of symptoms and in selected cases paves way for further treatments such as external beam radiation, chemotherapy, and surgery.

Keywords

Central airway obstruction • Therapeutic bronchoscopy • Tracheal stenosis • Lung cancer • Rigid bronchoscopy

S. Hadique, M.D. (✉)
Pulmonary and Critical Care Medicine, West Virginia University, 1 Medical Center Drive 4075A, HSN MS 9166, Morgantown, WV 26506, USA
e-mail: sarahhadique@gmail.com; shadique@hsc.wvu.edu

P. Jain, M.B.B.S., M.D., F.C.C.P.
Pulmonary and Critical Care, Louis A Johnson VA Medical Center, Clarksburg, WV 26301, USA

A.C. Mehta, M.B.B.S.
Respiratory Institute, Lerner College of Medicine, Cleveland Clinic, Cleveland, OH 44195, USA

A.C. Mehta and P. Jain (eds.), *Interventional Bronchoscopy: A Clinical Guide*, Respiratory Medicine 10, DOI 10.1007/978-1-62703-395-4_8, © Springer Science+Business Media New York 2013

Introduction

Central airway refers to the trachea, the mainstem and lobar bronchi. Obstruction of central airways results from a variety of malignant or nonmalignant causes (Table 8.1). The obstructing lesions are classified into endo-luminal, extrinsic, or a combination of both (Fig. 8.1) [1]. Primary lung cancer is the most common cause of central airway obstruction (CAO). The rising incidence of lung cancer suggests that interventional pulmonologists will continue to encounter increasing number of patients with advanced CAO in the future. Obstruction of the central airways causes a variety of symptoms such as dyspnea, cough, hemoptysis, wheezing, atelectasis, and post-obstructive pneumonia. Dyspnea in these patients is due to airflow limitation and increased work of breathing. In some of these patients the symptoms are acute in onset with severe respiratory distress and imminent suffocation. In other instances, the symptoms develop slowly, simulating the clinical features of asthma or chronic obstructive pulmonary disease (COPD). For this

Table 8.1 Causes of Malignant and nonmalignant central airway obstruction (CAO)

Malignant	Nonmalignant	
Primary lung tumors	*Acquired*	*Congenital*
Primary airway tumor	• Post endotracheal tube	• Tracheomalacia
• Squamous cell carcinoma	• Post tracheostomy	• Bronchomalacia
• Adenoid cystic carcinoma	• Thermal or chemical airway burns	• Vascular sling
• Mucoepidermoid cancer	• Foreign body	• Membranous web
• Carcinoid tumors	• Airway stents	• Relapsing polychondritis
Metastatic tumors	• Surgical anastomosis	
• Thyroid	• Post radiation fibrosis	
• Colon	*Systemic diseases*	
• Breast	• Tuberculosis	
• Renal	• Sarcoidosis	
• Melanoma	• Amyloidosis	
• Kaposi's sarcoma	• Fibrosing medisatinitis	
Adjacent tumor	• Wegners granulomatosis	
• Esophageal cancer	• HPV papillomatosis	
• Laryngeal cancer	*Miscellaneous*	
• Mediastinal tumors	• Mucous plug	
• Lymphoma	• Blood clot	
	• Hemartoma	
	• Epiglottitis	
	• Goiter	
	• Idiopathic	

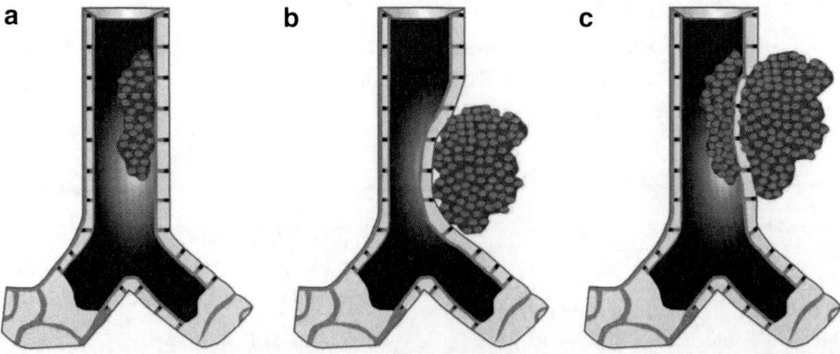

Fig. 8.1 Types of central airway obstruction: (**a**) endoluminal, (**b**) extrinsic, (**c**) mixed endoluminal and extrinsic

reason, physicians often fail to recognize the correct diagnosis in many patients with CAO in the early stages.

The management of CAO poses unique challenges and requires a multidisciplinary approach [2–4]. Having a dedicated airway team in place for rapid evaluation and treatment of these patients is very effective but such teams are available only at the centers of excellances [5]. Relief of CAO should be expeditious and should initially focus on securing the airway [6]. Once the airway is secured, a variety of airway interventions can be offered to restore the patency of central airways.

A variety of techniques such as mechanical debridement, balloon bronchoplasty, cryotherapy, laser photoresection, electrocautery and argon plasma coagulation, brachytherapy, photodynamic therapy, and stent placement are available to interventional bronchoscopist [7–9]. The choice of the intervention depends on the type and location of lesion, and the urgency of the procedure. In addition, the clinical stability, the nature of the underlying diagnosis, and the overall prognosis and quality of life also impact the choice of the preferred intervention. In the absence of large randomized controlled trials in this field to guide the therapy, the choice of therapy also depends on the availability of trained personnel and equipment at the facility, personal preference, and institution-specific protocols. In many instances a combination of procedures are employed to achieve optimal results.

In this chapter we review the diagnostic and therapeutic approach to CAO secondary to malignant conditions. We discuss the causes, clinical evaluation, imaging and the therapeutic options available to the interventional pulmonologists for the management of malignant CAO. We also highlight the current trends and recent developments in this area.

Causes of Central Airway Obstruction

Malignant airway obstruction can result from primary airway tumors, extension of adjacent malignancies or the metastatic disease to the airway (Table 8.1).

Lung cancer is the leading cause of malignant CAO. According to some estimates, CAO occurs in approximately 20–30 % of lung cancer patients and up to 40 % of lung cancer deaths are related to advanced local or regional disease [10]. Other common etiologies include esophageal, thyroid, and primary mediastinal malignancies. Many centrally located malignant tumors not only encase and compress the airways causing extrinsic compression but also invade the wall of the airway causing endoluminal disease. Mostly, the CAO in these patients results from a combination of both an endoluminal spread and an extrinsic compression [2].

Endobronchial metastasis is most frequently observed in patients with breast cancer, colorectal cancer, melanoma, and renal cell carcinoma [11]. According to postmortem studies, isolated endobronchial metastases without involvement of pulmonary parenchyma occur in up to 2 % of patients with extra-thoracic malignancies [12]. In contrast, patients with pulmonary metastasis are shown to have endobronchial lesions in 18–42 % of cases [13, 14]. On this background, physicians must have a low threshold to perform a diagnostic bronchoscopy when a patient known to have extra-thoracic malignancy develops cough, dyspnea, hemoptysis, or atelectasis.

Kaposi's sarcoma (KS) is the most common malignant complication of human immunodeficiency virus (HIV) infection. Pulmonary involvement may occur in up to 20 % of HIV-infected patients with cutaneous Kaposi's sarcoma [15]. In many instances, KS involves the airways and present with symptoms of CAO [16]. On bronchoscopy, multiple rounded cherry-red or purpuric raised lesions are seen throughout the airway mucosa, sometimes causing complete lobar or segmental endobronchial obstruction [17].

Primary airway tumors are less common and pose considerable diagnostic and therapeutic challenge. About 600–700 cases are estimated to occur in USA every year [2]. Nearly three-quarters of primary airway tumors of trachea and carina are squamous cell carcinoma and adenoid cystic carcinoma. In a 60-year review of tracheal tumors from MD Anderson Cancer Center in Texas, 74 patients were diagnosed with primary tracheal cancers. Among these, 34 (45.9 %) were squamous cell carcinomas, 19 (25.7 %) were adenoid cystic carcinomas, and the remaining 21 (28.4 %) were of other histologic types [18]. Squamous cell tracheal carcinoma usually develops in the sixth or seventh decade and is more common in men and smokers. In contrast, adenoid cystic carcinoma affects younger patients, is not related to smoking, and is equally distributed between men and women [19].

Carcinoid tumor is the most common tumor etiology distal to the carina [20]. Most patients with endobronchial carcinoids present with cough, hemoptysis, and unilateral wheeze and not with carcinoid syndrome.

Tracheal tumors are often slow growing and their symptoms and signs are insidious in onset. Patients are often misdiagnosed as adult onset asthma for several months before the correct diagnosis is established [21]. Physicians must be keenly aware of the possibility of tracheal tumors as the cause of dyspnea and wheezing that are not responsive to usual asthma therapies.

CAO can also be caused by many nonmalignant causes (Table 8.1). The most common nonmalignant cause among adults is formation of granulation tissue and fibrous stricture secondary to trauma induced by prolonged endotracheal intubation, or tracheostomy. Other common nonmalignant causes include foreign bodies and tracheobronchomalacia. The term "nonmalignant" is more appropriate than "benign" since the signs and symptoms caused by these lesions are as ominous and life-threatening as those caused by malignant CAO. The detailed discussion of nonmalignant CAO is beyond the realm of this chapter and has been reviewed elsewhere [22–25].

Clinical Assessment

The clinical presentation of airway obstruction depends on the severity and location of airway obstruction. Moreover, the patient's underlying health status and ability to compensate for decreased airflow will influence the extent to which the symptoms appear. The presentation can range from asymptomatic radiological abnormality to a life-threatening airway obstruction.

Dyspnea is the most common symptom. Early symptoms may go unnoticed because many patients become increasingly accustomed to their dyspnea on exertion or cough by imposing a gradual limitation to their physical activity. Dyspnea on exertion, typically, does not develop until the trachea is narrowed to about 8 mm or 50 % of diameter. Dyspnea at rest can be expected when the lumen is narrowed to about 5 mm or 25 % of diameter [26, 27]. Accordingly, the majority of patients who experience symptoms of CAO already have advanced airway disease at the time of presentation. Airway narrowing to such a critical degree further increases their susceptibility to develop complete airway obstruction from mucous plugging, blood clots, or airway inflammation. Hence, it is not surprising that acute respiratory distress is the presenting symptom in more than one-half of patients with CAO [25].

Hemoptysis is the second most common symptom, occurring in up to 50 % of patients with CAO [28]. Other symptoms of CAO are cough, wheezing, stridor, recurrent respiratory tract infections and atelectasis. Post-obstructive pneumonia can be found in approximately one-third of these patients on initial presentation. Symptoms of hoarseness or coughing with swallowing suggest vocal cord paralysis or laryngeal dysfunction, or esophageal cancer.

Many of these patients carry a diagnosis of asthma or COPD with recurrent exacerbation. Indeed some of these patients have already developed cushingoid features from prolonged and frequent use of corticosteroids. Any of the afore mentioned symptoms including atypical and medically refractory adult-onset asthma or frequent COPD exacerbation should raise the suspicion of a central airway pathology that requires further work up with radiographic imaging and a bronchoscopy.

A detailed history from the patient or the family provides useful information regarding the acuity of the problem and the performance status of the patient prior to the clinical presentation. Such information is helpful in predicting the treatment outcome for the individual patient. Although acute airway obstruction is first manifestation of malignancy in some patients, the majority of patients with malignant CAO are already known to have a thoracic tumor. Therefore, history of current or remote malignancy, and any history of receiving chemotherapy or radiation therapy must be sought. Since many patients with CAO are seriously ill with limited cardiopulmonary reserves, a meticulous assessment of operative risks is essential in every patient. A thorough evaluation for comorbid medical conditions like heart disease (which may influence anesthesia administration), coagulopathy, renal failure, obstructive sleep apnea, and cervical arthritis (which may pose difficulty with rigid bronchoscopy) are essential in formulation of appropriate treatment plan. It is also important to seek any prior history of problems during intubation or bronchoscopy as it will alert the treating team to maintain a heightened state of readiness to deal with difficult airways during the interventional procedure.

Physical examination may be unremarkable in early stages. Chest examination may reveal evidence of tracheal deviation, stridor, localized or diffuse wheezing, hoarseness, decreased breath sounds or signs of retained secretions, and obstructive pneumonia. In rare instances, patients may present with subcutaneous emphysema or superior vena cava syndrome with facial and upper extremity edema and dilated superficial veins over the chest wall. Patients with acute respiratory distress can be seen to use accessory muscles of respiration and often demonstrate signs of tachycardia, tachypnea, diaphoresis, and restlessness. Bradycardia, cyanosis, and obtundation are more ominous and suggest that the airway lumen is severely compromised. Immediate intervention is needed in these patients in order to avoid imminent asphyxia and death.

Pulmonary Function Tests

Many patients are too ill to perform pulmonary function tests in the acute setting. Forced expiratory maneuvers can worsen the airflow obstruction and should not be attempted in the presence of critical narrowing of large airways. In these patients, meticulous history and physical examination bolstered by chest imaging and bronchoscopy are sufficient for diagnosis and treatment planning.

In more stable patients, pulmonary function tests provide useful information. Spirometry has a low sensitivity for early detection of CAO. In contrast, flow-volume loop helps define the location of obstruction and provides invaluable clinical information [29]. A plateau in the inspiratory limb of the flow-volume loop indicates variable extra-thoracic obstruction, commonly caused by vocal cord paralysis, extra-thoracic goiter, and laryngeal tumors (Fig. 8.2a). Flattening of the expiratory limb of the loop indicates variable intra-thoracic obstruction (Fig. 8.2b). Fixed large

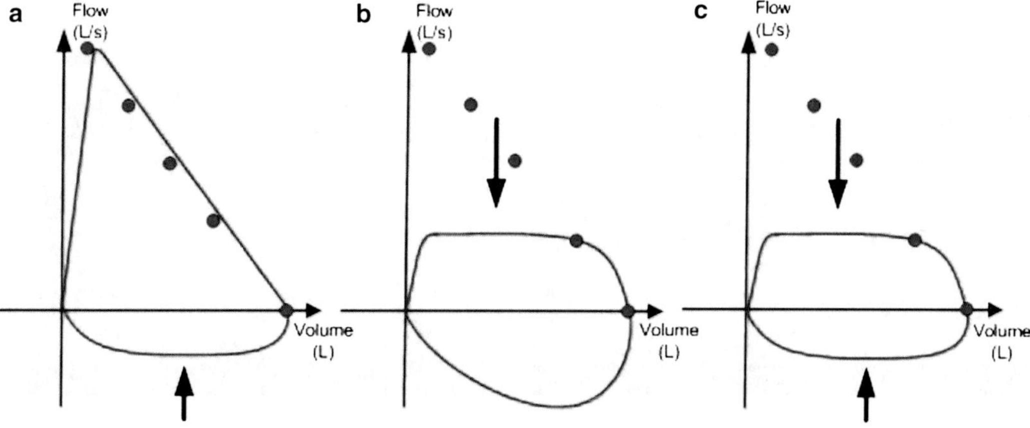

Fig. 8.2 Flow-volume loops showing (**a**) Variable extrathoracic obstruction, (**b**) Variable intrathoracic obstruction, (**c**) Fixed obstruction

airway obstruction due to tracheal stenosis or to tracheal compression by large tumors demonstrates flattening of both the inspiratory and expiratory phases of the flow (Fig. 8.2c) [30].

Chest Imaging

Imaging studies plays a pivotal role in the procedural preparation and bronchoscopic planning. Technological advancement in radiology, most notably in Computed Tomography (CT) imaging has revolutionized noninvasive imaging of the central airways. CT imaging should be obtained as much as possible but may not be feasible in acutely ill patients who are unable to hold breath or lay supine during the procedure [31].

Chest radiograph has low sensitivity but may suggest possibility of central airway or bronchial obstruction in some cases. A narrowing of the tracheal or bronchial air column, and tracheal distortion or significant deviation should raise the suspicion for CAO (Fig. 8.3). A chest radiograph may also disclose a mass or mediastinal lymphadenopathy. A more distal obstruction may be associated with the radiological findings of atelectasis, consolidation, effusions, and elevation of the hemi-diaphragm. Chest radiograph must also be obtained upon completion of interventional procedure to assess the results, and to rule out the procedure related adverse event such as pneumothorax or atelectasis. Postoperative chest radiograph is also useful for the future reference.

The advent of helical CT in 1991 and more recently, multidetector helical CT (MDCT) scanners have dramatically improved the quality of axial imaging and 2D or 3D reformation images by signifcantly reducing the motion artifacts. With the latest CT scanners, thin section images of the central airways can be obtained during a short breath hold. The most attractive feature of CT imaging is its ability to demonstrate the airway distal to the site of stenosis beyond which the bronchoscope cannot be passed. Intravenous contrast is not essential but is recommended for better assessment of enlarged paratracheal lymph nodes or thyroid mass.

Imaging of the central airways and related thoracic structures with axial CT plays a key role in initial assessment and treatment planning (Fig. 8.4). However, it has several limitations that must be considered. First, the true cranio-caudal extent of the disease is underestimated on axial images. second, it has a limited ability to detect subtle and early airway stenoses. Finally, axial images are unable to display complex 3D relationships between the obstructing lesion and the airway. Many of the aforementioned limitations of axial images are overcome by multiplanar and

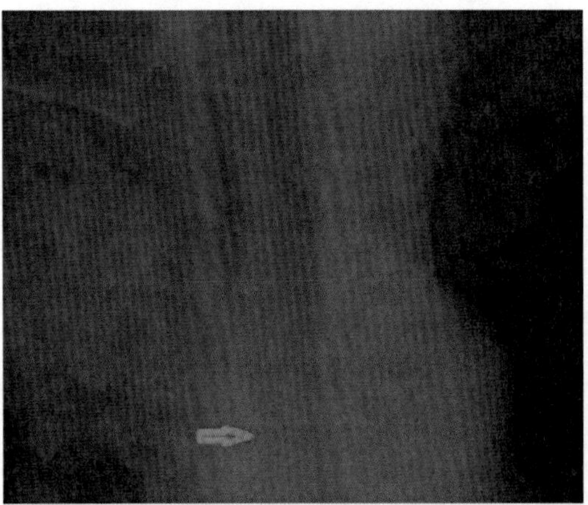

Fig. 8.3 Chest radiograph showing narrowing of lower part of trachea secondary to compression from a right upper lobe lung cancer

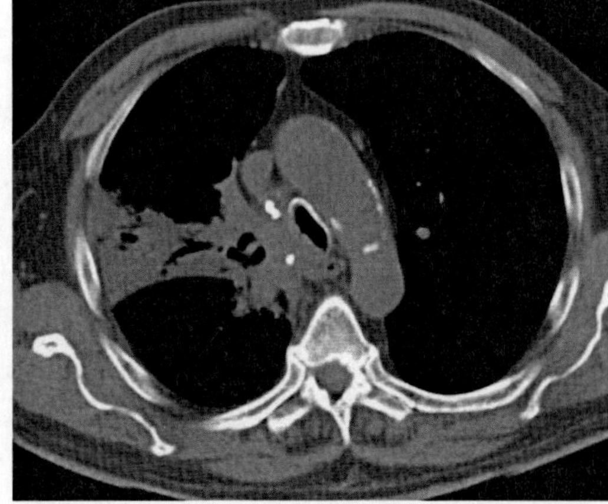

Fig. 8.4 Chest computed tomography (CT) showing narrowing and distortion of trachea from extrinsic compression

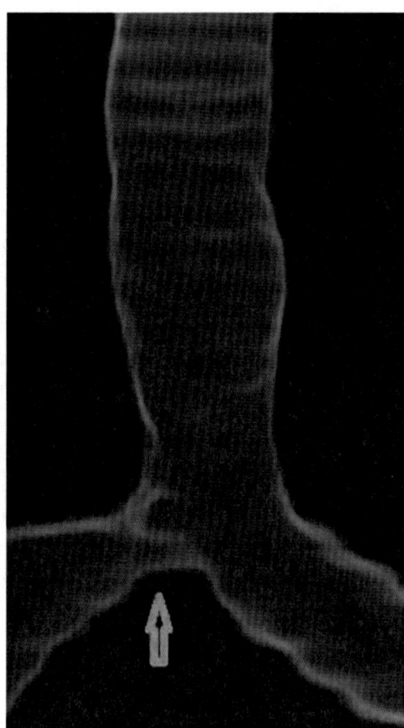

Fig. 8.5 External 3D rendered image showing narrowing of distal trachea and right main bronchus

3D reconstruction of CT images [32]. Axial imaging of the central airways and reformatted multiplanar images provide complimentary information [33]. Information from multidetector CT with 3D reconstruction is helpful in selecting the length and size of airway stent [34]. Several studies have also established the usefulness of MDCT in evaluation of stent related complications [35, 36]. In one such study, MDCT detected 29 of 30 (97 %) stent related complications diagnosed by bronchoscopy [36]. MDCT images with 3D reconstruction are also found useful in evalation of patient prior to other interventional therapies and surgery for CAO [37].

There are two fundamental types of 3D reconstruction: external rendering and internal rendering. External 3D rendered images demonstrate the external surface of the airway (Fig. 8.5) and its relationship to adjacent structures. Several studies have attested to the usefulness of external 3D rendered images prior to interventional procedures in patients with CAO. In one such study, addition of 3D external randering to axial imaging provided further information on the shape, length and degree of airway stenosis in one-third of patients with nonmalignant tracheobronchial stenosis and corrected the interpretation of axial CT in 10 % of patients [38].

Internal rendering uses the helical CT data to produce images of the internal lumen of the airway as seen during conventional bronchoscopy. Virtual bronchoscopy allows evaluation of airways beyond the high-grade lesions that are not accessible with standard bronchoscopy [39]. In one study, virtual bronchoscopy images of diagnostic quality could be obtained in 19 of 20 patients with high-grade airway stenosis but the subtle external compression was underestimated in 25 % of patients [40]. According to another report, virtual bronchoscopy has a sensitivity of 90–100 % for endoluminal or obstructive lesions, but only 16 % for mucosal lesions [41]. In a recent study, virtual bronchoscopy findings were compared with flexible bronchoscopy findings in 50 patients with tracheobronchial lesions. Virtual bronchoscopy was superior to flexible bronchoscopy in showing the airways distal to the obstructing lesion whereas flexible bronchoscopy was superior to virtual bronchoscopy in detecting the early tumor infiltration and subtle mucosal alterations [42]. The utility of virtual bronchoscopy is limited by false positive results since thick secretions or blood clots can be miskaten for endobronchial tumors [43]. Nevertheless, the false positive result with virtual bronchoscopy is more of a problem for the segmental bronchi than for the central airways where the majority of interventional procedures are needed [44].

Optical coherence tomography (OCT) is an imaging technique similar to ultrasound, but instead of using sound waves uses infrared light to obtain the images. Preliminary experience indicates that OCT has a higher spatial resolution than ultrasound and therefore provides a more detailed insight into the depth of airway invasion by the tumor [45]. Anatomic optical coherence tomography (aOCT) is a modification of OCT technology, designed to allow accurate real-time measurement of size and diameter of central airways. The aOCT unit is introduced through the working channel of the bronchoscope and is advanced beyond the obstructing lesion to assess the extent of stenosis. Images are obtained as the aOCT catheter is slowly retracted back towards the bronchoscope. The technique had been validated for measurement of diameter of airway models, excised pig airways, and normal human airways [46]. The clinical experience in CAO is limited to a single report in which useful information was obtained with aOCTin all three patients who underwent the procedure [47]. In one patient, aOCT guided the choice of stent, in the second patient, it assessed the extent of tumor obstructing the left main bronchus and in third patient it assessed the dynamic properties of the airway in presence of severe tracheobronchomalacia. There is potential for this technique to be used alongside CT imaging in evaluation of patients considered for therapeutic bronchoscopy but this is an area where further work is needed. The key question to be addressed is whether or not the added perspective with aOCT will translate into tangible benefits to these patients.

Bronchoscopy

Bronchoscopy gives the most essential information in the pre-interventional assessment of patients with CAO. Direct visualization not only identifies the lesion, its location, and the extent of airway involvement but also highlights the vascularity and fragility of the lesion (Fig. 8.6). In addition it provides tissue diagnosis and allows the operator to assess the extent of mucosal infiltration and any extrinsic compression of the airway by the tumor. It also permits the assessment of the diameter of the stricture for the appropriate choice of the stent [48]. Bronchoscopy in these patients is not without risks. There is potential for patients to develop complete airway obstruction due to physical presence of the bronchoscope in the critically narrowed central airways. Local bleeding and mucosal trauma during bronchoscopy may further compromise the airway lumen increasing the risk of sudden development of ventilatory failure and asphyxiation. Therefore, it is essential that the procedure is performed with utmost care by the most experienced operator with ready access to full resuscitation capabilities.

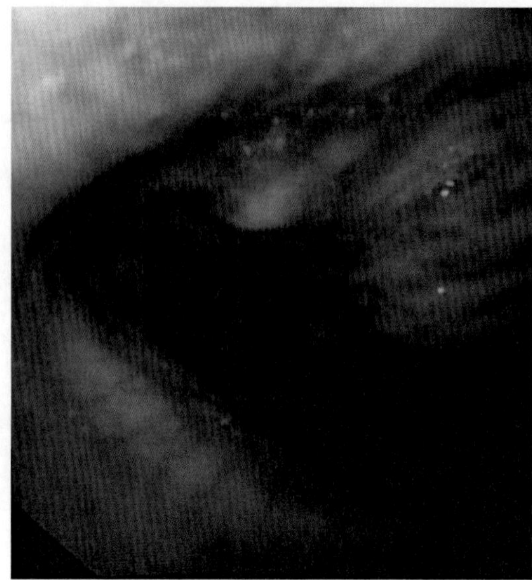

Fig. 8.6 Bronchoscopic image showing significant narrowing and distortion of trachea from external compression and infiltration of tumor from right side

In some instances, the standard bronchoscope cannot be negotiated through the critically stenosed airways. In these patients, examination of distal airways can be accomplished using ultrathin bronchoscopes, which have a diameter of 2.8–3.5 mm. Successful inspection of distal airway with ultrathin bronchoscopes has been possible in more than 80 % of cases in which standard bronchoscope could not be passed beyond the obstructing lesion [49, 50].

Choice of a flexible or rigid bronchoscope for interventional procedure is an important consideration. Many of those with an in-depth knowledge in this field prefer rigid scope for therapeutic bronchoscopy in majority of patients with CAO. Unfortunately, the availability of rigid bronchoscopy is limited to a handful of tertiary care centers. Only a few pulmonologists have received any training or have any experience in rigid bronchoscopy. However, this trend seems to be changing. In fact it is the greater appreciation of rigid bronchoscope in management of CAO that is behind the revival of this forgotten skill in recent times [51].

Rigid bronchoscope has several advantages over flexible bronchoscope in therapeutic bronchoscopy (Table 8.2) [52]. It allows better airway

Table 8.2 Comparison of rigid and flexible bronchoscope for therapeutic bronchoscopy

	Rigid bronchoscope	Flexible bronchoscope
Availability	Limited	Unlimited
Airway protection	++	None
Working channel	Wide	Narrow
Suction capability	Superior	Limited
Control of bleeding	More effective	Less effective
Anesthesia	General	Conscious sedation
Reach	Limited to trachea and main stem bronchus	Also suitable for lobar and segmental bronchi
Mechanical debulking	Rapid	Less effective and more time consuming
Unique capabilities	Silicone stent placement and microdebrider	Ultrathin bronchoscopy and EBUS
Risk of fire during LPR	Lower	Higher

protection and concurrent ventilation. It has a wider working channel, which does not occlude the airway and permits efficient suctioning and instrumentation. In some patients immediate restoration of airway lumen can be achieved via a rigid bronchoscope as the barrel can be used to dilate the narrowed airway, and to core out the lesion. Rigid bronchoscope is more useful than flexible bronchoscope if the procedure is complicated by massive hemorrhage. Finally, some interventions such as placement of silicone stent and debulking with microdebrider can only be accomplished using a rigid bronchoscope.

The usefulness of therapeutic bronchoscopy with the rigid bronchoscope was illustrated in retrospective review of 32 patients with central airways obstruction who required admission to the intensive care unit prior to the intervention. Emergent interventions such as dilatation, laser photoresection, or silicone stent insertion were performed in the operating room under general anesthesia. Immediate extubation was possible in 10 of 19 (52.6 %) patients who were receiving mechanical ventilation prior to the therapeutic bronchoscopy and 20 of 32 (62.5 %) could be transferred to a lower level of care immediately after intervention [53].

Unlike rigid bronchoscopy, flexible bronchoscopy is performed under conscious sedation and is more widely available. Many interventional procedures such as laser photoresection, electrocautery, argon plasma coagulation, cryotherapy, photodynamic therapy, and metal stent insertion can be performed using flexible bronchoscope. However, flexible bronchoscopy carries significant risk in presence of severe CAO. As discussed above, the presence of bronchoscope may convert incomplete CAO into complete airway obstruction. Furthermore, relaxation of respiratory muscle and central nervous system depression due to sedative medications may cause the airway to become more unstable during flexible bronchoscopy. It is therefore essential to have immediate access to advance airway management, including ready availability of rigid bronchoscopy in these cases. If such facilities are not available, transferring the patient to a specialized center with a dedicated airway team should be given a serious consideration after the initial resuscitation.

Endobronchial ultrasound (EBUS) is rapidly emerging as an important adjunct to bronchoscopy in management of patients with CAO. EBUS allows better evaluation of submucosal and peri-bronchial tumors, the true extent of which is difficult to determine during bronchoscopic examination. EBUS is highly accurate in estimating depth of invasion of the tracheobronchial wall in patients with endobronchial tumors. In one study, EBUS findings were confirmed in 23 of 24 (95.8 %) of such patients upon examination of the surgical specimens. In the single case in which the findings were different, lymphocytic infiltration between the cartilage rings was misinterpreted as tumor infiltration [54]. In another study, EBUS was helpful in selecting appropriate candidates with centrally located early-stage lung cancer for photodynamic therapy with curative intent [55]. Based on the evidence of extra-cartilaginous spread of tumor on EBUS, the investigators chose alternative therapies to nine patients who were initially thought to be appropriate candidates for PDT. The estimated depth of tumor invasion by EBUS was accurate in six of the nine surgical specimens. EBUS is also found useful prior to placement of airway stents. Miyazawa and associates studied the functional outcome of patients after placement of an airway stent at choke point which were detected using flow-volume loop, flexible bronchoscopy, EBUS, CT, and ultrathin bronchoscopy [56]. Choke point is the area of greatest flow limitation and is usually found where the airways are maximally stenosed. All patients with extrinsic compression from non-operable lung cancer in this study had balloon dilation followed by airway stent placement using rigid bronchoscope. These interventions provided immediate improvement in dyspnea and flow-volume loops in all study subjects. Patients with extensive stenosis showed partial response and repeat evaluation showed that the choke point had migrated downstream from the initially stented segment. EBUS showed presence of cartilage destruction at the new choke points. Additional stenting in these areas was followed by improvement in dyspnea, flow-volume loop, and pulmonary function tests. The study illustrates the potential role of EBUS in improving the functional results of airway stent placement in patients with CAO.

EBUS is also found useful in patients undergoing therapeutic bronchoscopy for advanced CAO. Herth and associates performed EBUS in 1,174 of 2,446 therapeutic bronchoscopies over a 3-year period [57]. EBUS was used in conjunction with mechanical tumor debridement, airway stent placement, laser photoresection, argon plasma coagulation, brachytherapy, foreign body removal and endoscopic abscess drainage. Overall, guidance from EBUS influenced the therapeutic approach in 43 % of cases. The most common management changes were adjustment of size of the stent and termination of procedure after finding a large blood vessel in close proximity. In some instances EBUS findings suggested need for surgical interventions rather than endoscopic therapy. No patient in the EBUS group experienced severe bleeding or fistula formation after completion of the procedure.

Anesthesia and Ventilation

Appropriate anesthesia management is a crucial part of interventional bronchoscopy. An in-depth discussion on this subject is beyond the scope of this chapter and readers are referred to several excellent reviews for details [58, 59]. The majority of patients who need urgent intervention for central airway stenosis are at high-risk of developing anesthesia-related complications due to associated severe respiratory distress, hypoxemia, pulmonary sepsis, and superior vena cava obstruction. Many of these patients are in class IV or V risk category of the American society of anesthesiologists classification of physical status (Table 8.3). Availability of experienced anesthesia personnel for airway management and for monitoring oxygenation, ventilation, and circulation is very helpful and is strongly recommended during therapeutic bronchoscopy in these patients.

Table 8.3 American Society of Anesthesiologists (ASA) classification of physical status

ASA class	Description
Class I	A normal, healthy patient
Class II	A patient with mild systemic illness
Class III	A patient with severe systemic disease that limits activity but is not incapacitating
Class IV	A patient with incapacitating systemic disease that is a constant threat to life
Class V	A moribund patient not expected to survive 24 h with or without operation
E	In the event of an emergency operation, precede the number with an "E"

Aggressive supportive therapy must be started while interventional procedure is being planned. Many patients experience symptomatic relief with administration of humidified oxygen and inhaled bronchodilators. Although used commonly, systemic steroids have no proven value in these patients. Temporary benefit has been reported with inhalation of 70 % helium and 30 % oxygen (heliox) symptomatic patients with severe CAO [60].

Several interventional procedures such as cryotherapy, electrocautery, APC, and airway stenting in noncritical patients can be performed under conscious sedation using flexible bronchoscope. In some instances, deep sedation or general anesthesia is needed for patient comfort and better control of cough. General anesthesia is also needed during flexible bronchoscopy for the procedures such as laser photoresection that require patients to remain still for a prolonged period of time. Airway can be established with a size-8 or larger endotracheal tube or a laryngeal mask airway in these patients. Rigid bronchoscopy is always carried out under general anesthesia. The rigid bronchoscope is the most reliable airway for the anesthesiologists to maintain the ventilation during complex and prolonged interventional bronchoscopy procedures.

The intubation can be performed with the patient either awake with a topical anesthetic agent or with an inhalational or intravenous agent with or without non-depolarizing muscle relaxants. Loss of airway control has been reported using all types of induction. It is essential to have the trained operators and the equipment in a state of readiness at the time of induction, should an urgent rigid bronchoscopy is needed to secure the airway [61].

Some anesthesiologists prefer intravenous agents because of rapid and smooth induction with less airway irritation [62]. Others prefer inhalational agents such as halothane [63] or sevoflurane for induction in these patients [64]. Many of the inhalational agents have a bronchodilator effect that is helpful in patients with concomitant reactive airway disease.

Maintenance of anesthesia can also be accomplished with either inhalational agents of with intravenous agents. Recent trend is to use total intravenous anesthesia (TIVA) for these procedures [65]. Continuous administration of intravenous agents to maintain anesthesia is possible during suctioning, dilation and stenting whereas administration of inhalational agent must be interrupted during these procedures [66]. Propofol is the most preferred intravenous agent due to its short onset of action (30 s) and rapid recovery time of 15 min after a 2 h infusion. Remifentanil is the preferred narcotic agents due to its rapid onset (60 s) and short duration of action (3–10 min). Long acting opioids must be avoided to prevent postoperative respiratory depression.

Ventilation can be difficult to maintain in many patients with high-grade CAO. Positive pressure ventilation can be delivered during flexible bronchoscopy through the side-port of the adapter over the endotracheal tube (ETT). The bronchoscope is placed through a self-sealing diaphragm of the adapter that minimized the loss of tidal volume. Because the presence of bronchoscope invariably increases the resistance to airflow, a minimum of size 8 and preferably larger ETT is recommended for therapeutic bronchoscopy.

A rigid bronchoscope has a side arm adapter that allows administration of anesthetic agent and assisted ventilation during therapeutic bronchoscopy. An eyepiece occludes the proximal end of bronchoscope and allows controlled ventilation, but the gas leak cannot be prevented whenever the eyepiece is removed, thus placing the operators at some risk of inhalation of anesthetic agents during the procedure.

High frequency jet ventilation (HFJV) allows uninterrupted ventilation during rigid bronchoscopy. A small 2.0-mm catheter can provide a safe level of oxygenation. The HFJV catheter is typically placed beyond the stenosis in patients with tracheal obstruction [67]. There is a potential for development of dynamic hyperinflation during HFJV because the resistance to airflow is more pronounced during the expiration than during inspiration. However, the airway pressures (Paw) with HFJV during rigid bronchoscopy generally does not exceed the safe limits and is unlikely to cause severe lung distension or barotrauma in subjects with normal lungs [68].

The anesthesiologist and bronchoscopist must be ready to manage the complications of the procedure such as massive hemorrhage and barotrauma, and perforation of the airways. A thoracic surgeon on standby is always prudent, although emergent thoracotomy is seldom needed [69]. Careful monitoring is essential during the immediate postoperative period, as there is danger of redevelopment of CAO from mucous plugs, edema, aspiration, blood clots, sloughed tissue and migrated stents.

Airway fire is an important concern during laser photoresection, electrocautery, and argon plasma coagulation. The predisposing factors include use of flammable anesthetic agents, high FiO_2 during procedures, and presence of combustible material such as ETT in the airway. The risk of endobronchial ignition can be reduced by decreasing the FiO_2 to at or below 0.4 and holding the jet ventilation for a few seconds during these procedures [70, 71].

Management of Central Airway Obstruction

All patients with CAO should be identified as high risk patients. A recent database has reported a complication rate of 19.8 % and a 30-day mortality of 7.8 % after the therapeutic bronchoscopy, reflecting the severity of illness and poor underlying health status [72]. The importance of having an experienced and dedicated airway team in place for managing such challenging patients cannot be overstated.

At the outset, the goals of the therapy must be defined for every individual patient. The fundamental purpose of therapeutic bronchoscopy is palliation of symptoms. There can be no doubt that a successful procedure in these patients is highly effective in achieving the relief of symptoms and in improving the quality of life. For example, in a prospective study, 85 % of participants experienced improvement in dyspnea and 65 % of participants experienced improvement in quality of life after undergoing therapeutic bronchoscopy for advanced CAO related to malignancy [73]. Similar results were reported in another study in which 6-min walk distance increased by 99.7 m, FEV1 increased by 448 ml, and FVC increased by 416 ml at 30-day after undergoing bronchoscopic intervention for advanced malignant airway obstruction [74]. More importantly, the majority of patients also experienced improvement in dyspnea after the procedure. Temporary control of hemoptysis has been achieved in up to 94 % of patients with central airway tumors undergoing therapeutic bronchoscopy [75].

On the other hand, it is debatable whether therapeutic bronchoscopy improves the overall survival of patients with malignant CAO. This question has fueled much discussion but remains largely unanswered due to lack of prospective randomized trials. Performing a prospective, blinded, randomized study on such patient population is neither feasible nor ethical. In the absence of high quality evidence from prospective randomized trial, the majority of information in this context has been obtained from extrapolation of data from case series, retrospective studies, and comparison with historical control [75, 76]. Notwithstanding, we argue that survival is an inappropriate end point for an intervention which is primarily designed to relieve the unpleasant and highly distressing symptoms of choking and asphyxia. Furthermore, expecting improvement in the overall survival with the local relief in obstructive lesions alone is unrealistic since most patients with malignant CAO have not only an advanced and inoperable malignancy but also suffer from serious comorbidities such as advanced COPD and coronary artery disease.

Still, it is encouraging to note that many patients who initially present with advanced CAO are able to receive additional anticancer therapies after experiencing improvement in symptoms and Karnofsky performance status with therapeutic bronchoscopy [77]. Control of pulmonary sepsis after interventional treatment is helpful in improving the ability of many of these patients to withstand the cancer chemotherapy. In one study, there was no difference between the survival rates of NSCLC patients who required therapeutic bronchoscopy for CAO before receiving chemotherapy and the patients who received chemotherapy for advanced lung cancer but had no

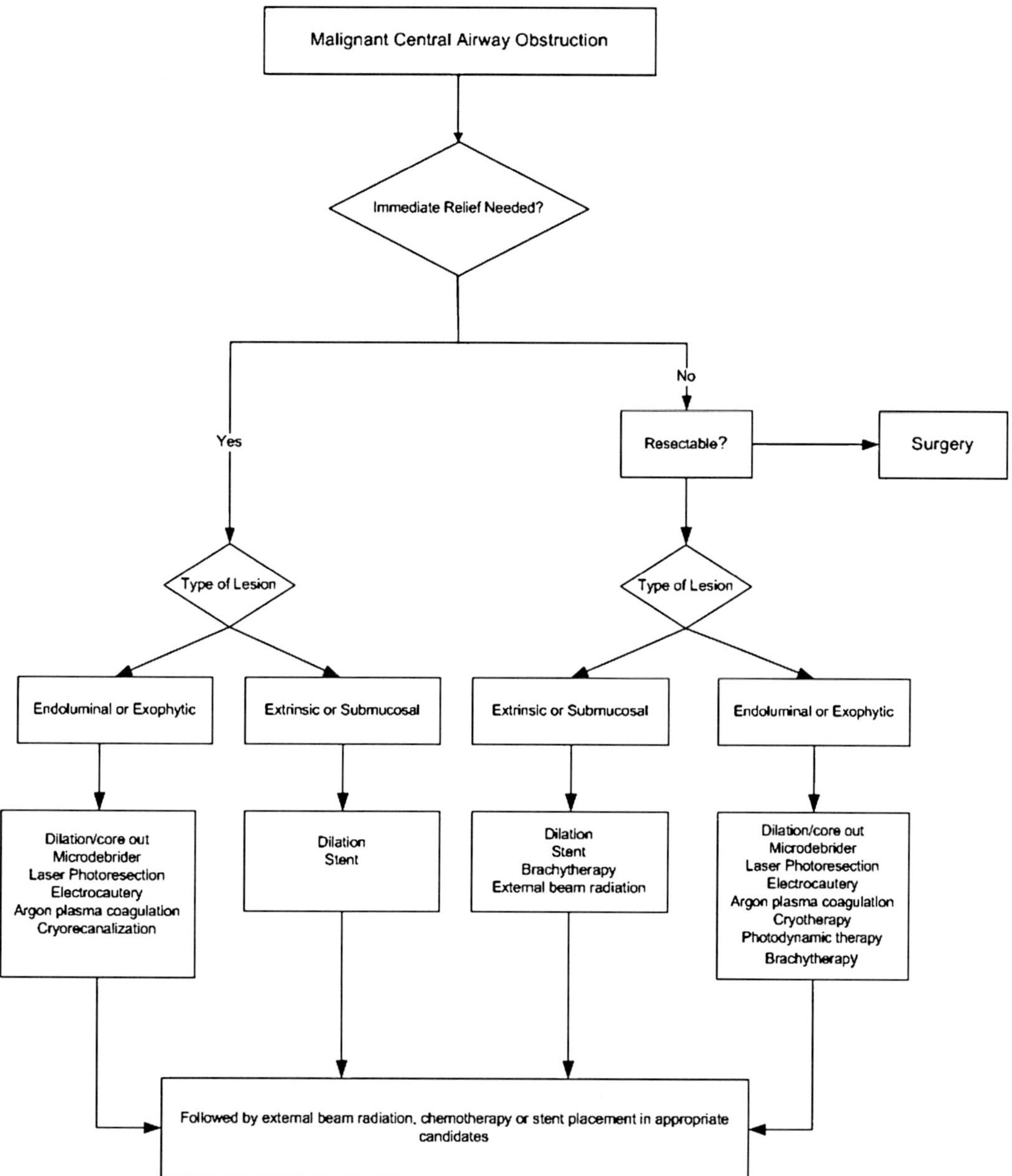

Fig. 8.7 Treatment algorithm for malignant central airway obstruction

evidence of CAO at initial presentation [78]. In some reports, the early and rapid palliation with endoscopic therapy and subsequent administration of chemotherapy has allowed some of these patients to undergo surgery with curative intent [79, 80]. In highly selected patients, longer survival has been possible after the surgical treatment. For example, the 3-year survival after induction chemotherapy and surgery was 52 % whereas the median survival after palliative treatment alone was 12.1 months in one study [80].

A simplified treatment algorithm is summarized in Fig. 8.7. Broadly, the ablative techniques are categorized into those with immediate effects and those with delayed effects. Mechanical debulking, laser photoresection (LPR), electrocautery and argon plasma coagulation (APC) and cryorecanalization have an immediate effect [81] whereas cryotherapy, brachytherapy and photodynamic therapy (PDT) have delayed effects [82] and are more suitable when urgent relief in symptoms is not essential. Airway stents are mainly indicated for extrinsic compression and their successful deployment immediately improves the airway diameter. Balloon bronchoplasty is particularly effective in preparing stenotic airways for stent placement, in expanding metallic stents after insertion, and in the placement of brachytherapy catheters that would otherwise be impeded by high-grade stenoses. In majority of instances, combination of several interventional procedures is needed for the most optimal results. In the following section, we briefly discuss the scientific basis, clinical application, complications and limitations of various interventional procedures used in management of patients with malignant CAO.

Mechanical Debulking

Mechanical debulking using rigid bronchoscope is an effective method to achieve rapid recanalization of central airways. In this technique, the beveled end of the rigid bronchoscope is used as a chisel to shave off large parts of the obstructing endobronchial tumors. The procedure is also referred to as "core out." This technique is most suitable for patients with an intrinsic tumor involving tracheal or main-stem bronchi causing critical airway stenosis. Rigid bronchoscope is ideally suited for this procedure because of its ability to control airways, better suction capability, ability to introduce forceps of larger size to grasp the tumor fragments, and ability to manage hemorrhage more effectively as compared to the flexible bronchoscope.

The majority of patients undergoing this procedure have acute respiratory distress due to critical airway stenosis. The airway team must be in attendance, ready to perform rigid bronchoscopy to secure the airway before any attempt is made to initiate anesthesia induction. In many instances, there is no time for imaging procedures. Still, it is important to visualize and assess the lesion and examine the distal airways before performing the procedure. Also, the accumulated secretions and blood must be removed from the airways as much as possible to improve the visibility. A flexible bronchoscope introduced via rigid scope is used for this purpose. It is imperative that the axis of airway is determined before making any attempt to core-out the lesion. The mechanical coring out of the tumor is accomplished by engaging the base of the tumor with the tip of bronchoscope and dissecting off the lesion. In order to reduce the risk of perforation of airways or adjacent blood vessels, the operator must keep the rigid bronchoscope parallel to the axis of the airway throughout the procedure. The tumor fragments are removed using graspers, suction and in some instances with the assistance of cryotherapy probe. Flexible bronchoscope should be used to remove the tumor fragments downstream from the lesion obstructing the proximal airways. Bleeding is rarely severe and can be managed by irrigation with ice-cold saline, topical application of epinephrine, and applying direct pressure using the rigid bronchoscope. Argon plasma coagulation may be used if oozing of blood persists despite the aforementioned measures. Balloon tamponade may be needed to control bleeding from distal airways. In some instances, initial devascularization of tumor with application of thermal energy may reduce the risk of bleeding after the core-out procedure.

Most patients undergoing this procedure experience an immediate relief in symptoms. For example, in one study, a significant improvement in endoscopic appearance, subjective symptoms and radiological findings was achieved in 51 of 56 patients undergoing this procedure [63]. Successful debulking of tumor in this study was followed by surgical intervention in 16 (29 %) of patients and other interventions such as external beam radiation therapy or chemotherapy in 34 (62 %) of patients.

The main advantages of debulking with rigid bronchoscope are low cost and immediate results. A successful procedure paves way for additional interventions in more controlled and secure settings at a future date. The most obvious limitation of the procedure is the availability of operators trained in rigid bronchoscopy. Mechanical debulking has also been described using a rotating airway microdebrider, which is an electrically powered instrument with a rotating blade and suction capability. It is used in conjunction with either rigid bronchoscopy or suspension laryngoscopy. Preliminary experience is encouraging, but more studies are needed before it can be recommended for general use [83, 84].

Balloon Bronchoplasty

Balloon dilatation is a simple technique in which a pressurized balloon is used to provide immediate relief in symptoms due to CAO. In malignant tracheobronchial stenosis, balloon dilation is most commonly used for dilating airways before placement of stents in patients with predominantly extrinsic compression [85]. It is also used for dilation of previously placed airway stents and for opening folded Dumon's stents [86]. Balloon dilation has also been used to facilitate placement of brachytherapy catheter across the obstructing lesion. Balloon dilation also has an established role in management of airway stenosis secondary to a variety of benign causes such as post lung transplantation anastomotic strictures, post-intubation tracheal stenosis, and tuberculosis [87–89].

In the past, balloon dilation was accomplished using rigid bronchoscopes or with guide-wires under fluoroscopy guidance [85]. However, several studies have established the feasibility and safety of the procedure in non-critically ill patients using flexible bronchoscope under conscious sedation [88, 90]. Here, the deflated balloon is introduced via the working channel, placed across the obstruction, and is inflated using a pressure syringe device under direct vision. The inflation diameters of balloons vary from 4 to 20 mm and the length of balloons vary from 4 to 8 cm. In many instances, the operator has to use several balloons of increasing diameter to achieve the desired results.

Immediate relief in symptoms is achieved in the majority of patients undergoing airway balloon dilation [87, 90]. In many instances, there is resolution of post-obstructive pneumonia and atelectasis. In one series, an average of 10 % improvement in FEV1 was found 1 month after the procedure [91]. Effective dilation of airways clearly facilitates airway stent placement and allows effective application of other modalities such as brachytherapy in many patients. Balloon dilation has a useful role in management of patients with benign airway stenosis who are not suitable for surgery or have failed prior surgical attempts. The procedure is inexpensive and the technique is easy to learn. Unfortunately, despite excellent initial results, the benefits are not sustained and a majority of patients either require further airway dilation or need an additional procedure such as stent placement for relief of symptoms [87, 88, 91]. Generally, the procedure is safe and no major complications are encountered but rarely, it is complicated by bleeding, airway perforation and pneumomediastinum. In one study, superficial mucosal tears occurred in 60 patients and deep mucosal tears occurred 4 of 124 patients undergoing balloon dilation [92]. All mucosal tears healed without any adverse clinical consequences. Most experts believe that sequential balloon dilation is less traumatic to the airways than the mechanical dilation with the rigid bronchoscopes.

Electrocautery

Electrocautery has become a popular option for immediate palliation of malignant CAO because of its ability to restore airway lumen with rapid ablation of tumors. Electrocautery uses the electrical energy to heat the tissues to achieve desired results such as coagulative necrosis at low temperatures or tissue vaporization at high temperature. The electrical energy is delivered to the endobronchial tissue using a variety of probes applied through rigid or flexible bronchoscope. Owing to the difference in the voltage, there is flow of electrons from the probe to the target tissue. Heat is generated as electrons flow through the tissues with high electrical impedance. The biological effect on the tissues depend on the amount of heat generated, which in turn depends on the type of current, surface area of contact, power, duration of contact, and tissue characteristics. In coagulation mode, low voltage, low power and high current settings are used to cause coagulative necrosis, as the tissue temperature approaches 70 °C. In contrast, the cutting mode involves application of high voltage and low current to causes the tissue temperature to approach 200 °C, which causes vaporization or carbonization. In many instances, a blend of coagulation and cutting mode is used to achieve desired results. A good correlation has been found between the visible changes on the mucosal surface and the histological extent of coagulation necrosis after application of electrocautery [93]. Highly vascular lesions require higher settings due to "heat sink" effect. Lesions covered by secretions or fluids of any kind also require higher energy as they offer much less resistance to the flow of electrons.

The technique requires a high frequency electrical generator, insulated bronchoscope and an array of accessory instruments to deliver the electrical energy to the tissues. A grounding plate is applied in the close proximity of the treatment site to complete the circuit. Placing grounding plate away from the treatment site may require higher setting to complete the circuit and increase posiibiltiy of detouring the current to the metallic prosthesis, if present.

The electrocautery accessories include polypectomy wire snare, coagulation probe, cutting knife and hot biopsy forceps. The choice of accessory depends on the endoscopic appearance of the tumor. Snare is most useful for the removal of pedunculated lesion. Here, the snare is looped over the lesion and tightened slowly as electrocautery is activated to provide a combination of cutting and coagulation mode at the base of the lesion. The tissue is severed by the heat generated by the electrical current and not by the mechanical force of the snare. Coagulation probe is useful for sessile or flat lesions. Cutting blade is used for making radial cuts on concentric web-like strictures in the trachea or main-stem bronchi. Mechanical debulking may be needed in association with a combination of coagulation, cutting and vaporization to achieve rapid airway recanalization. The tissue pieces are removed with biopsy forceps, suction, or cryoprobe. It is essential to the remove the blood and carbonized tissue and debris on a frequent basis in order to maintain the operative field as clean as possible.

Several studies have established the usefulness of electrocautery for rapid palliation of CAO. Sutedja and associates performed bronchoscopic electrocautery in patients with locally advanced central lung cancers using flexible bronchoscope and conscious sedation [94]. A greater than 75 % opening of airway diameter was achieved in 11 patients and dyspnea improved in 8 of 17 study patients. Coulter and Mehta performed a total of 47 electrocautery procedures in 38 patients with central airway tumors or benign web like lesions using flexible bronchoscope [95]. Successful results were achieved in 89 % of procedures, thus obviating need for laser photoresection (LPR). One must note that no patient included in this series was in extremis and to be included in the study, the patients were required to have a <50 % luminal obstruction and a tumor size had to be <2 cm in greatest dimension. Nonetheless, the investigators found electrocautery to be an attractive alternative to LPR in a carefully selected patient population. A large retrospective study from Duke Medical Center has recently addressed the efficacy and safety of electrocautery in patients with benign or malignant airway obstruction [96]. In this study, 117 electrocautery procedures were performed in 94 patients over a 5-year period. Rigid bronchoscope was used in 62 %. Endoscopic improvement was achieved in 94 % of patients. Symptoms improved in 71 % of patients. Radiological improvement was also reported in a significant proportion of patients. These results clearly establish the important role of electrocautery in palliative treatment of advanced CAO. In some instances, electrocautery has also been used to treat occult central airway cancers that are not suitable for radical surgery [97].

Electrocautery achieves results similar to LPR in a significant proportion of carefully selected patients with CAO [98]. Its main advantages over LPR are lower cost and ability to perform the procedure under conscious sedation using flexible bronchoscope. In fact, electrocautery has replaced LPR to become the first-line heat therapy for CAO in many institutions. The procedure is generally safe and major complications are seldom encountered [99]. However, there are several drawbacks. There is risk of endobronchial fire if appropriate precautions are not taken. To reduce the risk of fire, the FiO_2 must be maintained ≤0.4 during the procedure and one must make sure that there are no combustible sources such as endobronchial tubes or silicone stents within the airways. The procedure cannot be performed if high-flow oxygen is needed to maintain adequate oxygenation. The procedure should be avoided in patients with permanent pacemaker or defbrillator. Electrocautery is not suitable for control of airway hemorrhage and it loses its effectiveness in the presence of significant airway bleeding.

Argon Plasma Coagulation

Argon plasma coagulation (APC) is a noncontact form of electrosurgical technique used in management of CAO and hemoptysis from a visible endobronchial source [100]. Plasma, sometimes considered a fourth state of matter, is a gas of charged particles with special physical properties. Plasma is produced in the endobronchial tree when a high-frequency, high-voltage current delivered to a tungsten-tip electrode ionizes the argon delivered through the Teflon catheter at a rate of 0.3–2 L/min. Argon plasma emerges from the catheter tip as a spray of monopolar current seeking and causing the coagulative necrosis of the nearest grounded tissue. Similar to the standard electrocautery, a grounding pad is placed in close proximity of the treatment site to complete the circuit. The passage of electrical current through the bronchial mucosa leads to tissue heating, dessication and coagulation. The electrical resistance increases as the tissue coagulates, which suppresses the further current flow, thereby limiting the depth of coagulation to about 2 mm after about 2 s of application. The self-limiting effect of APC on tissue coagulation limits its efficacy in rapid palliation of large and bulky endobronchial tumors, but at the same time also reduces the risk of perforation of tracheobronchial wall. A further advantage of APC is its ability to reach the lesions located lateral to the probe or around the bends and corners that are not suitable for LPR.

Patients with predominantly intraluminal lesions located in the trachea or main-stem bronchus, with a patent distal lumen and functional lung are the most suitable candidates for APC treatment. APC is delivered to the endobronchial tissue through the flexible bronchoscope. In unstable patients, it is better to secure the airways with a rigid bronchoscope or endotracheal tube, and use the artificial airway to introduce the flexible bronchoscope into the tracheobronchial tree. Standard flexible bronchoscopy technique is sufficient in a stable patient. The electrical current is generated by a high-frequency current generator. The diameter of the flexible probe varies from 1.5 to 2.3 mm and it is introduced into the airways through the working channel of the bronchoscope. In order to prevent thermal damage to the instrument, the tip of the APC probe should be pushed several centimeters beyond the distal end of bronchoscope. One must make sure that the probe tip is within 1 cm of target lesion before the plasma spray is generated. An argon flow of 0.8–1 L/min and a power setting of 30 W are suitable initial settings. Argon plasma should be applied in bursts of 1–3 s to achieve the suitable results. In debulking an endobronchial tumor, the coagulated tissue and the eschar formed with the application of APC needs to be removed on a regular basis using biopsy forceps or cryoprobe. Further APC is applied on the viable underling tissue and the cycle is repeated till desired results are obtained.

Several case-series have addressed the usefulness of APC in management of airways diseases. Reichle and associates performed 482 APC procedures in 364 patients for a variety of indications [100]. APC was performed for management of central airway tumors in 186 patients. The airways patency could be restored in 67 % of patients. Rigid bronchoscope was used for application of APC in 90 % of these patients.

The procedure was performed for control of hemoptysis arising from a visible endobronchial source in 119 patients. Adequate hemostasis could be achieved in 118 of these patients. In 34 patients, the investigators successfully used APC to restore the patency of airway stents, which were occluded due to in-growth of cancer or granulation tissue. Similarly, Morice and associates performed 70 APC procedures in 60 patients for management of neoplastic airway obstruction and for control of hemoptysis [101]. All except four procedures were performed under conscious sedation without endotracheal intubation. All 31 patients with hemoptysis experienced complete resolution of airway bleeding. From the mean pretreatment airway obstruction of 76 %, the mean residual obstruction was reduced to 18 % after completion of the procedure. All patients undergoing APC for CAO experienced improvement in symptoms. Similar experience with APC has been reported by others for both malignant and benign CAO [102–104].

The main advantages of APC are low cost and excellent efficacy in control of superficial hemorrhage from endobronchial lesions. Ability to deliver argon plasma through a standard flexible bronchoscope is another attractive feature. However, the technique may not be suitable for bulky endobronchial tumors causing a critical airway stenosis. Further, there is risk of endobronchial fire if the FiO_2 cannot be maintained at a concentration ≤0.4 during the procedure. In addition, a recent report has drawn attention to three cases of gas embolism after the APC procedure over a 3 year period for an estimated incidence of 1.5–2 % [105]. The risk of gas embolism can be minimized by maintaining the argon flow to as low as possible during the procedure.

Laser Photoresection

Laser photoresection (LPR) is a highly effective technique for immediate relief of CAO. Even though the application of LPR has declined since the availability of electrocautery and APC, it still maintains a useful role in clinical practice. The acronym laser stands for light amplification by stimulated emission of radiation. Laser is an artificially produced electromagnetic radiation that does not exist in nature. Laser is produced by exciting the electrons of a substance to higher energy level. When the electrons fall back to the ground energy level, the packets of energy called photons are released that constitute the laser beam. The substance used for producing laser is called medium. The wavelength of laser depends on the medium used. Laser differs from ordinary light in three important ways. (1) As compared to the white light, which is a mix of wavelengths varying from 390 to 800 nm, laser light is monochromatic with all waves having the same wavelength. (2) The crests and troughs of all laser waves are in phase with each other—a property is called coherence. (3) The laser waves travel in the same direction in a narrow beam with minimal divergence. This property is called collimation. Due to these properties, the energy carried with laser light can be carried in form a narrow beam that can be focused on the target with intense power.

Due to these unique properties, laser has found many medical uses. Laser energy can cut, coagulate or vaporize the biological tissues. In interventional bronchoscopy, it is mainly used in management of CAO. Neodymium:yattrium-aluminum-garnet (Nd:YAG) is the most commonly used medium for production of laser during bronchoscopy. Nd:YAG laser has a wavelength of 1064 nm, which is in infrared zone, invisible to human eye. Thus, it needs to be carried with a pilot red light so that the operator can visualize the laser beam as it is applied in the tracheobronchial tree. Because Nd:YAG laser is poorly absorbed by quartz material, it can be delivered to the tracheobronchial tree with the flexible bronchoscope. Penetration of up to 10 mm can be achieved with Nd:YAG since it is poorly absorbed by hemoglobin as well as the water content of the tissue. Nd:YAG laser causes coagulation of tissues at low power settings and vaporization of tissues at high-power settings. Precise cutting of tissues, which is feasible with CO_2 laser, cannot be achieved with Nd:YAG laser. More recently, many interventional bronchoscopists have started to

Table 8.4 Factors affecting the outcome of laser photoresection

Factors	Favorable	Unfavorable
Location	Trachea and right or left main-stem bronchi	Lobar and segmental bronchi
Type of lesion	Predominantly endobronchial	Predominantly extrinsic
Endoscopic appearance	Exophytic	Submucosal
Length of lesion	<4 cm	>4 cm
Distal lumen	Visible and free of tumor	Not visible or diffusely infiltrated with the tumor
Duration of atelectasis	<4–6 weeks	>4–6 weeks
Mediastinal anatomy	Normal	Distorted
Pulmonary vascular supply	Intact	Compromised due to infiltration or compression by the tumor
Hemodynamic status	Stable	Unstable
Performance status	Good	Poor
Cardiopulmonary reserve	Adequate to withstand anesthesia	Inadequate
Oxygen requirement	≤40 %	>40 %
Coagulation profile	Normal	Abnormal

use Neodymium:yttrium-aluminum-perovskite (Nd:YAP) laser during bronchoscopy, as it is cheaper, more portable and has better coagulating properties than Nd:YAG laser. Preliminary studies show it to be as effective as Nd:YAG laser in management of malignant CAO.

Palliation of unresectable and symptomatic exophytic central airway tumor is the most common indication for the use of LPR. Bronchoscopic management of subglottic and tracheal stenosis is the most common nonmalignant indication. Less commonly, LPR has also been used for management of endobronchial granuloma, broncholiths, and inflammatory polyps. In palliative treatment of central airway tumors, it is important to recognize the factors that are associated with favorable or unfavorable results from LPR (Table 8.4). Most important among these are the location of the obstructing lesion and the status of airways beyond the obstruction. Lesions located in the trachea and main-stem bronchi are more suitable for LPR than the lesions in more distal location. The success rate is considerably lower for the tumors located in the lobar and segmental bronchi. Most suitable for LPR are tumors that are <4 cm in length with patent and tumor-free distal airways. LPR would be futile if the distal airway and the lung parenchyma are diffusely infiltrated with the tumor. Removal of obstructing mass from the proximal airways would not lead to any meaningful benefit to the patient in this situation. Certain findings on chest CT provide useful information regarding the outcome of LPR. Direct infiltration or compression of the corresponding pulmonary artery by the tumor mass on chest CT is a contraindication to LPR because restoration of airway patency could lead to worsening of dead-space ventilation and may actually cause worsening rather than improvement in dyspnea and hypoxemia. Similarly, to avoid creating a fistula, LPR should not be attempted if the CT shows contiguous involvement of the esophagus and bronchus with the tumor. Extreme caution is also warranted if there is significant distortion of mediastinal anatomy and a large thoracic vessel is seen in close proximity to the target lesion. LPR is contraindicated in patients with extrinsic airway compression.

LPR can be performed using either a rigid or a flexible bronchoscope. The end results and the complication rates are similar with both types of scopes [106]. Therefore, the choice is largely a matter of personal preference and training. Operators proficient in rigid bronchoscopy prefer to use the rigid scope because of its ability to perform mechanical debulking and superior suction capability [107]. Using rigid bronchoscope also improves the ability to manage a major bleeding complication during the procedure. Accordingly, rigid bronchoscope is always preferred over the flexible bronchoscope for highly vascular lesions. In many centers, majority of LPR procedures are performed with the flexible bronchoscope, which is introduced through an endotracheal tube or laryngeal mask airway. An important advantage of using flexible bronchoscope is in treatment of distal tumors affecting the lobar bronchi that are difficult to reach with the rigid scope. However, the duration of LPR is significantly longer with the flexible bronchoscope because removal of debris and debulking of tumor with the biopsy forceps is more time consuming. Also, compared to the rigid technique, the risk of endobronchial fire is significantly higher with the flexible technique because the bronchoscope, endotracheal tube, and laser fiber are flammable, whereas the rigid bronchoscope is nonflammable.

When using the rigid bronchoscope, it is customary to coagulate the tumor with low power settings followed by mechanical debulking with the bevel of the rigid bronchoscope [108]. After removing the main bulk of the tumor, laser can be used to further vaporize the residual tumor and to control the bleeding. With the flexible technique, a combination of mechanical debulking with the biopsy forceps and laser photocoagulation is used to achieve the similar results. To minimize the risk of airway perforation, the laser beam must always be fired parallel to the wall of the airway and not directly at it [109]. The laser tip must be kept 3–4 mm away from the target at all times. Smoke, debris, blood, and respiratory secretions must be removed on a regular basis to keep the operative field as clean as possible. Inspired oxygen should be limited to ≤40 % at all times to reduce the risk of endobronchial fire. For LPR with the flexible bronchoscope, the authors have developed general guidelines, designated as "rule of four" to achieve the optimal results and to minimize the complications with the procedure (Table 8.5).

Table 8.5 Mehta's rule of four for application of Nd:YAG Laser with flexible bronchoscope

Length of lesion	<4 cm
Duration of atelectasis	<4 weeks
Initial setting	
• Power (noncontact)	40 W
• Pulse duration	0.4 s
Distances	
• Endotracheal tube to lesion	>4 cm
• Fiber tip to lesion	4 mm
• Distal end of scope to fiber tip	4 mm
Fraction of inspired oxygen	≤0.4
Number of pulses between cleaning	<40
Procedure time	<4 h
Total number of laser treatments	<4
Life expectancy	>4 weeks
Laser team	≥4

Immediate improvement in airway caliber and relief in symptoms is reported in 70–90 % of patients undergoing LPR [110–114]. The success rate depends on the location of tumor in the tracheobronchial tree. For example, Cavaliere and associates achieved successful results in more than 90 % of tumors involving trachea or main-stem bronchi, compared to 50–70 % success in tumors involving the lobar bronchi [108]. Similarly, Hermes and associates reported the success rates of 95 % for tumors involving trachea, 80 % for tumors involving main-stem bronchi, and 68 % involving lobar bronchi [115]. Successful LPR has led to a dramatic improvement in symptoms of critical airway stenosis and impending asphyxia in many patients with CAO [116, 117]. In one report, 9 of the 17 patients with inoperable central airway tumors who required ventilator assistance for acute respiratory failure were extubated after successful LPR and many of them were able to receive further treatments for lung cancer [118]. Successful LPR is also associated with control of hemoptysis, and improvement in pulmonary functions, pulmonary ventilation and perfusion, radiological findings of atelectasis, Karnofsky performance status, and quality of life [119–121]. Many patients have undergone surgery and have received additional palliative treatment for lung cancer after experiencing relief of CAO with LPR [122]. The effect of LPR on survival remains speculative due to lack of prospective randomized studies. However, some authors have reported a better survival for patients undergoing successful LPR compared with the historical control [123]. For instance, in one report, no patient in the historical control group survived beyond 7 months whereas the survival rates were 60 % and 28 % at 7 months and 1 year respectively after LPR [113]. Survival is also reported to be longer in patients with successful LPR than in patients with unsuccessful treatment [124]. However, this may have been related to a higher tumor burden in patients who failed to achieve good results with initial LPR. In one study, the survival of patients receiving emergent Nd:YAG laser therapy was significantly longer than that of historical control subjects who received only emergent external beam radiation therapy [125]. In addition, according to one study, patients who undergo brachytherapy in combination with Nd:YAG laser have a better survival than those who undergo only laser photoresection [126].

A review of 14 case series has reported procedure related complications in up to 4.4 % of patients undergoing LPR [127]. Careful selection of patients and the experience of operator are important factors affecting the complication rate and patient outcome. In a large series, complications included massive hemorrhage in 1 %, and pneumothorax in 0.4 % of patients undergoing LPR [111]. Fatal outcome has been reported in up to 1–2 % of patients in some series [112, 116]. Massive hemorrhage due to perforation of major thoracic vessel by the laser beam is the most serious complication of LPR [113]. Such an event defies all local measures to control bleeding and is rapidly fatal in majority of cases. Airway fire is another serious but less common complication. Prevention of fire hazard is of utmost importance [128, 129]. The risk of airway fire can be reduced by maintaining the FiO_2 to ≤0.4, using single pulse setting on laser, keeping the scope and laser fiber as clean as possible, and avoiding use of combustible anesthetic gas during the procedure. Silicone tubes are more resistant to fire than standard PVC endotracheal tubes. The risk of fire can also be lowered by maintaining maximum possible distance between the endotracheal tube and the surgical field [128]. Patients with airway thermal injury must be kept under surveillance for future development of granulation tissue and airway stenosis [128, 130]. The equipment for LPR is expensive and is not universally available [131]. All personnel involved in LPR need thorough education and training in laser safety issues. The procedure is perhaps best performed by a dedicated airway team with an experienced anesthetist.

Cryotherapy

Exposing biological tissues to the cycles of freezing and thawing causes cellular injury and death. Bronchoscopic cryotherapy uses nitrous oxide gas and rigid or flexible probes to freeze the endobronchial tissues. Cooling is governed by Joule-Thompson principle according to which, there is decrease in temperature with expansion of gas as it moves from an area of high pressure to an area of low pressure. Nitrous oxide used for this technique is stored at room temperature under high pressure in cylinders. Rapid decrease in pressure as the gas is released from the tip of the probes causes rapid cooling to a temperature below −70 °C that causes the tissue surrounding the probe to freeze within a period of few seconds.

There are several mechanisms of cell injury when exposed to cycles of freezing and thawing. The intracellular ice crystals damage vital cell organelles such as mitochondria. Extracellular ice crystals cause osmotic injury and cellular dehydration due to alteration of ion concentration across the biological membranes. Tissues exposed to freezing and thawing also display delayed ischemic injury due to vasoconstriction, platelet aggregation and vascular thrombosis that develop 6–12 h after the procedure. Further, it is speculated that cryotherapy also induces immunological injury to the tissues through activation of natural killer cells.

The extent of cellular death depends on speed of freezing and thawing. Maximum damage is observed when the tissue is frozen at a rapid speed and thawed at a slow speed. Cellular injury decreases with the distance from the center of application. Other important determinants of ultimate effect are the number of freeze-thaw cycles and the water content of the tissue treated with cryotherapy. Because of their low water content, fibrous tissue, and cartilage are inherently resistant to cryodestruction, which explains a very low likelihood of airway perforation after cryotherapy.

Both rigid and flexible cryoprobes are available and the choice is a matter of personal preference. An important difference is in the process of thawing, which is active with the rigid technique and passive with the flexible technique. Due to this reason, the procedure with flexible probe requires a longer duration as compared to the procedure performed with the rigid instrument. Cryotherapy with flexible technique is performed under conscious sedation. Flexible cryoprobe is advanced through the working channel. The tip of the probe is applied tangentially onto the infiltrating tumors or is directly driven into the tumor mass in exophytic lesions. Freezing is activated using a foot pedal and is continued for a period of 20–30 s until an ice ball is seen surrounding the probe. The tissue starts to thaw as soon as the foot is removed from the pedal. Typically, 1–3 freeze-thaw cycles, each lasting for about 60 s are applied at each area. Probe is then moved 5 mm away and the same procedure is carried out at an adjacent part of tumor. Entire tumor must be covered as much as possible. At the end of the procedure, the tumor appears unchanged. In conventional cryotherapy, no attempt should be made to mechanically remove any parts of tumor at the completion of the procedure. Immediate bleeding is seldom a problem. Delayed necrosis of tumor occurs over next 5–10 days. A clean up bronchoscopy is needed at this time to remove the necrotic tissue with the biopsy forceps and the bronchoscopic suction. Sometimes, large parts of tumor are eliminated by spontaneous expectoration.

Cryotherapy is suitable for destruction of both exophytic tumors as well as the tumors with a predominant submucosal and infiltrative growth. Overall response rate is reported to be in the range of 75–80 % [132–134]. Majority of patients experience improvement in dyspnea, exercise capacity, pulmonary functions and performance status [135–137]. Hemoptysis is reported to resolve in up to 90 % of patients [138]. However, because the maximum effects of cryotherapy are delayed for several days, it cannot be used for immediate debulking of large airway tumors causing acute and severe CAO. Cryotherapy is suitable for treatment of highly vascular tumors such as adenoid cystic carcinoma and bronchial carcinoids [139]. Cryotherapy has also been used in treatment of carcinoma-in-situ and micro-invasive cancers. For instance, in one study, 35 patients with early lung cancer were treated with cryotherapy. Complete response rate at 1 year was 91 %. Ten patients (28 %) developed recurrence of tumors within 4 years of treatment [140]. Cryotherapy can be used for control of granulation tissue that develops after placement of airway stent. Cryotherapy has also been used for removal of airway foreign bodies and obstructing blood clot. A organic foreign body with high water content is most suitable for removal with this technique. A small clinical study has suggested synergistic effect of cryotherapy and external beam radiation therapy for the treatment of unresectable lung cancers [141]. Independent studies by others are needed to validate these data. Animal studies have also suggested an exciting possibility of synergy between cryotherapy and chemotherapy in non-small-cell lung cancer model [142, 143]. Humans studies are yet to address these findings.

Bronchoscopic cryotherapy has an excellent safety record. Complications such as bleeding, bronchospasm and cardiac arrhythmia are seldom encountered. There is minimal, if any risk of airway perforation. There is no risk of airway fire, and the procedure can be performed regardless of need for high-flow oxygen therapy. The initial setup and the individual procedure are less expensive than most other bronchoscopic interventional procedures. The main downside is the delay in treatment response that makes it an unsuitable choice when immediate results are desired. Recently, a novel extension of cryotherapy technique called cryorecanalization has been developed that is effective in immediate relief of CAO.

Cryorecanalization

The flexible cryoprobes used in the past were not designed to withstand the traction needed for extraction of large pieces of tumors. New design of cryoprobes have a greater freezing power and a more stable joint between the gas channel and the tip, which is able to withstand traction of up to 50 N without showing structural disintegration. Use of these probes allows immediate recanalization of obstructed airways. The probe is 2.3 mm in diameter and can be used with any standard therapeutic bronchoscope. The procedure is performed under conscious sedation with endotracheal intubation. The cryoprobe is introduced through the working channel and is guided into the tumor. The probe tip is cooled for a period of 5–20 s. Once the ice ball forms, the frozen tumor is extracted from the surrounding tissue by pulling the probe and the bronchoscope as a unit. The frozen tissue attached to the cryoprobe tip is removed from the airways along with the bronchoscope. The attached tumor is removed from the tip by placing it in water bath. The process is repeated till most of the tumor is extracted and the airway patency is restored. The results are immediate. No clean up bronchoscopy is needed.

Hetzel and associates performed cryorecanalization in 60 patients using this technique [144]. Complete recanalization was achieved in 37 (61 %) of study patients. Additional 13 patients (22 %) experienced partial recanalization. Significant endobronchial bleeding requiring argon plasma coagulation to achieve hemostasis was needed in 6 (10 %) patients. The same investigators have recently updated their experience with cryorecanalization and have reported successful results in 205 (91 %) of 225 patients [145]. In this study, the procedure was least effective in patients who had a long segment of airway stenosis secondary to an infiltrative tumor. Mild bleeding, treated with ice cold saline or topical epinephrine was encountered in 9 (4 %) of patients. Moderate bleeding requiring balloon blocker or APC for control was encountered in 18 (8 %) of patients.

Cryorecanalization has several advantages. It is an inexpensive procedure, and does not needed rigid bronchoscopy or general anesthesia. There is no need for clean up bronchoscopy. The results are immediate. The duration of procedure is generally shorter than that needed for LPR. However, safety is a concern. Airway bleeding is the most important consideration. The operators must be ready to manage the bleeding complications, which may be expected in as many as 10 % of patients.

Photodynamic Therapy

Photodynamic therapy uses a photosensitizing agent followed by exposure to nonthermal laser of appropriate wavelength to destroy the central airway tumors. Porfimer sodium (Photofrin) is the most commonly used photosensitizing agent for this purpose. After an intravenous administration, porfimer sodium is cleared from most organs within a period of 72 h but is preferentially retained in the endobronchial tumor, liver, spleen and skin for a longer period of time. Tumor selectivity is fundamentally a function of difference in the concentration of this agent between the tumor cells and the normal bronchial mucosa. Porfimer sodium is a light absorbing molecule that produces highly reactive singlet oxygen species in a Type II photooxidation reaction when exposed to the light of the wavelength that corresponds to its absorption spectrum. Intracellular generation of highly reactive oxygen species causes direct cytotoxic injury to the tumor cells [146]. Endothelial injury and tissue ischemia also contribute to regression of tumor. There is also evidence of immunological and complement mediated injury to the tumor cells [147]. Typically, the regression of the tumor occurs after a delay of several days. Accordingly, PDT is not suitable for immediate relief of symptoms due to CAO.

Porfimer sodium is administered at an intravenous dose of 2 mg/kg. Approximately 48 h later, flexible bronchoscopy is performed and the tumor is exposed to the light in order to activate the photosensitizing agent. The light used for this purpose is in red region of spectrum with a wavelength of 630 nm that can penetrate to a depth of 5–10 mm below the surface of the tumor [148]. Potassium titanyl phosphate (KTP) pumped dye laser is the most commonly used light source. Being a nonthermal laser, it can be carried via a quartz fiber and is suitable for use with flexible bronchoscope. Standard laser precautions, such as eye protection are essential, but there is no risk of endobronchial fire. Illumination can be achieved with two different techniques. Cylindrical diffusers distribute the light circumferentially in 360°. These are used for interstitial illumination of tumor in which the tip of the quartz fiber is placed directly into the tumor. In contrast, microlens has a forward emitting light, which is suitable for surface treatment of a flat or superficial tumor. The light energy of 200 J/cm, corresponding to 400 mW/cm length of diffuser for 500 s is recommended for the initial treatment session [149, 150]. The light exposure time for this dose lasts for a period of about 8 min. Necrotic tumor and debris accumulates at the site of treatment over a period of 48 h after the initial treatment session. Some patients may develop atelectasis and post-obstructive pneumonia and may require an emergent bronchoscopy. A clean up bronchoscopy is indicated 48 h after the initial session to remove the necrotic tumor, mucus, and debris. At times, the necrotic tumor tends to have a gelatinous consistency and may be difficult to remove [151]. Use of rigid scope or cryoprobe may be needed for airway clearance in those cases. After removal of necrotic tumor and mucus, the airways should be reevaluated for the presence of residual tumor. Re-illumination may be performed if residual tumor is found. There is no need to administer photosensitizing agents at this time since the tumors are known to retain the porfimer sodium up to a period of 7 days.

PDT has an established role in palliative treatment of advanced central airway cancers. Patients with advanced stage non-resectable and predominantly intraluminal central tumor are the most suitable candidates for PDT. A successful PDT in these patients is associated with a significant relief in symptoms, decrease in endobronchial obstruction and improvement in pulmonary function tests. In one series, PDT was performed in 100 patients with inoperable lung cancer [149]. Endobronchial obstruction decreased from 86 to 18 %, and FVC and FEV1 improved by 430 ml and 280 ml respectively. The median survival after PDT was significantly longer for patients with a WHO performance score of ≤2 than for those with performance score of >2. Others have reported similar results with PDT in advanced central lung cancer [152, 153]. Photodynamic therapy has also been used in combination with other treatment modalities such as LPR [154] and brachytherapy [155] with favorable clinical response in patients with malignant CAO. Although sequential therapies were separated by a period of 4–6 weeks in these studies, further work is needed to determine the most effective sequence and the most optimal interval between different bronchoscopic modalities in these patients. Few studies have compared the results of LPR with those of PDT in head-to head comparison. Compared to LPR, the clinical response with PDT is delayed but the benefits last for a longer period of time [156]. In a randomized study, patients treated with PDT had a longer time until treatment failure and better median survival than in patients treated with LPR [157]. However, this study was limited by a small sample size and difference in the tumor staging at the time of randomization, with the PDT group having fewer patients with advanced central lung cancer. Several studies have also established the usefulness of PDT in treatment of patients with early stage central airway lung cancer who are not suitable for surgical treatment [158, 159]. In fact, PDT has been suggested as the option of first choice for treatment of these patients according to the 2003 ACCP evidence-based clinical practice guidelines for lung cancer [160].

The most common adverse effects associated with PDT are respiratory symptoms such as cough, expectoration of necrotic tumor, dyspnea and atelectasis [161]. In some instances, an emergent bronchoscopy is needed. Nonfatal hemoptysis is reported in up to 18 % of patients. An important side effect of PDT is skin photosensitivity. However, it is preventable and in one series, only 4 % of patients undergoing PDT experienced mild skin photosensitivity [149].

PDT has several advantages over other bronchoscopic techniques for the treatment of CAO. The procedure is technically easy and is performed under conscious sedation using flexible bronchoscope. The procedure has an excellent safety record. There is low risk of airway perforation and hemorrhage. There is no risk of endobronchial fire. However, several limitations of PDT must also be highlighted. The procedure is expensive. There is need for repeat clean up bronchoscopy.

Some patients require rigid bronchoscopy for airway toilet. Most importantly, photosensitivity seriously limits the outdoor activities for a period of nearly 6 weeks, which may be unacceptable to the patient. The patients must wear protective clothes and eyewear and must avoid direct exposure to sun light for a period of 4–6 weeks. This is an important drawback for patients with a limited life expectancy.

Brachytherapy

Brachytherapy refers to a technique in which irradiation source is placed within or close proximity to the target to deliver the maximum dose to the tumor while sparing the normal surrounding tissues. In case of central airway tumors, the irradiation source is placed directly inside the endobronchial tree close to the tumor with the assistance of flexible bronchoscope. The radiation dose to the surrounding tissue is dictated by inverse square law, according to which, the dose rate decreases as a function of the inverse square of the distance from the center of the source. Accordingly, this mode of radiation therapy allows the tumor to receive significantly higher radiation doses than the surrounding healthy structures such as lung parenchyma and mediastinum. Typically, it requires up to 3 weeks for the tumor to regress after the application of radiation therapy. Therefore, brachytherapy is not suitable for immediate relief of obstructive symptoms.

The fundamental goal of brachytherapy is palliation of symptoms such as cough, dyspnea and hemoptysis in patients with central airway tumor who cannot undergo curative surgery. Brachytherapy is most useful for endobronchial tumors with a significant component of submucosal and peribronchial disease. Brachytherapy is a useful option for recurrent tumors after patient has already received maximally tolerated external beam radiation therapy. To be able to offer brachytherapy, the bronchoscopists should be able to pass the catheter beyond the obstructing lesion. In patients with near-total stenosis, partial recanalization of airway is needed using other techniques such as LPR, electrocautery or balloon dilation before brachytherapy can be offered. Brachytherapy is suitable for control of tumor located external to cartilage and the bronchial wall that cannot be treated with aforementioned bronchoscopic techniques. Treatment is also effective against endobronchial metastasis. Brachytherapy is not suitable for predominantly extrinsic airway compression where airway stent is the most logical choice. Caution is also warranted if there is imminent danger of development of fistula between the bronchial wall and the surrounding structures.

The dose delivered to the tumor depends on the choice of radioactive source and the dwelling time. The dose is calculated at a distance of 10 mm from the source axis. The low dose rate (LDR), intermediate dose rate (IDR), and high dose rate (HDR) treatments imply a dose of <2 Gy/Hr, 2–12 Gy/Hr and >12 Gy/Hr respectively to a target at a distance of 10 mm. The majority of centers have adopted high dose rate brachytherapy, which uses Iridium-191 (Ir-192) as the radiation source. The American Brachytherapy Society recommends either three weekly fractions of 7.5 Gy each, two weekly fractions of 10 Gy each, or four weekly fractions of 6 Gy each when using HDR brachytherapy as the primary modality for palliation of symptoms [162]. Each treatment sessions lasts for a period of 5–30 min and is easily administered on an outpatient basis.

Brachytherapy requires a close collaboration between the bronchoscopist and the radiation oncologist. The role of the bronchoscopist is to identify a suitable candidate and place an afterloading catheter into the tracheobronchial tree to facilitate local delivery of radiation source. Radiation oncologist is involved in the calculation of radiation dose and in actual delivery of radiation to the tumor by placing the radiation seeds inside the afterloading catheter in locations appropriate to the tumor. Bronchoscopy is performed through the nose under conscious sedation and topical anesthesia. During bronchoscopy, fluoroscopic guidance is used for placement of radio-opaque markers on the skin corresponding to the distal and the proximal end of the tumor to assist the radiation oncologist in delineation of the irradiation length. An afterloading catheter of 2–3 mm external diameter with a guide wire is placed beyond the distal end of the tumor and the bronchoscope is withdrawn. The afterloading catheter is secured at the nose. The radiation oncologist now places the dummy seeds consisting of radio-opaque markers into the catheter and obtains orthogonal chest radiographs to simulate the pathway of the radiation source. Once the final treatment plan is made, the patient is transferred to a shielded room and dummy seeds are removed. The radiation seeds are then introduced through the afterloading catheter and advanced into the intended location under computer control. Irradiation length is defined by the first and the last dwell point of the radiation seeds, as guided by the skin markers placed by the bronchoscopist. It is usual to extend the radiation field to 1-cm at beyond each end of the tumor. Catheter is removed after the radiation dose is delivered and the patient is discharged after a short period of observation. The use of HDR with afterloading technique eliminates any risk of radiation exposure to the medical personnel.

Brachytherapy is shown to be effective for palliation of both previously untreated [163–165] and treated [166] lung cancer patients with CAO. Studies have shown improvement in symptoms as well as bronchoscopic findings [164]. Cough is reported to improve in 20–70 %, dyspnea in 25–80 % and hemoptysis in 70–90 % of patients [167]. As expected, bronchoscopic response to brachytherapy is shown to correlate with resolution of symptoms [168]. Atelectasis is said to resolve in 25 % of patients [166]. Studies have also shown improvement in quality of life, pulmonary functions and ventilation-perfusion scans after brachytherapy [169, 170]. Survival benefit with brachytherapy has not been shown. However, in a randomized study, the symptom free period increased from 2.8 months with LPR alone to 8.5 months with a combination of LPR and HDR brachytherapy [171]. For the patients who have not received prior treatment, the duration of response and survival is better with external beam radiation therapy than with brachytherapy [172]. Therefore, brachytherapy should not be chosen as the first line therapy over EBRT for these patients. However, brachytherapy can be offered to the patients who have already received maximally allowable EBRT and have developed recurrence of cancer. The combination of external beam radiation and brachytherapy has been compared with external beam radiation alone in patients with inoperable central airway cancers. In one such study, for patients with an obstructing tumor of main-stem bronchus, the re-expansion of collapsed lung was observed in 57 % of patients with the combination therapy as compared to 35 % of patients with external beam radiation therapy alone [173]. Moreover, the radiation exposure to normal lung parenchyma could be decreased by 32 % in a study in which adjunctive brachytherapy was added to the EBRT for the local control of tumor [174].

Brachytherapy is a therapeutic option for occult early stage central lung cancers if surgery cannot be performed. Complete endoscopic response in 60–90 % and 5-year survival rate of 30–80 % is reported with brachytherapy in these patients [163, 175, 176]. A median survival of nearly 2 years has been achieved with brachytherapy in patients with central lung cancers not eligible for surgery in recent case series [177, 178]. Brachytherapy has also been used in management of excessive granulation tissue in lung transplant recipients [179–182].

Endobronchial brachytherapy is associated with many side effects. Of most concern are hemoptysis and formation of airway fistula. Fatal hemoptysis has been reported in 5–10 % of patients undergoing brachytherapy [163, 164, 178]. Persistence of malignancy after brachytherapy, direct contact between the brachytherapy applicator and airway wall, presence of major blood vessel in vicinity and concomitant LPR are associated with higher risk of massive hemorrhage after brachytherapy [183, 184]. A dose of >10 Gy per fraction is also associated with higher risk of bleeding complications [185]. Brachytherapy for upper lobe tumors has been associated with higher risk of hemoptysis in some studies. This is most likely due to close proximity of the pulmonary artery with the anterior segment of the right upper lobe and apical-posterior segment of the left upper lobe respectively [186].

In some instances, bleeding is simply a reflection of natural progression of the disease. Radiation bronchitis and airway stenosis occurs in up to 10 % of patients after brachytherapy [187]. The histological changes vary from mucosal inflammation to severe bronchial wall fibrosis. The risk of radiation bronchitis is associated with large cell lung cancer histology, prior LPR, concomitant external beam radiation therapy and application of brachytherapy for curative purpose [188].

Brachytherapy has several advantages over other bronchoscopic techniques. For a bronchoscopist, it is a straightforward procedure. Brachytherapy can be offered for the lesions located at obtuse angles and in the segmental bronchi, which are not suitable and in many instances off-limits for LPR. The procedure retains effectiveness for the peribronchial tumors as well. The main disadvantages are potential for serious adverse effects and high cost of the equipment needed to deliver radiation source to the endobronchial location. Accordingly, the facilities of brachytherapy are limited to large tertiary care centers. Moreover, a close collaboration between the bronchoscopists and the radiation oncologist is needed, which can cause interdisciplinary scheduling conflicts.

Airway Stents

Airway stents have a critical role in maintaining airway patency in patients with extrinsic airway compression [189–191]. Successful deployment of airway stents is associated with immediate relief in dyspnea and asphyxia. In many instances, stent placement has allowed successful weaning and extubation in ventilator dependent patients [192]. Frequently, stents are placed for the management of extrinsic airway compression after the intra-luminal component of the tumor is treated with other bronchoscopic techniques such as LPR or electrocautery [193]. For a detailed discussion on airway stent, readers are referred to Chap. 9.

External Beam Radiation

External beam radiation therapy has an important place in treatment of advanced and inoperable lung cancer. In a recent study of 1,250 patients, palliation of symptoms was achieved in 68 % for hemoptysis, 54 % for cough, 51 % for pain, and 38 % for dyspnea [194]. However, the results are delayed and mucosal edema and inflammation from radiation therapy have a potential to cause worsening of symptoms in the patients who already have a critically narrowed central airways. External beam radiation in such patients can only be offered once the airway lumen is restored with the bronchoscopic techniques. Several studies have established the usefulness of external beam radiation in management of atelectasis due to obstructing endobronchial tumors. Radiological response and aeration of the collapsed lung has been reported in 21–74 % of patients with external beam radiation therapy [195–197]. In one of these studies, 71 % of patients who received radiation within 2 weeks of developing atelectasis had a complete re-expansion of their lungs, whereas only 23 % of those who received radiation therapy after 2 weeks had a similar response [197].

Multimodality Treatment

It cannot go unnoticed from the aforementioned discussion that a single modality of bronchoscopic therapy will not be sufficient for every patient with malignant CAO. A comprehensive treatment plan is needed in majority of these patients to achieve the most satisfactory results. Several recent case-series have established the value of such multi-modality therapy that combines interventional bronchoscopy with external beam radiation, chemotherapy and surgery for most effective palliation and treatment of patients with advanced CAO [5, 75, 96, 198–200]. Multimodality treatment has been reported to reestablish satisfactory airway lumen in up to 95 % of patients with CAO [96, 199]. In majority of patients included in these studies, a combination of mechanical debulking and thermal ablation with laser or electrocautery was used for endobronchial component of tumors and airway stenting was used for extrinsic airway compression. There is suggestion that multimodality treatment confers a modest survival advantage to these patients as compared to single modality treatment. For example, in one report, compared with Nd:YAG treatment alone, multimodality treatment prolonged survival by 4.9 months in NSCLC patients with CAO. In another study, 3-year survival rate was 2.3 % in patients treated with single modality treatment and 22 % in patients who received multimodality therapy [198]. Although we are aware of limitations of survival analysis on retrospective data, these results further underscore the need to have a team of dedicated health care providers with expertise in different modes of therapies to achieve the desired results in patients with malignant CAO.

Conclusion

Multiple options exist for management of patients with CAO. Selection of a technique in an individual patient depends upon the severity and type of CAO, rapidity with which the relief is needed, availability of expertise, patient preference and the cost. Regardless, it is important to realize that the fundamental aim of bronchoscopic interventions is to palliate distressing symptoms such as dyspnea, and hemoptysis to improve quality of remaining life and not essentially prolongation of survival. Many of the bronchoscopic techniques are costly and in some instances provide a limited, if any meaningful benefit to the patient. Hence, patients with limited expected survival of <3 months due to an advanced and metastatic cancer or a serious and terminal systemic disease should be subjected to these procedures with great caution. This is especially true if adequate palliation of symptoms can be achieved with nonbronchoscopic means. Furthermore, it is important to realize that majority of these patients are fragile with limited cardiorespiratory reserves. Therefore, it is essential that every effort is made to avoid major procedure-related complications. Most bronchoscopic modalities are expensive and should be chosen keeping the cost of medical care in mind. We cannot overstate that approach to these patients should be cautious, conservative and cost effective.

References

1. Lee P, Kupeli E, Mehta AC. Therapeutic bronchoscopy in lung cancer. Laser therapy, electrocautery, brachytherapy, stents and photodynamic therapy. Clin Chest Med. 2002;23:241–56.
2. Ernst A, Feller-Kopman D, Becker HD, Mehta AC. Central airway obstruction. Am J Respir Crit Care Med. 2004;169:1278–97.
3. Freitag L. Interventional endoscopic treatment. Lung Cancer. 2004;45 Suppl 2:S235–8.
4. Williamson JP, Phillips MJ, Hillman DR, Eastwood PR. Managing obstruction of the central airways. Intern Med J. 2010;40:399–410.
5. Stephens KE, Wood DE. Bronchoscopic management of central airway obstruction. J Thorac Cardiovasc Surg. 2000;119:289–96.
6. Theodore PR. Emergent management of malignancy related acute airway obstruction. Emerg Med Clin North Am. 2009;27:231–41.
7. Folch E, Mehta AC. Airway interventions in the tracheobronchial tree. Semin Respir Crit Care Med. 2008;29:441–52.
8. Brodsky JB. Bronchoscopic procedures for central airway obstruction. J Cardiothorac Vasc Anesth. 2003;17:638–46.
9. Gorden JA, Ernst A. Endoscopic management of central airway obstruction. Semin Thorac Cardiovasc Surg. 2009;21:263–73.
10. Dela Cruz CS, Tanoue LT, Matthay RA. Lung cancer: epidemiology, etiology, and prevention. Clin Chest Med. 2011;32:605–44.
11. Sorensen JB. Endobronchial metastases from extrapulmonary solid tumors. Acta Oncol. 2004;43:73–9.
12. Braman SS, Whitcomb ME. Endobronchial metastasis. Arch Intern Med. 1975;135:543–7.
13. Kiryu T, Hoshi H, Matsui E, et al. Endotracheal/endobronchial metastasis. Chest. 2001;119:768–75.
14. Shepherd MP. Endobronchial metastatic disease. Thorax. 1982;37:362–5.
15. Ognibene FP, Shelhamer JH. Kaposi's sarcoma. Clin Chest Med. 1988;9:459–65.
16. Garay SM, Belenko M, Fazzini E, Schinella R. Pulmonary manifestations of Kaposi's sarcoma. Chest. 1987;91:39–43.
17. Zibrak JD, Silvestri RC, Costello P, Marlink R, Jensen WA, Robins A, et al. Bronchoscopic and radiologic features of Kaposi's sarcoma involving the respiratory system. Chest. 1986;90:476–9.
18. Webb BD, Walsh GL, Roberts DB, Sturgis EM. Primary tracheal malignant neoplasms: the

University of Texas MD Anderson Cancer Center experience. J Am Coll Surg. 2006;202:237–46.
19. Honings J, Gaissert HA, Van Der Heijden HFM, et al. Clinical aspects and treatment of tracheal malignancies. Acta Otolaryngol. 2010;130:763–72.
20. Zimmer W, DeLuca SA. Primary tracheal neoplasms: recognition, diagnosis and evaluation. Am Fam Physician. 1992;45:2651–7.
21. Gaissert HA, Grillo HC, Shadmehr MB, et al. Long term survival after resection of primary adenoid cystic and squamous cell carcinoma of trachea and carina. Ann Thorac Surg. 2004;78:1889–97.
22. Murgu SD, Colt HG. Tracheobronchomalacia and excessive dynamic airway collapse. Respirology. 2006;11:388–406.
23. Marel M, Pekarek Z, Spasova I, et al. Management of benign stenosis of the large airways in the University hospital in Prague, Czech Republic, in 1998–2003. Respiration. 2005;72:622–8.
24. Perotin JM, Jeanfaivre T, Thibout Y, et al. Endoscopic management of idiopathic tracheal stenosis. Ann Thorac Surg. 2011;92:297–302.
25. Brichet A, Verkindre C, Dupont J, et al. Multidisciplinary approach to management of post intubation tracheal stenosis. Eur Respir J. 1999;13: 888–93.
26. Hollingsworth HM. Wheezing and stridor. Clin Chest Med. 1987;8:231–40.
27. Geffin B, Grillo HC, Cooper JD, Pantoppidan H. Stenosis following tracheostomy for respiratory care. JAMA. 1971;216:1984–8.
28. Jabbardarjani H, Kiani A, Karimi S, Kharabian S, Masjedi MR. Role of endoscopic treatments in patients with adenoid cystic carcinoma. J Bronchol. 2007;14:251–4.
29. Stoller JK. Spirometry: a key diagnostic test in pulmonary medicine. Cleve Clin J Med. 1992;59:75–8.
30. Acres JC. Clinical significance of pulmonary function tests: upper airway obstruction. Chest. 1981;80:207–11.
31. Boiselle PM, Ernst A. Recent advances in central airway imaging. Chest. 2002;121:1651–60.
32. Boiselle PM, Reynolds KF, Ernst A. Multiplanar and three-dimensional imaging of the central airways with multidetector CT. Am J Roentgenol. 2002;179: 301–8.
33. Boiselle PM. Multislice helical CT of the central airways. Radiol Clin North Am. 2003;41:561–74.
34. Lee KS, Lunn W, Feller-Kopman D, Ernst A, Hatabu H, Boiselle PM. Multislice CT evaluation of airway stents. J Thorac Imaging. 2005;20:81–8.
35. Fettetti GR, Kocier M, Calaque O, et al. Follow up after stent insertion in the tracheobronchial tree: role of helical computed tomography in comparison with flexible bromchoscopy. Eur Radiol. 2003;13: 1172–8.
36. Dialani V, Ernst A, Sun M, et al. MDCT detection of airway stent complications: comparison with bronchoscopy. Am J Roentgenol. 2008;191:1576–80.
37. LoCicero III J, Costello P, Campos CT, et al. Spiral CT with multiplanar and three-dimensional reconstructions accurately predicts tracheobronchial pathology. Ann Thorac Surg. 1996;62:811–7.
38. Remy-Jardin M, Remy J, Artaud D, Fribourg M, Duhamel A. Volume rendering of the tracheobronchial tree: clinical evaluation of bronchographic images. Radiology. 1998;208:761–70.
39. Haponik EF, Aquino SL, Vining DJ. Virtual bronchoscopy. Clin Chest Med. 1999;20:201–17.
40. Fleiter T, Merkle EM, Aschoff AJ, et al. Comparison of real time virtual and fiberoptic bronchoscopy in patients with bronchial carcinoma: opportunities and limitations. Am J Roentgenol. 1997;169:1591–5.
41. Finkelstein SE, Schrump DS, Nguyen DM, Hewitt SM, Kunst TF, Summers RM. Comparative evaluation of super high-resolution CT scan and virtual bronchoscopy for the detection of tracheobronchial malignancies. Chest. 2003;124:1834–40.
42. Allah MF, Hussein SRA, Al-Asmar ABH, et al. Role of virtual bronchoscopy in the evaluation of bronchial lesions. J Comput Assist Tomogr. 2012;36: 94–9.
43. De wever W, Vendecaveye V, Lanciotti S, Verschakelen JA. Multidetector CT-generated virtual bronchoscopy: an illustrated review of the potential clinical indications. Eur Respir J. 2004;23: 776–82.
44. Hoppe H, Dinkel HP, Walder B, von Allmen G, Gugger M, Vock P. Grading airway stenosis down to the segmental level using virtual bronchoscopy. Chest. 2004;125:704–11.
45. Whiteman SC, Yang Y, Gey van Pittius D, et al. Optical coherence tomography: real time imaging of bronchial airways microstructures and detection of inflammatory/neoplastic morphologic changes. Clin Cancer Res. 2006;12:813–8.
46. Williamson JP, Armstrong JJ, McLaughlin RA, et al. Measuring the airway dimensions during bronchoscopy using anatomical optical coherence tomography. Eur Respir J. 2010;35:34–41.
47. Williamson JP, McLaughlin RA, Phillips MJ, Armstrong JJ, Becker S, Walsh JH, et al. Using optical coherence tomography to improve diagnostic and therapeutic bronchoscopy. Chest. 2009;136: 272–6.
48. Colt HG. Functional evaluation before and after interventional bronchoscopy. In: Bollinger CT, Mathur PN, editors. Interventional bronchoscopy. Basel, Switzeland: S. Krager; 2000. p. 55–64.
49. Schuurmans MM, Michaud GC, Diacon AH, Bolliger CT. Use of ultrathin bronchoscope in the assessment of central airway obstruction. Chest. 2003;124:735–9.
50. Oki M, Saka H. Thin bronchoscope for evaluating stenotic airways during stenting procedure. Respiration. 2011;82:509–14.
51. Helmers RA, Sanderson DR. Rigid bronchoscopy. the forgotten art. Clin Chest Med. 1995;16:393–9.

52. Ayers ML, Beamis Jr JF. Rigid bronchoscopy in the twenty-first century. Clin Chest Med. 2001;22: 355–64.
53. Colt HG, Harrell JH. Therapeutic rigid bronchoscopy allows level of care changes in patients with acute respiratory failure from central airways obstruction. Chest. 1997;112:202–6.
54. Kurimoto N, Murayama M, Yoshioka S, Nishisaka T, Inai K, Dohi K. Assessment of usefulness of endobronchial ultrasonography in determination of depth of tracheobronchial tumor invasion. Chest. 1999; 115:1500–6.
55. Miyazu Y, Miyazawa T, Kurimoto N, Iwamoto Y, Kanoh K, Kohno N. Endobronchial ultrasonography in the assessment of centrally located early-stage lung cancer before photodynamic therapy. Am J Respir Crit Care Med. 2002;165:832–7.
56. Miyazawa T, Miyazu Y, Iwamoto Y, Ishida A, Kanoh K, Sumiyoshi H, et al. Stenting at the flow-limiting segment in tracheobronchial stenosis due to lung cancer. Am J Respir Crit Care Med. 2004;169: 1096–102.
57. Herth F, Becker HD, LoCicero 3rd J, Ernst A. Endobronchial ultrasound in therapeutic bronchoscopy. Eur Respir J. 2002;20:118–21.
58. Sarkiss M. Anesthesia for bronchoscopy and interventional pulmonology: from moderate sedation to jet ventilation. Curr Opin Pulm Med. 2011;17: 274–8.
59. Conacher ID, Paes LL, McMohan CC, Morritt GN. Anesthetic management of laser surgery for central obstruction: a 12-year case series. J Cardiothorac Vasc Anesth. 1998;12:153–6.
60. Milner QJW, Abdy S, Allen JG. Management of severe tracheal obstruction with helium/oxygen and a laryngeal mask airway. Anesthesia. 1997;52: 1087–9.
61. Brodsky JB. Anesthetic considerations for bronchoscopic procedures in patients with central-airway obstruction. J Bronchol. 2001;8:36–43.
62. McMahon CC, Rainey L, Fulton B, Conacher ID. Central airway compression. Anaesthetic and intensive care consequences. Anaesthesia. 1997;52: 158–62.
63. Mathisen DJ, Grillo HC. Endoscopic relief of malignant airway obstruction. Ann Thorac Surg. 1989;48: 469–75.
64. Watters MP, McKenzie JM. Inhalational induction with sevoflurane in an adult with severe complex central airways obstruction. Anaesth Intensive Care. 1997;25:704–6.
65. Purugganan R. Intravenous anesthesia for thoracic procedures. Curr Opin Anaesthesiol. 2008;21:1–7.
66. Choudhury M, Saxena N. Total intravenous anaesthesia for tracheobronchial stenting in children. Anaesth Intensive Care. 2002;30:376–9.
67. El-Baz N, Jensik R, Faber LP, Faro RS. One-lung high-frequency ventilation for tracheoplasty and bronchoplasty: a new technique. Ann Thorac Surg. 1982;34:564–71.
68. Biro P, Layer M, Becker HD, Herth F, Wiedemann K, Seifert B, et al. Influence of airway-occluding instruments on airway pressure during jet ventilation for rigid bronchoscopy. Br J Anaesth. 2000;85: 462–5.
69. Plummer S, Hartley M, Vaughan RS. Anaesthesia for telescopic procedures in the thorax. Br J Anaesth. 1998;80:223–34.
70. Macdonald AG. A brief historical review of non-anaesthetic causes of fires and explosions in the operating room. Br J Anaesth. 1994;73:847–56.
71. Denton RA, Dedhia HV, Abrons HL, Jain PR, Lapp NL, Teba L. Long-term survival after endobronchial fire during treatment of severe malignant airway obstruction with the Nd:YAG laser. Chest. 1988;94: 1086–8.
72. Ernst A, Simoff M, Ost D, Goldman Y, Herth FJF. Prospective risk-adjusted morbidity and mortality outcome analysis after therapeutic bronchoscopy procedures. Results of a multi-institutional outcomes database. Chest. 2008;134:514–9.
73. Amjadi K, Voduc N, Cruysberghs Y, et al. Impact of interventional bronchoscopy on quality of life in malignant airway obstruction. Respiration. 2008;76: 421–8.
74. Oviatt PL, Stather DR, Michaud G, MacEachern P, Tremblay A. Exercise capacity, lung function, and quality of life after interventional bronchoscopy. J Thorac Oncol. 2011;6:38–42.
75. Hans CC, Prasetyo D, Wright GM. Endobronchial palliation using Nd:YAG laser is associated with improved survival when combined with multimodal adjuvant treatments. J Thorac Oncol. 2007;2: 59–64.
76. Razi SS, Levovics RS, Schwartz G, et al. Timely airway stenting improves survival in patients with malignant central airway obstruction. Ann Thorac Surg. 2010;90:1088–93.
77. Venuta F, Rendina EA, Dr Giacomo T, et al. Endoscopic treatment of lung cancer invading the airway before induction chemotherapy and surgical resection. Eur J Cardiothorac Surg. 2001;20:464–7.
78. Chhajed PN, Baty F, Pless M, Somandin S, Tamm M, Brutsche MH. Outcome of treated advanced non-small cell lung cancer with and without central airway obstruction. Chest. 2006;130:1803–7.
79. Daddi G, Puma F, Avenia N, Santoprete S, Casadei S, Urbani M. Resection with curative intent after endoscopic treatment of airway obstruction. Ann Thorac Surg. 1998;65:203–7.
80. Venuta F, Rendina EA, De Giacomo T, et al. Nd:YAG laser resection of lung cancer invading the airway as a bridge to surgery and palliative treatment. Ann Thorac Surg. 2002;74:995–8.
81. Bolliger CT, Suteja TG, Strausz J, Freitag L. Therapeutic bronchoscopy with immediate effects:laser, electrocautery, argon plasma coagulation, and stents. Eur Respir J. 2006;27:1258–71.
82. Vergnon JM, Huber RM, Moghissi K. Place of cryotherapy, brachytherapy, and photodynamic therapy

in therapeutic bronchoscopy of lung cancers. Eur Respir J. 2006;28:200–18.

83. Lunn W, Garland R, Ashiku S, Thurer RL, Feller-Kopman D, Ernst A. Microdebrider bronchoscopy: a new tool for the interventional bronchoscopist. Ann Thorac Surg. 2005;80:1485–8.
84. Lunn W, Bagherzadegan N, Munjampappi SK, Feller-Kopman D, Ernst A. Initial experience with a rotating airway microdebrider. J Bronchol. 2008;15: 91–4.
85. Hautmann H, Gamarra F, Jurgen K, Huber RM. Fiberoptic bronchoscopic balloon dilatation in malignant tracheobronchial stenosis. Chest. 2001; 120:43–9.
86. Noppen M, Schlesser M, Meysman M, Peche R, Vincken W. Bronchoscopic balloon dilatation in the combined management of postintubation stenosis of trachea in adults. Chest. 1997;112:1136–40.
87. Lee KH, Ko GY, Song HY, Shim TS, Kim WS. Benign tracheobronchial stenosis: long term clinical experience with balloon dilation. J Vasc Interv Radiol. 2002;13(9 pt 1):909–14.
88. Sheski FD, Mathur PN. Long-term results of fiberoptic bronchoscopic balloon dilation in the management of benign tracheobronchial stenosis. Chest. 1998;114:796–800.
89. DeGarcia J, Culebras M, Alverez A, et al. Bronchoscopic balloon dilatation in the management of bronchial stenosis following lung transplantation. Respir Med. 2007;101:27–33.
90. Mayse ML, Greenheck J, Friedman M, Kovitz KL. Successful bronchoscopic balloon dilation on non-malignant tracheobronchial obstruction without fluoroscopy. Chest. 2004;126:634–7.
91. Shitrit D, Kuchuk M, Zismanov V, et al. Bronchoscopic balloon dilation of tracheobronchial stenosis: long-term follow-up. Eur J Cardiothorac Surg. 2010;38:198–210.
92. Kim JH, Shin JH, Song HY, et al. Tracheobronchial laceration after balloon dilation for benign strictures. Incidence and clinical significance. Chest. 2007;131:1114–7.
93. van Boxem TJ, Westerga J, Venmans BJ, Postmus PE, Suteja G. Tissue effects of bronchoscopic electrocautery: bronchoscopic appearance and histologic changes of bronchial wall after electrocautery. Chest. 2000;117:887–91.
94. Sutedja K, van Kralingen, Schramel FMNH, Postmus PE. Fiberoptic bronchoscopic electrosurgery under local anesthesia for rapid palliation in patients with central airway malignancies: a preliminary report. Thorax. 1994;49:1243–6.
95. Coulter TD, Mehta AC. The heat is on. Impact of endobronchial electrosurgery on the need for Nd-YAG laser photoresection. Chest. 2000;118: 516–21.
96. Wahidi MM, Unroe MA, Adlakha N, Beyea M, Shofer SL. The use of electrosurgery as the primary ablation modality for malignant and benign airway obstruction. J Thorac Oncol. 2011;6:1516–20.
97. van Boxem TJ, Venmans BJ, Schramel FM, et al. Radiographically occult lung cancer treated with fiberoptic eloectrocautery: a pilot study of simple and inexpensive technique. Eur Respir J. 1998;11: 169–72.
98. Sutedja T, van Boxem TJ, Schramel FM, et al. Endobronchial electrocautery is an excellent alternative for Nd:YAG laser to treat airway tumors. J Bronchol. 1997;4:101–5.
99. Horinouchi H, Miyazawa T, Takada K, et al. Safety study of endobronchial electrosurgery for tracheobronchial lesions. Multicenter prospective study. J Bronchol. 2008;15:228–32.
100. Reichle G, Freitag L, Kullman HJ, Prenzel R, Macha HN, Farin G. Argon plasma coagulation in bronchology: a new method-alternative or complimentary? J Bronchol. 2000;7:109–17.
101. Morice RC, Ece T, Keus L. Endobronchial argon plasma coagulation for treatment of hemoptysis and neoplastic airway obstruction. Chest. 2001;119: 781–7.
102. Okada S, Yamauchi H, Ishimori S, satoh S, Sugawara H, Tanaba Y. Endoscopic surgery with a flexible bronchoscope and argon plasma coagulation for tracheobronchial tumors. J Thorac Cardiovasc Surg. 2001;121:180–3.
103. Crosta C, Spaggiari L, De Stefano A, et al. Endoscopic argon plasma coagulation for palliative treatment of malignant airway obstruction: early results in 47 cases. Lung Cancer. 2001;33:75–80.
104. Keller CA, Hinerman R, Singh A, Alverez F. The use of endoscopic argon plasma coagulation in airway complications after solid organ transplantation. Chest. 2001;119:1968–75.
105. Reddy C, Majid A, Michaud G, et al. Gas embolism following bronchoscopic argon plasma coagulation. A case series. Chest. 2008;134:1066–9.
106. Chan AL, Tharratt RS, Siefkin AD, Albertson TE, Volz EG, Allen RP. Nd:YAG laser bronchoscopy. Rigid or fiberoptic mode? Chest. 1990;98:271–5.
107. Brutinel WM, Cortese DA, Edell DA, McDougall JC, Prakash UB. Complications of Nd:YAG laser therapy. Chest. 1989;94:902–3.
108. Cavaliere S, Venuta F, Foccoli P, Toninelli C, La Face B. Endoscopic treatment of malignant airway obstructions in 2,008 patients. Chest. 1996;110: 1536–42.
109. Dumon JF, Shapshay S, Bourcereau J, et al. Principles of safety in application of neodymium-YAG laser in bronchology. Chest. 1984;86:163–8.
110. Dumon JF, Reboud E, Garbe L, Aucomte F, Meric B. Treatment of tracheobronchial lesions by laser photoresection. Chest. 1982;81:278–84.
111. Cavaliere S, Foccoli P, Farina PL. Nd:YAG loaser bronchoscopy. A five year experience with 1396 applications in 1000 patients. Chest. 1988;94: 15–21.
112. Kvale PA, Eichenhorn MS, Radke JR, Miks V. YAG laser photoresection of lesions obstructing the central airways. Chest. 1985;87:283–8.

113. Brutinel WM, Cortese DA, McDougall JC, Gillio RG, Bergstralh EJ. A two-year experience with the neodymium-YAG laser in endobronchial obstruction. Chest. 1987;91:159–65.
114. Hujala K, Sipila J, Grenman R. Endotracheal and bronchial laser surgery in the treatment of malignant and benign lower airway obstruction. Eur Arch Otorhinolaryngol. 2003;260:219–22.
115. Hermes A, Heigener D, Gatzemeier U, Schatz J, Reck M. Efficacy and safety of bronchoscopic laser therapy in patients with tracheal and bronchial obstruction: a retrospective single institution report. Clin Respir J. 2012;6:67–71.
116. Toty L, Personne C, Colchen A, Vourch G. Bronchoscopic management of tracheal lesions using the neodymium yttrium aluminum garnet laser. Thorax. 1981;36:175–8.
117. George PJM, Garrett CPO, Hetzel MR. Role of neodymium YAG laser in the management of tracheal tumors. Thorax. 1987;42:440–4.
118. Stanopoulos IT, Beamis JF, Martinez FJ, Vergos K, Shapshay SM. Laser bronchoscopy in respiratory failure from malignant airway obstruction. Crit Care Med. 1993;21:386–91.
119. Hetzel MR, Nixon C, Edmondstone WM, et al. Laser therapy in 100 tracheobronchial tumors. Thorax. 1985;40:341–5.
120. Gilmartin JJ, Veale D, Cooper BG, Keavey PM, Gibson GJ, Morritt GN. Effects of laser treatment on respiratory function in malignant narrowing of central airways. Thorax. 1987;42:578–82.
121. George PMJ, Clarke G, Tolfree S, Garrett CPO, Hetzel MR. Changes in regional ventilation and perfusion of lung after endoscopic laser treatment. Thorax. 1990;45:248–53.
122. Venuta F, Rendina EA, De Giacomo T, et al. Nd:YAG laser resection of lung cancer invading the airway as bridge to surgery and palliative treatment. Ann Thorac Surg. 2002;74:995–8.
123. Eichenhorn MS, Kvale PA, Miks VM, et al. Initial combination therapy with YAG laser photoresection and irradiation for inoperable non-small cell carcinoma of lung. A preliminary report. Chest. 1986;89: 782–5.
124. Gelb AF, Epstein JD. Neodymium-yttrium aluminum garnet laser in lung cancer. Ann Thorac Surg. 1987;43:164–7.
125. Desai SJ, Mehta AC, VanderBurg MS, Golish JA, Ahmad M. Survival experience following Nd:YAG laser photoresection for primary bronchogenic carcinoma. Chest. 1988;94:939–44.
126. Shea JM, Allen RP, Tharratt RS, Chan AL, Seifkin AD. Survival of patients undergoing Nd:YAG laser therapy compared with Nd:YAG laser therapy and brachytherapy for malignant airway disease. Chest. 1993;103:1023–31.
127. Moghissi K, Dixon K. Bronchoscopic Nd:YAG laser treatment in lung cancer, 30 year on: an institutional review. Lasers Med Sci. 2006;21:186–91.
128. Casey KR, Fairfax WR, Smith SJ, Dixon JA. Intratracheal fire ignited by the Nd:YAG laser during treatment of tracheal stenosis. Chest. 1983;84: 295–6.
129. Krawtz S, Mehta AC, Wiedemann HP, et al. Nd:YAG laser induced endobronchial burn. Management and long term follow-up. Chest. 1989;95:916–8.
130. Ilgner J, Falter F, Westhofen M. Long-term follow up after laser induced endotracheal fire. J Laryngol Otol. 2002;116:213–5.
131. van Boxem T, Muller M, Venmans B, Postmus B, Suteja T. Nd:YAG laser vs. bronchoscopic electrocautery for palliation of symptomatic airway obstruction: a cost-effectiveness study. Chest. 1999;116:1108–12.
132. Walsh D, Maiwand MO, Nath A, Lockwood P, Lloyd M, Saab M. Bronchoscopic cryotherapy for advanced bronchial carcinoma. Thorax. 1990;45:509–13.
133. Mathur PN, Wolfe KM, Busk MF, Briet M, Datzman M. Fiberoptic bronchoscopic cryotherapy in the management of tracheobronchial obstruction. Chest. 1996;110:718–23.
134. Lee SH, Choi WJ, Sung SW, et al. Endoscopic cryotherapy of lung and bronchial tumors: a systemic review. Korean J Intern Med. 2011;26:137–44.
135. Marasso A, Gallo E, Massagglia GM, Onoscuri M, Bernardi V. Cryosurgery in bronchoscopic treatment of tracheobronchial stenosis. Indications, limits, personal experience. Chest. 1993;103:472–4.
136. Maiwand MO. Cryotherapy for advanced carcinoma of the trachea and bronchi. Br Med J. 1986;293: 181–2.
137. Asimakopoulos G, Beeson J, Evan J, Maiwand MO. Cryosurgery for malignant endobronchial tumors. Analysis of outcome. Chest. 2005;127:2007–14.
138. Maiwand MO. The role of cryosurgery in palliation of tracheobronchial carcinoma. Eur J Cardiothorac Surg. 1999;15:764–8.
139. Bertoletti L, Elleuch R, Kaczmarek D, Jean-Francois R, Vergnon JM. Bronchoscopic cryotherapy treatment of isolated endoluminal typical carcinoid tumors. Chest. 2006;130:1405–11.
140. Deygas N, Froudarakis M, Ozenne G, Vergnon JM. Cryotherapy in early superficial bronchogenic carcinoma. Chest. 2001;120:26–31.
141. Vergnon JM, Schmitt T, Alamartine E, Barthelemy JC, Fournel P, Emonot A. Initial combined cryotherapy and irradiation for unresectable non-small cell lung cancer. Preliminary results. Chest. 1992;102: 1436–40.
142. Forest V, Hadjeres R, Bertrand R, Jean-Francois R. Optimization and molecular signaling of apoptosis in sequential cryotherapy and chemotherapy combination in human A549 lung cancer xenografts in SCID mice. Br J Cancer. 2009;100:1896–902.
143. Forest V, Peoch M, Campos L, Guyotat D, Vergnon JM. Benefits of a combined treatment of cryotherapy and chemotherapy on tumor growth and late cryo-induced angiogenesis in a non-small cell lung cancer model. Lung Cancer. 2006;54:79–86.

144. Hetzel M, Hetzel J, Schumann C, Marx N, Babiak A. Cryorecanalization: a new approach for the immediate management of acute airway obstruction. J Thorac Cardiovasc Surg. 2004;127:1427–31.
145. Schumann C, Hetzel M, Babiak A, et al. Endobronchial tumor debulking with a flexible cryoprobe for immediate treatment of malignant stenosis. J Thorac Cardiovasc Surg. 2010;1309:997–1000.
146. Edell ES, Cortese DA. Photodynamic therapy: its uses in management of bronchogenic carcinoma. Clin Chest Med. 1995;16:455–63.
147. Cecic I, Minchinton AI, Korbelik M. The impact of complement activation on tumor oxygenation during photodynamic therapy. Photochem Photobiol. 2007; 83:1049–55.
148. Dougherty TJ, Marcus SL. Photodynamic therapy. Eur J Cancer. 1992;28A:1734–42.
149. Moghissi K, Dixon K, Stringer M, Freeman T, Thorpe A, Brown S. The place of bronchoscopic photodynamic therapy in advanced unresectable lung cancer: experience on 100 cases. Eur J Cardiothorac Surg. 1999;15:1–6.
150. Ernst A, Garland R, Beamis JF. Photodynamic treatment in lung cancer. J Bronchol. 1996;6:285–8.
151. Mehrishi S, Ost D. Photodynamic therapy. J Bronchol. 2002;9:218–22.
152. McCaughan JS, Williams TS. Photodynamic therapy for endobronchial malignant disease: a prospective fourteen year study. J Thorac Cardiovasc Surg. 1997; 114:940–7.
153. Ernst A, Freitag L, Feller-Koppman D, LoCicero J, Ost D. Photodynamic therapy for endobronchial obstruction is safely performed with flexible bronchoscopy. J Bronchol. 2003;10:260–3.
154. Moghissi K, Dixon K, Hudson E, Stringer M, Brown S. Endoscopic laser therapy in malignant tracheobronchial obstruction using sequential Nd:YAG laser and photodynamic therapy. Thorax. 1997;52:281–3.
155. Freitag L, Ernst A, Thomas M, Prenzel R, Wahlers B, Macha HN. Sequential photodynamic therapy (PDT) and high dose brachytherapy for endobronchial tumor control in patients with limited bronchogenic carcinoma. Thorax. 2004;59:790–3.
156. Moghissi K, Dixon K, Parsons RJ. A controlled trial of Nd:YAG laser versus photodynamic therapy for advanced malignant bronchial obstruction. Laser in Med Sci. 1993;8:269–73.
157. Diaz-Jimenez JP, Martinez-Bellarin JE, Llunell A, Farrero E, Rodriguez A, Castro MJ. Efficacy and safety of photodynamic therapy versus Nd:YAG laser resection in NSCLC with airway obstruction. Eur Respir J. 1999;14:800–5.
158. Moghissi K, Dixon K, Andrew J, Thorpe C, Stringer M, Oxtoby C. Photodynamic therapy in early central lung cancer: a treatment option for patients ineligible for surgical resection. Thorax. 2007;62:391–5.
159. Corti L, Toniolo L, Boso C, et al. Long-term survival of patients treated with photodynamic therapy for carcinoma in situ and early non-small cell lung carcinoma. Lasers Surg Med. 2007;39:394–402.
160. Mathur PN, Edell E, Sutedja T, Vergnon JM. Treatment of early non-small cell lung cancer. Chest. 2003;123:176–80.
161. Moghissi K, Dixon K. Is bronchoscopic photodynamic therapy a therapeutic option in lung cancer? Eur Respir J. 2003;22:535–41.
162. Nag S, Kelly JF, Horton JL, et al. Brachytherapy for carcinoma of the lung. Oncology (Winston Park). 2001;15:371–81.
163. Ozkok S, Karakoyun-Celik O, Goksel T, et al. High dose rate endobronchial brachytherapy in the management of lung cancer: response and toxicity evaluation in 158 patients. Lung Cancer. 2008;62:326–33.
164. Kelly JF, Delclos ME, Morice RC, et al. High dose rate brachytherapy effectively palliates symptoms due to airway tumors: the 10-year M.D. Anderson cancer center experience. Int J Radiat Oncol Biol Phys. 2000;48:697–702.
165. Anacak Y, Mogulcok N, Ozkok S, et al. High dose rate endobronchial brachytherapy in combination with external beam radiation therapy for Stage III non-small cell lung cancer. Lung Cancer. 2011;34:253–9.
166. Hernandez P, Gursahaney A, Roman T, et al. High dose rate brachytherapy for the local control of endobronchial carcinoma following external radiation. Thorax. 1996;51:354–8.
167. DuRand IA, Barber PV, Goldring J, et al. British Thoracic Society guidelines for advanced diagnostic and therapeutic flexible bronchoscopy in adults. Thorax. 2011;66:iii1–21.
168. Guarnaschelli JN, Jose BO. Palliative high dose rate endobronchial brachytherapy for recurrent carcinoma: The University of Louisville experience. J Palliat Med. 2010;13:981–9.
169. Goldman JM, Bulman AS, Rathemell AJ, Carey BM, Muers MF, Joslin CA. Physiological effect of endobronchial radiotherapy in patients with major airway occlusion by carcinoma. Thorax. 1993;48:110–4.
170. Mallick I, Sharma SC, Behera D. Endobronchial brachytherapy for symptom palliation in non-small cell lung cancer- analysis of symptom response, endoscopic improvement and quality of life. Lung Cancer. 2007;55:313–8.
171. Chella A, Ambrogi MC, Ribechini A, et al. Combined Nd:YAG laser/HDR brachytherapy versus Nd:YAG laser only in malignant central airway involvement: a prospective randomized study. Lung Cancer. 2000;27:169–75.
172. Stout R, Barber P, Burt P, et al. Clinical and quality of life outcomes in the first United Kingdom randomized trial of endobronchial brachytherapy (intraluminal radiotherapy) vs external beam radiotherapy in palliative treatment of inoperable non-small cell lung cancer. Radiother Oncol. 2000;56: 323–7.
173. Langendijk H, de Jong J, Tjwa M, et al. External irradiation versus external irradiation plus endobronchial brachytherapy in inoperable non-small cell

lung cancer: a prospective randomized study. Radiother Oncol. 2001;58:257–68.
174. Bastin KT, Mehta MP, Kinsella TJ. Thoracic volume radiation sparing following endobronchial brachytherapy: a quantitative analysis. Int J Radiat Oncol Biol Phys. 1993;25:703–7.
175. Fuwa N, Matsumoto A, Kamata M, et al. External irradiation and intraluminal irradiation using middle dose rate iridium in patients with roentgenographically occult lung cancer. Int J Radiat Oncol Biol Phys. 2001;49:965–71.
176. Marsiglia H, Baldeyrou P, Lartigau E, et al. High dose rate brachytherapy as sole modality for early stage endobronchial carcinoma. Int J Radiat Oncol Biol Phys. 2000;47:665–72.
177. Hennequin C, Bleichner O, Tredaniel J, et al. Long-term results of endobronchial brachytherapy: a curative treatment? Int J Radiat Oncol Biol Phys. 2007; 67:425–30.
178. Guilcher MA, Prevost B, Sunyach MP, et al. High dose rate brachytherapy for non-small cell carcinoma: a retrospective study of 226 patients. Int J Radiat Oncol Biol Phys. 2011;79:1112–6.
179. Halkos ME, Godette KD, Lawrence EC, Miller JI. High dose rate brachytherapy in the management of lung transplant airway stenosis. Ann Thorac Surg. 2003;76:381–4.
180. Brenner B, Kramer MR, Katz A, et al. High dose rate brachytherapy for non-malignant airway obstruction: new treatment option. Chest. 2003;124: 1605–10.
181. Madu CN, Machuzak MS, Sterman DH, et al. High dose rate brachytherapy for the treatment of benign obstructive endobronchial granulation tissue. Int J Radiat Oncol Biol Phys. 2006;66:1450–6.
182. Tendulkar RD, Fleming PA, Reddy CA, Gildea TA, Machuzak M, Mehta AC. High dose rate endobronchial brachytherapy for recurrent airway obstruction from hyperplastic granulation tissue. Int J Radiat Oncol Biol Phys. 2008;70:701–6.
183. Hara R, Itami J, Aruga T, et al. Risk factors for massive hemoptysis after endobronchial brachytherapy in patients with tracheobronchial malignancies. Cancer. 2001;92:2623–7.
184. Gollis SW, Ryder WD, Burt PA, et al. Massive hemoptysis, death and other morbidity associated with high dose rate intraluminal radiotherapy for carcinoma of bronchus. Radiother Oncol. 1996;39: 105–16.
185. Langendijk JA, Tjwa MK, de Jong JM, et al. Massive hemoptysis after radiotherapy in inoperable non-small cell lung carcinoma: is endobronchial radiotherapy really a risk factor? Radiother Oncol. 1998; 49:175–83.
186. Bedwinek J, Petty A, Bruton C, et al. The use of high dose rate endobronchial brachytherapy to palliate symptomatic endobronchial recurrence of previously irradiated bronchogenic carcinoma. Int J Radiat Oncol Biol Phys. 1991;22:23–30.
187. Speiser B, Spratling I. Remote afterloading brachytherapy for local control of endobronchial carcinoma. Int J Radiat Oncol Biol Phys. 1993;25: 579–89.
188. Speiser B, Spratling I. Intermediate dose rate remote afterloading brachytherapy for intraluminal control of bronchogenic carcinoma. Int J Radiat Oncol Biol Phys. 1990;18:1443–8.
189. Saad CP, Murthy S, Krizmaniach G, Mehta AC. Self-expandable metallic airway stents and flexible bronchoscopy. Long-term outcome analysis Chest. 2003;124:1993–9.
190. Husain SA, Finch D, Ahmad M, Morgan A, Hetzel MR. Long term follow up of ultraflex metallic stents in benign and malignant airway obstruction. Ann Thorac Surg. 2007;83:1251–6.
191. Wood DE, Liu YH, Vallieres E, Karmey-Jones R, Mulligan MS. Airway stenting for malignant and benign tracheobronchial stenosis. Ann Thorac Surg. 2003;76:167–74.
192. Noppen M, Stratakos G, Amjadi K, et al. Stenting allows weaning and extubation in ventilator or tracheostomy dependency secondary to benign airway disease. Respir Med. 2007;101:139–45.
193. Breitenbucher A, Chhajed PN, Brtusche MH, Mordasini C, Schilter D, Tamm M. Long term follow up and survival after ultraflex stent insertion in the management of complex malignant airway stenosis. Respiration. 2008;75:443–9.
194. Reinfuss M, Mucha-Malecka A, Walasek T, et al. Palliative thoracic radiotherapy in non-small cell lung cancer. An analysis of 1250 patients. Palliation of symptoms, tolerance and toxicity. Lung Cancer. 2011;71:344–9.
195. Majid OA, Lee S, Khushalani S, Seydel HG. The response of atelectasis from lung cancer to radiation therapy. Int J Radiat Oncol Biol Phys. 1986;12: 231–2.
196. Chetty KG, Moran EM, Sassoon CS, Viravathana T, Light RW. Effect of radiation therapy on bronchial obstruction due to bronchogenic carcinoma. Chest. 1989;95:582–4.
197. Reddy SP, Marks JE. Total atelectasis of the lung secondary to malignant airway obstruction. Response to radiation therapy. Am J Clin Oncol. 1990;13: 394–400.
198. Santos RS, Raftopoulos Y, Keenan RJ, Hala A, Maley RH, Landreneau RJ. Bronchoscopic palliation of primary lung cancer. Single or multimodality therapy? Surg Endoscopy. 2004;18:931–6.
199. Jeon K, Kim H, Yu CM, et al. Rigid bronchoscopic intervention in patients with respiratory failure caused by malignant central airway obstruction. J Thorac Oncol. 2006;1:319–23.
200. Neyman K, Sundest A, Espinoza A, Kongerud J, Fosse E. Survival and complications after interventional bronchoscopy in malignant central airway obstruction. A single center experience. J Bronchol Intervent Pulmonol. 2011;18:233–8.

Airway Stents

9

Pyng Lee and Atul C. Mehta

Abstract

Stenting is commonly used as a method of palliation for patients with central airway obstruction due to malignancy. Stents are also used to maintain airway patency following dilatation of post-inflammatory and infectious strictures, for airway dehiscence after lung transplantation as well as in the management of tracheo-bronchomalacia. Covered stents can be applied to seal fistulas between trachea or bronchi and the esophagus, and dehiscence of pneumonectomy stump. Careful patient selection, characteristics of the airway stenosis, physician's expertise, and availability of equipment determine the type of stent used. Placement of tube stents requires rigid bronchoscopy and dilatation of strictures beforehand while metal stents can be applied using a flexible bronchoscope. Advantages and disadvantages of commonly used airway stents, techniques as well as the complications associated with stent placement are discussed.

Keywords

Airway stents • Covered stents • Central airway obstruction • Rigid bronchoscopy

Introduction

A stent is a hollow, cylindrical prosthesis that maintains luminal patency and provides support for a graft or anastomosis. It is named after Charles Stent, a British dentist who developed the first dental splints in the nineteenth century. Airway stenting has been practiced for over a century and the indications for stent placement are to protect the airway lumen from tumor or granulation tissue ingrowth, counterbalance the extrinsic pressure exerted on the airway, or both

P. Lee, M.D. (✉)
Yong Loo Lin School of Medicine, National University of Singapore, NUHS Tower Block, Level 10, 1E Kent Ridge Road, Singapore 119228, Singapore

Division of Respiratory and Critical Care Medicine, National University Hospital, NUHS Tower Block, Level 10, 1E Kent Ridge Road, Singapore 119228, Singapore
e-mail: pynglee@hotmail.com

A.C. Mehta, M.B.B.S.
Respiratory Institute, Lerner College of Medicine, Cleveland Clinic, Cleveland, OH 44195, USA

A.C. Mehta and P. Jain (eds.), *Interventional Bronchoscopy: A Clinical Guide*, Respiratory Medicine 10,
DOI 10.1007/978-1-62703-395-4_9, © Springer Science+Business Media New York 2013

[1]. The covering of the stent provides the barrier effect, while dynamic and static properties determine the splinting effect [2].

The first stents were implanted surgically by Trendelenburg [3] and Bond [4] for the treatment of airway strictures, which quickly progressed to endoscopic application by Brunings and Albrecht in 1915 [5]. In 1965, Montgomery designed a T-tube with an external side limb made of silicone and rubber for subglottic stenosis. Silicone has become the most commonly used material for stents [6]; however, the designs of the silicone stents at that time abolished the innate mucociliary mechanisms essential to clear the airway of secretions. The real breakthrough came when Dumon presented a dedicated tracheobronchial prosthesis that can be introduced with the rigid bronchoscope [7]. These straight stents are made of silicone with studs on the outer wall that allow ciliary action, are relatively inexpensive, and can be easily removed and exchanged when needed. An important factor limiting their widespread use is the need for rigid bronchoscopy, and based on ACCP survey only 5 % of pulmonologists in North America are trained in rigid bronchoscopy [8]. Moreover, silicone stents are poorly tolerated in the subglottis and tend to migrate when deployed for complex tracheal strictures. These disadvantages have led to modifications of metal stents originally developed for the vascular system for use in the tracheobronchial tree [9, 10]. Although metal stents are easy to apply with the flexible bronchoscope they cause significant granulation tissue ingrowth around the struts, and epithelialization into the airway wall makes their removal difficult and challenging [10]. Metal and tube stents can be used for malignant strictures, whereas in benign diseases silicone and hybrid stents are preferred to avoid long term complications associated with their metal counterparts. Therefore, an ideal stent is one that is easy to insert and remove, that can be customized to fit the dimensions and shape of the stricture, that reestablishes luminal patency by resisting compressive forces but sufficiently elastic to conform to airway contours without causing ischemia or erosion into adjacent structures, that is not prone to migration, that is biocompatible, nonirritating, and that does not precipitate infection, promote granulation tissue, nor interferes with airway ciliary action necessary to clear secretions, and that is affordable. The search for an ideal stent has become the holy grail of interventional pulmonologists, radiologists, thoracic surgeons and otolaryngologists involved in the management of patients with central airway obstruction.

Indications for Airway Stenting (Table 9.1)

Approximately 30 % of patients with lung cancer will present with central airway obstruction, of which 35 % will die as a result of asphyxia, hemoptysis, and postobstructive pneumonia [11]. Airway stenting is a valuable adjunct to other bronchoscopic techniques (see Chap. 8) and the indications are to reestablish patency of the

Table 9.1 Indications for airway stenting

Malignant neoplasm

1. Airway obstruction from extrinsic bronchial compression or submucosal disease
2. Obstruction from endobronchial tumor when patency is <50 % after bronchoscopic laser therapy
3. Aggressive endobronchial tumor growth and recurrence despite repetitive laser treatments
4. Loss of cartilaginous support from tumor destruction
5. Sequential insertion of airway and esophageal stents for tracheoesophageal fistulas

Benign airway disease

1. Fibrotic scar or bottleneck stricture following
    (a) Post-traumatic: intubation, tracheostomy, laser, balloon bronchoplasty
    (b) Post-infectious: endobronchial tuberculosis, histoplasmosis-fibrosing mediastinitis, herpes virus, diphtheria, klebsiella rhinoscleroma
    (c) Post-inflammatory: Wegener's granulomatosis, sarcoidosis, inflammatory bowel disease, foreign body aspiration
    (d) Post-lung transplantation anastomotic complications
2. Tracheobronchomalacia
    (a) Diffuse: idiopathic, relapsing polychrondritis, tracheobronchomegaly (Mounier-Kuhn syndrome)
    (b) Focal: tracheostomy, radiation therapy, post-lung transplantation
3. Benign tumors
    (a) Papillomatosis
    (b) Amyloidosis

compressed or stenosed airway, to support weakened cartilages in tracheo-bronchomalacia as well as seal tracheobronchial esophageal fistula [11, 12]. Although primary tumor resection and airway reconstruction provide the most reliable treatment option, most central airway obstructions due to malignancy are advanced at the time of diagnosis. Therefore, therapeutic bronchoscopy coupled with airway stenting not only results in rapid relief of symptoms and improved quality of life, it also allows time for adjuvant chemoradiotherapy that might lead to prolonged survival [1, 11–14]. Contrary to previous perception, malignant airway obstruction is not a poor prognostic sign if treated appropriately. Chhajed and coworkers demonstrated no survival difference between patients with malignant central airway obstruction treated with laser, stent or both followed by chemotherapy (8.2 months) versus those without airway obstruction on palliative chemotherapy (median 8.4 months) [15].

Benign strictures secondary to post-intubation injury, inflammatory and infectious disease may require stenting if the patient's underlying disease or associated comorbidity prohibits definitive surgical repair. Lung transplant recipients who develop airway dehiscence in the immediate postoperative period may benefit from placement of endobronchial stents. The Cleveland clinic experience of using uncovered metal stent as alternative treatment for high grade anastomotic dehiscence after lung transplantation has demonstrated not only satisfactory airway healing, stent removal is also not difficult if performed within 8 weeks of placement, before epithelialization with the airway wall occurs [16].

Types of Stents

A myriad of stents are available and the biomechanical properties depend on the materials used as well as how they are constructed. They are divided into three groups: (1) tube (polymer): Montgomery T-tube, Dumon, Polyflex, Noppen, Hood; (2) metal (covered or uncovered): Gianturco, Palmaz, Ultraflex; and (3) hybrid (silicone reinforced by metal rings): Orlowski, Dynamic (Figs. 9.1 and 9.2). Tube stents are inexpensive and can be repositioned and removed without difficulty. Their disadvantages include stent migration, granuloma formation, mucus plugging, unfavorable wall to inner diameter thickness; insufficient flexibility to conform to irregular airways; difficult to position in distal airways; interference with mucociliary clearance, and need

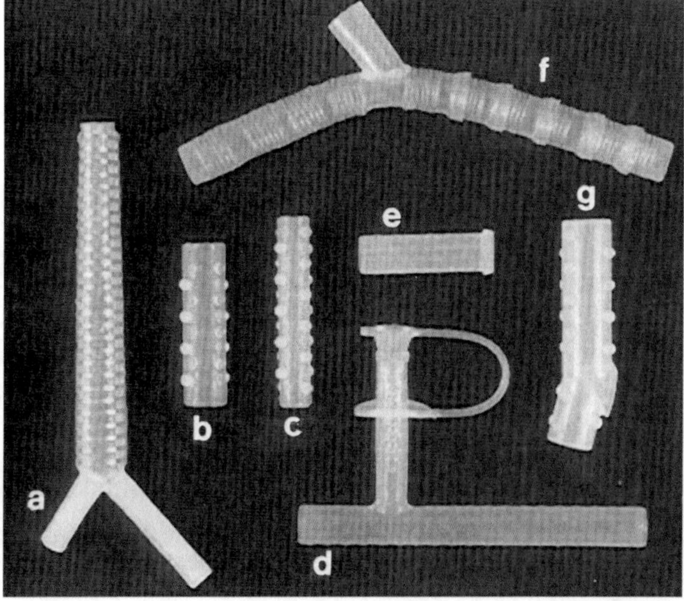

Fig. 9.1 Types of tube and hybrid stents. (**a**) Rusch stent, (**b**) Dumon tracheal stent, (**c**) Dumon bronchial stent, (**d**) Montgomery T-tube, (**e**) Hood bronchial stent, (**f**) Orlowski stent, (**g**) Hood custom tracheobronchial stent

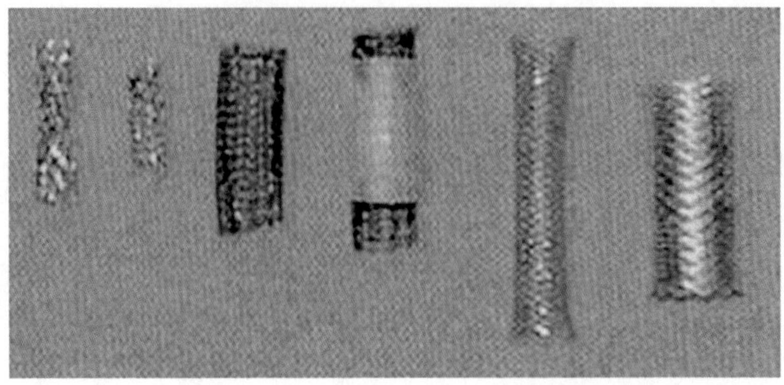

Fig. 9.2 Types of metallic stents. From *left* to *right*: Palmaz stent, Strecker stent, uncovered Ultraflex stent, covered Ultraflex stent, uncovered Wallstent, covered Wallstent

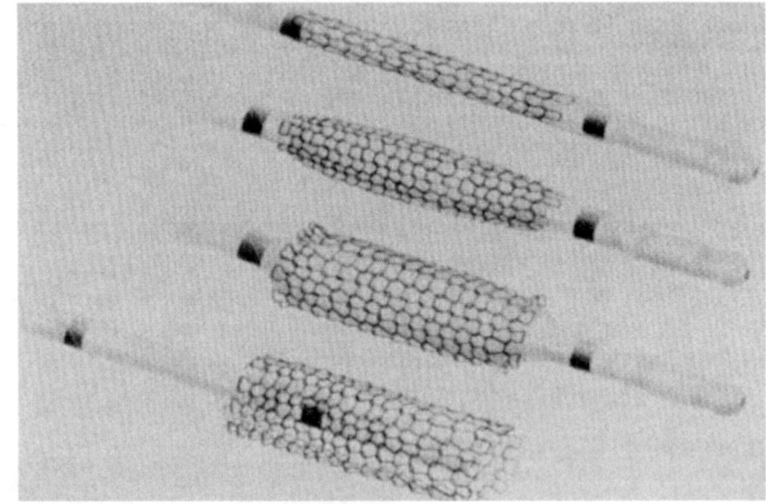

Fig. 9.3 Balloon expandable Palmaz and Strecker stents. A balloon expandable stent consists of a stent balloon assembly and relies on the balloon to dilate the stent to its correct diameter

for rigid bronchoscopy for placement. Rigid bronchoscopy poses a major obstacle since pulmonologists' training in this technique has dramatically declined worldwide [8].

Metal stents have gained popularity because of ease of insertion. They can be deployed at an outpatient setting with flexible bronchoscopy [17, 18], and are categorized by the method of deployment. A balloon-expandable stent relies on the balloon to dilate it to its correct diameter at the target site (Fig. 9.3) while self-expanding stent has a shape memory to assume its predetermined configuration after release from delivery catheter (Fig. 9.4). Other advantages include their radiopaque nature that allows radiographic identification, greater airway cross-sectional diameters, ability to conform to tortuous airways, preservation of mucociliary clearance, and ventilation when placed across a lobar bronchial orifice. Major disadvantages as indicated above are granulation tissue formation within the stent, infection, and difficulty in removal or repositioning following epithelialization which occurs in 6–8 weeks (Fig. 9.5a, b).

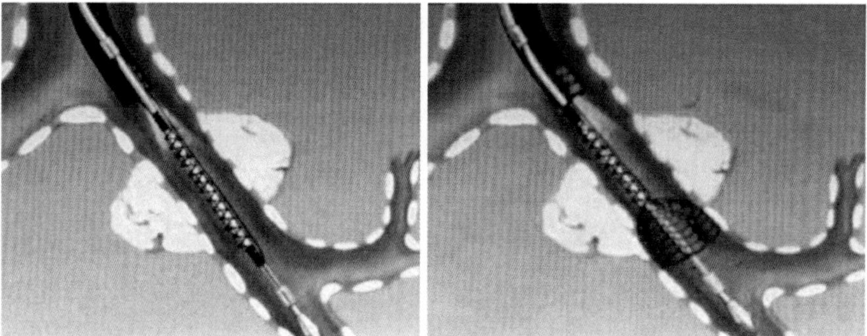

Fig. 9.4 Self-expanding ultraflex stent deployment system: Ultraflex stent is mounted on introduction catheter with crochet knots, pulling the thread releases stent

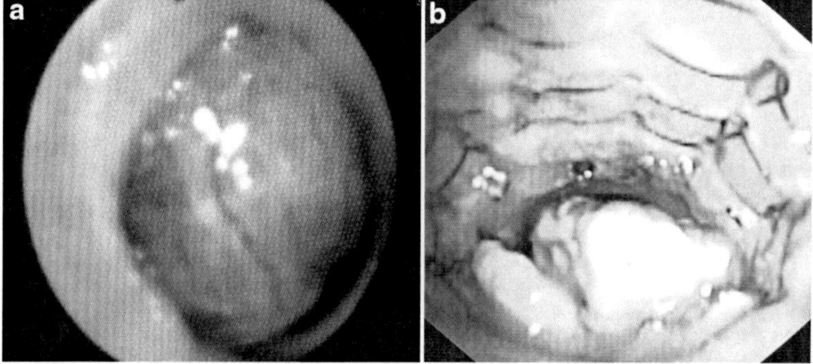

Fig. 9.5 Stent-related complications. (**a**) Obstructing granuloma distal to silicon Dumon stent (**b**) Obstructing granuloma distal to Ultraflex stent with *Pseudomonas* infection

Choice of Stent (Table 9.2)

Besides the site, shape and length of stricture, presence or absence of tracheobronchial malacia or fistula determine choice of stent. Proper sizing of the stent in relation to the dimensions of the trachea or bronchus is of utmost importance to avoid complications such as migration, mucus plugging, granulation, and tumor ingrowth. Tube stent placement requires specialized equipment, training and competency in rigid bronchoscopy, while metal stents can be inserted via flexible bronchoscopy in an outpatient setting. The ease of placement should not lead to the erroneous choice of the easiest stent over the best one for a given condition. The endoscopist should consider the patient's prognosis and airway pathology before deciding type of stent and its dimensions notably if the stent will confer benefit or prohibit curative surgical procedure later as well as expertise, equipment and team to place the stent. Tube stents are preferred for benign strictures since they are easy to remove and replace with minimal mucosal damage which might preclude subsequent surgery. In malacia secondary to relapsing polychondritis or tracheomegaly syndrome, uncovered metal stents are preferred as they do not interfere with mucociliary clearance and have low migration rate [19, 20]. In expiratory dynamic airway collapse associated with chronic obstructive pulmonary disease, a removable stent is considered only after standard therapy including noninvasive ventilation fails [21] while both covered metal and tube stents can be applied for malignant stenoses [11, 14, 15, 17, 18] and tracheoesophageal fistulae (Fig. 9.6) [22, 23].

Table 9.2 Comparison of the Dumon stent and the covered Ultraflex stent

Characteristics	Dumon stent	Covered Ultraflex stent
Mechanical considerations		
High internal to external diameter ratio	–	+++
Resistant to recompression when deployed	+	++
Radial force exerted uniformly across stent	+	++
Absence of migration	–	++
Suitable for use in tortuous airways	–	+++
Removable	+++	–
Dynamic expansion	–	++
Can be customized	+++	–
Tissue–stent interaction		
Biologically inert	++	++
Devoid of granulation tissue	+	–
Tumor ingrowth	++	+
Ease of use		
Can be deployed with FB	–	+++
Deployed under local anesthesia with conscious sedation	–	++
Radiopaque for position evaluation	–	+++
Can be easily repositioned	++	–
Cost		
Inexpensive	+	–

–: poor; +: fair; ++: good; +++: best

Stent Insertion Techniques

Prior to stent insertion, dilatation of the stricture to its optimal diameter should be attempted with rigid bronchoscope, bougie or balloon. Tumor tissue should be removed either with laser or electrocautery, and the largest possible prosthesis should be selected as it can be opened with balloon or forceps. Rigid bronchoscopy is employed for tube stents and flexible bronchoscopy for metal stents.

Tube Stents

Montgomery T-Tube

Since its inception the Montgomery T-tube has undergone only slight modifications, and continues to be used for the treatment of subglottic and tracheal stenosis [6]. Early acrylic models were replaced by silicone rubber and are available in different diameters and variable lengths for the three limbs. The prerequisite for this stent is a tracheostomy and can be placed during tracheostomy procedure or rigid bronchoscopy. The limb protruding out of the tracheostoma is left open for cricoid or glottic stenosis, unplugged for bronchial toilet or closed for speech. Migration is rarely encountered as one limb is fixed in the tracheostoma. High mucosal pressure is not required to hold the stent in position and therefore blood and lymphatic flow to the sensitive upper trachea is not compromised, thereby making the Montgomery T-tube safe for high tracheal stenosis.

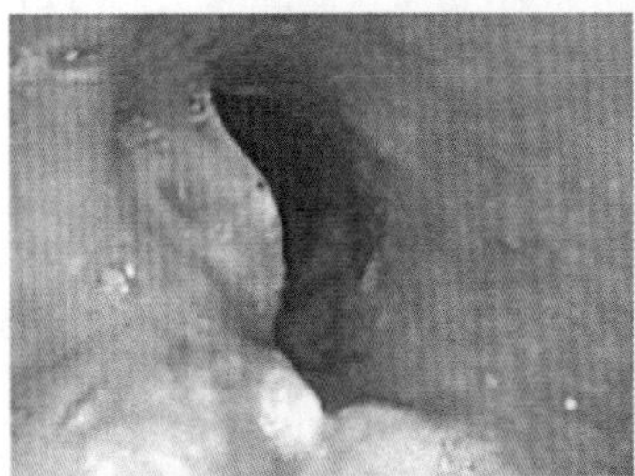
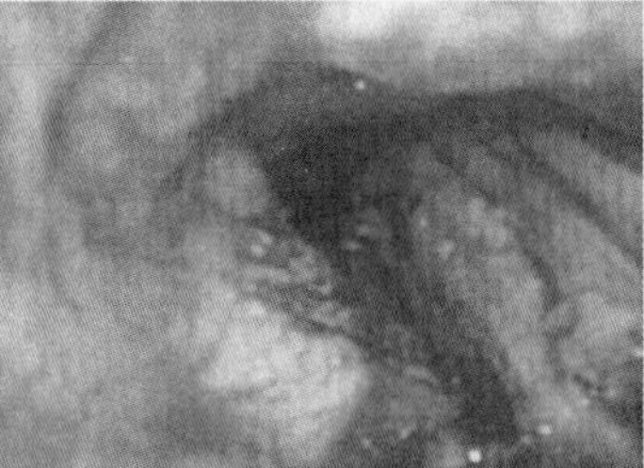
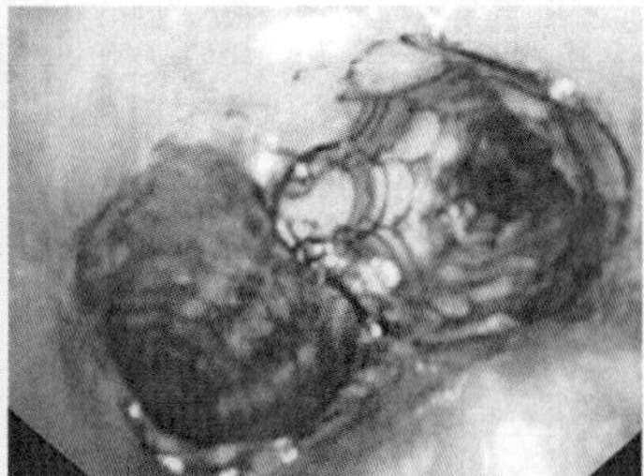

Fig. 9.6 Tracheoesophageal fistula of left main bronchus with infiltration of right main bronchus by esophageal carcinoma. Two covered self-expanding metallic stents are placed via flexible bronchoscopy

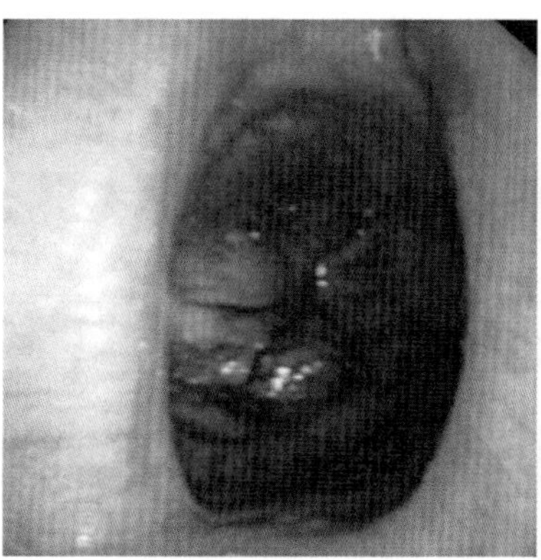

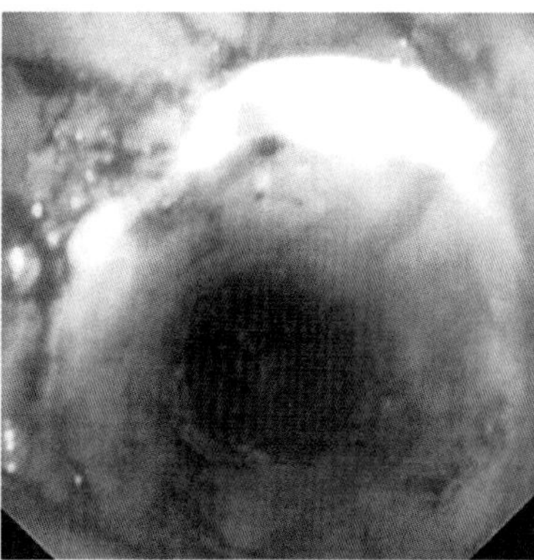

Fig. 9.7 (**a**) Adenoid cystic carcinoma of trachea with near total obstruction. (**b**) Laser photoresection of tumor and silicone stent insertion via rigid bronchoscopy

Dumon Stent

A dedicated tracheobronchial prosthesis made of silicone with studs, and deployed using rigid bronchoscope and stent applicator set (Dumon-Efer, France) was first described by Dumon [7]. In many instances, Dumon stent is placed after restoring the patency of airway with laser photoresection (Fig. 9.7). In a multicenter trial, 1,574 stents were deployed in 1,058 patients, out of which 698 were for malignant airway obstruction. Stent migration occurred in 9.5 %, granuloma formation in 8 % and stent obstruction by mucus in 4 % during 4 months follow up for malignant strictures and 14 months for benign disease [24]. Similar complication rates were observed by Diaz-Jimenez [25] and Cavaliere [11]. Since its introduction, the Dumon stent (Novatech, France) has become the most frequently used stent worldwide, and is regarded as the "gold standard" by many experts. Different diameters and lengths are available for stenoses of the trachea, mainstem bronchus and bronchus intermedius of adults and children. A recent addition is a bifurcated model known as Dumon Y stent (Tracheobronxane Y, Novatech, Grasse, France) which can be applied to palliate lower tracheal and/or main carinal stenoses (Fig. 9.8). The Dumon stent is not ideal for tracheo-bronchomalacia or to bridge tracheoesophageal fistula since good contact pressure between the airway wall and the studs is required to prevent migration.

Noppen Stent

The Noppen stent is made of Tygon (Reynders Medical Supplies, Belgium) and has outer wall shaped like cock-screw and needs a special introducer. A study demonstrated lower migration rate with Noppen stents for benign tracheal stenoses [26].

Polyflex Stent

The Polyflex stent (Boston Scientific, USA) is a self-expanding stent made of cross-woven polyester threads embedded in silicone. Incorporation of tungsten makes the stent radiopaque. It has a thinner wall to inner diameter compared with Dumon or Noppen stent, and with the pusher system it is deployed via rigid bronchoscopy. Different lengths and diameters are available, and are indicated for benign or malignant strictures as well as tracheobronchial fistulae. The tapered models can be used for sealing stump fistulae. However, the smooth outer surface is prone for migration. In a series of 12 patients where 16 Polyflex stents were used for anastomotic stenoses after lung transplantation, tracheal stenoses, tracheobronchomalacia, tracheobronchopathia osteochondroplastica, relapsing polychondritis, and bronchopleural fistula, migration rate was alarmingly high at 75 % and occurred as early as 24 h to 7 months of deployment [27].

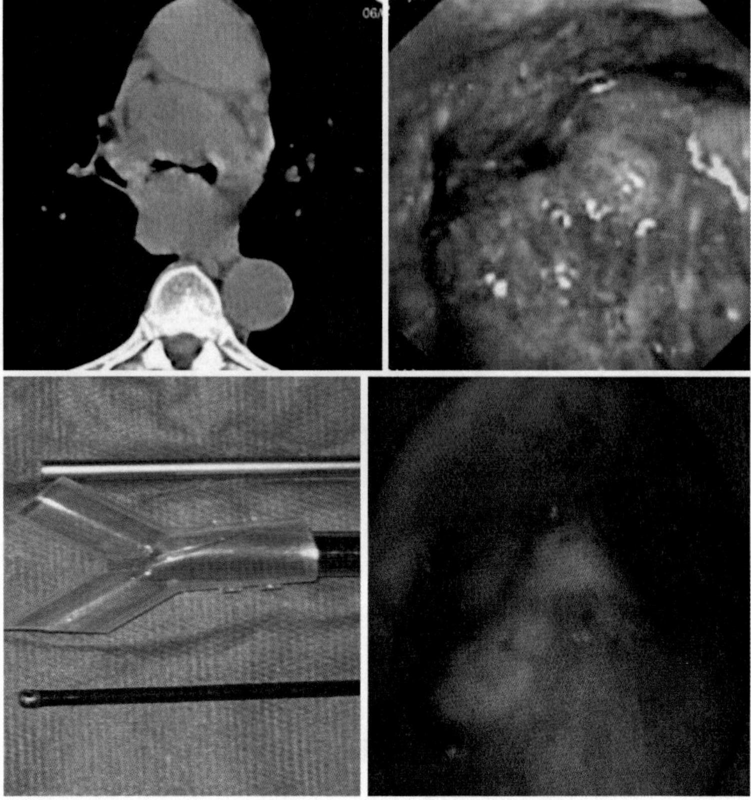

Fig. 9.8 Dumon Y stent placed via rigid bronchoscopy to relieve compression of the main carina by bulky lymph nodes due to metastases

The authors have since abandoned Polyflex stent in their practice.

Dynamic Stent

The dynamic stent (Rüsch Y stent, Rüsch AG Duluth, GA) is a bifurcated silicone stent that is constructed to simulate the trachea. It is reinforced anteriorly by horseshoe shaped metal rings that resemble tracheal cartilages and a soft posterior wall that behaves like the membranous trachea by allowing inward bulge during cough. Stent fracture from fatigue and retained secretions are rarely encountered, and the stent is used for strictures of the trachea, main carina, and/or main bronchi; tracheobronchomalacia; tracheobronchomegaly and esophageal fistula. Placement of dynamic bifurcated stent is facilitated with dedicated forceps and rigid laryngoscope (Fig. 9.9).

Metal Stents

Balloon Expandable Stents

Palmaz and Strecker stents can be dilated to 11–12 mm, and are restricted to children. The Palmaz stent is not indicated for adults as it exhibits plasticity without radial force and any strong external force from vigorous cough or compression from enlarging tumor or vascular structure can cause collapse, obstruction, and migration [28]. The Strecker stents are available 20–40 mm and used in adults for precise stenting of short segment stenoses as they do not foreshorten on deployment [29]. Palmaz and Strecker stents are uncovered and therefore unsuitable for malignant strictures, and may become loose following response to chemoradiotherapy.

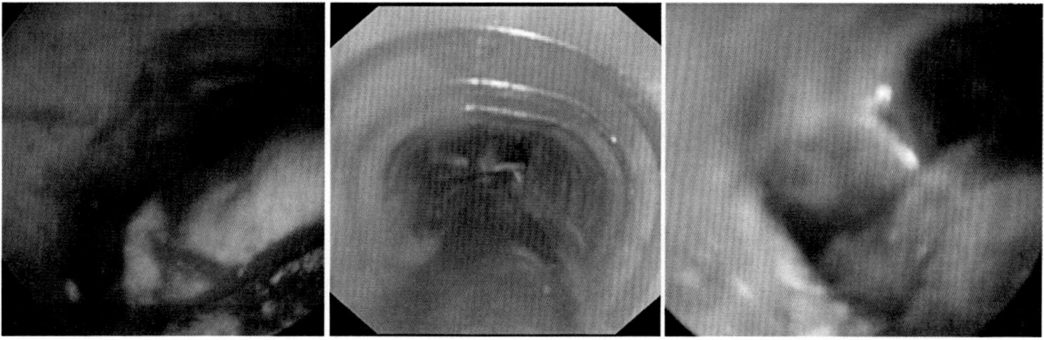

Fig. 9.9 Rusch Y stent reinforced anteriorly by metal rings to simulate tracheal cartilages with soft posterior wall like membranous trachea for carinal compression

Self-Expanding Stents

Ultraflex stens (Boston Scientific, USA) are most commonly used self-expanding stents that exert uniform radial force which stabilizes the stent and reduces the risk of mucosal perforation. They are available in covered and uncovered forms. The Ultraflex is made of nitinol (Fig. 9.10), an alloy with shape memory that deforms at low temperature and regains its original shape at higher temperatures. Miyazawa and coworkers deployed 54 Ultraflex stents in 34 patients with inoperable malignant airway stenoses. Immediate relief of dyspnea was achieved in 82 % of patients. Retained secretions and migration were not observed; stent removal and repositioning was possible and the Ultraflex stent was safe for subglottic stenosis [30]. They could also be placed satisfactorily without fluoroscopy thereby minimizing radiation exposure [31]. Common complications included infectious tracheobronchitis (15.9 %); obstructing granuloma (14.6 %) requiring multiple interventions to restore airway patency; tumor ingrowth (6.1 %); migration in four patients treated with Wallstents; and metal mesh fatigue in one patient after 2 years [32].

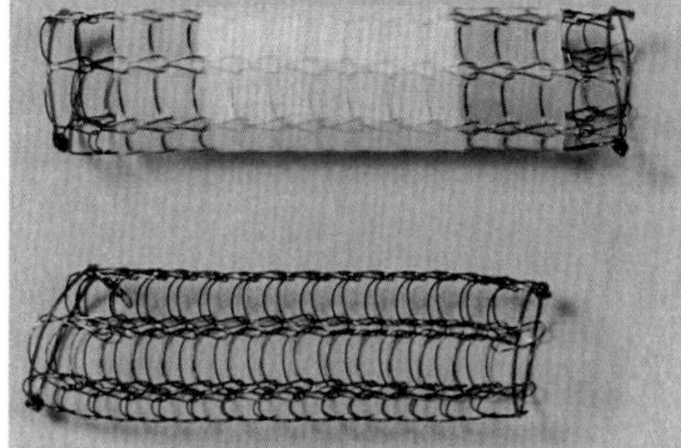

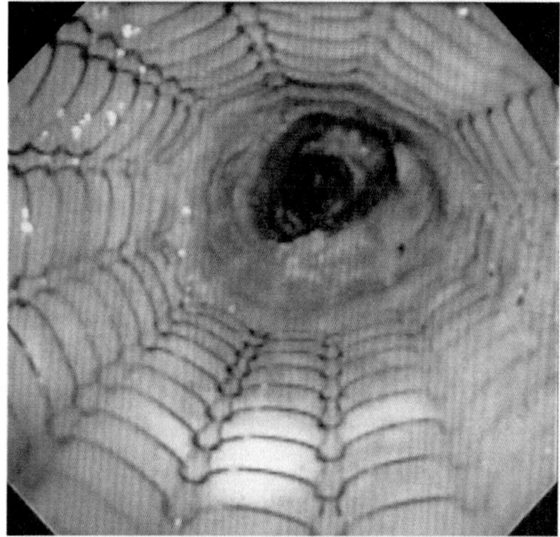

Fig. 9.10 Covered and uncovered Ultraflex stents

Alveolus Stent

Alveolus stent (Fig. 9.11) (Alveolus Inc, Charlotte, NC) is a polyurethane-covered metal stent designed for use in non-neoplastic airway strictures as it can be easily removed. It can be deployed with rigid and flexible bronchoscopy. Accurate sizing for the stent is achieved with Alveolus stent-sizing device (Alveolus Inc, Charlotte, NC) introduced through

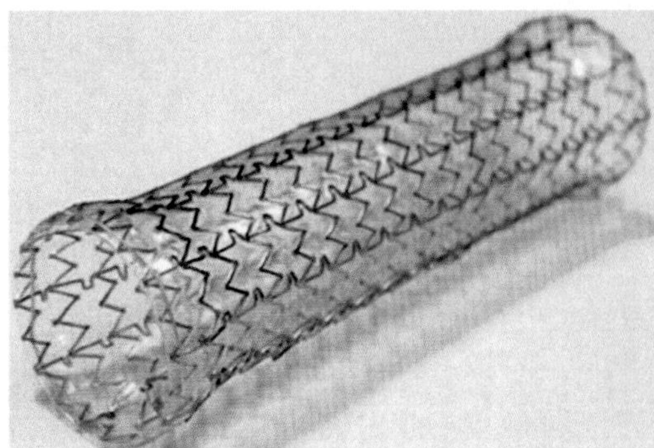

Fig. 9.11 Hybrid stent (Alveolus) that can be deployed with flexible or rigid bronchoscope without foreshortening

the working channel of therapeutic flexible bronchoscope. The sizing device has a measuring tool on one end and a handle on the other. When the internal wire is retracted from the handle, the wings of the measurement device open and are capable of measuring diameters from 6 to 20 mm. Once tissue contact is made, the color bars that code for specific lumen diameters will show which aid the bronchoscopists in the selection of appropriate stents. Alveolus stent is laser constructed from a single piece of nitinol with concentric rings held in position by nitinol strands. Due to its structure, it is amenable to length modification and does not foreshorten with deployment [33]. Despite its advantages, stent collapse causing hemoptysis and dyspnea has been reported [34].

Stent Alert Card

Following the procedure, a stent alert card detailing the type and dimensions of the stent and location within the tracheobronchial tree should be given to the patient. It should also indicate appropriate size of endotracheal tube to use if emergent intubation is required with the stent in situ. The search for the ideal stent continues.

References

1. Bolliger CT, Sutedja TG, Strausz J, Freitag L. Therapeutic bronchoscopy with immediate effect: laser, electrocautery, argon plasma coagulation and stents. Eur Respir J. 2006;27:1258–71.
2. Freitag L. Tracheobronchial stents. In: Bolliger CT, Mathur PN, editors. Interventional bronchoscopy, Progress in respiratory research, vol. 30. Basel, Switzerland: Karger; 2000. p. 171–86.
3. Trendelenburg F. Beitrage zu den Operationen an den Luftwegen. Langenbecks Arch Chir. 1872;13:335.
4. Bond CJ. Note on the treatment of tracheal stenosis by a new T-shaped tracheostomy tube. Lancet. 1891;I: 539–40.
5. Brunings W, Albrecht W. Direkte Endoskopie der Luft und Speisewege. Stuttgart: Enke; 1915. p. 134–8.
6. Montgomery WW. T-tube tracheal stent. Arch Otolaryngol. 1965;82:320–1.
7. Dumon JF. A dedicated tracheobronchial stent. Chest. 1990;97:328–32.
8. Colt HG, Prakash UB, Offord KP. Bronchoscopy in North America: survey by the American Association for Bronchology. J Bronchol. 2000;7:8–25.
9. Dasgupta A, Dolmatch BC, Abi-Saleh WJ, et al. Self-expandable metallic airway stent insertion employing flexible bronchoscopy: preliminary results. Chest. 1998;114:106–9.
10. Lemaire A, Burfeind WR, Toloza E, et al. Outcomes of tracheobronchial stents in patients with malignant airway disease. Ann Thorac Surg. 2005;80:434–8.
11. Cavaliere S, Venuta F, Foccoli P, et al. Endoscopic treatment of malignant airway obstruction in 2008 patients. Chest. 1996;110:1536–42.
12. Colt HG, Harrell JH. Therapeutic rigid bronchoscopy allows level of care changes in patients with acute respiratory failure from central airways obstruction. Chest. 1997;112:202–6.
13. Bolliger CT, Probst R, Tschopp K, Soler M, Perruchoud AP. Silicone stents in the management of inoperable tracheobronchial stenoses. Indications and limitations. Chest. 1993;104:1653–9.
14. Lee P, Kupeli E, Mehta AC. Therapeutic bronchoscopy in lung cancer. Laser therapy, electrocautery, brachytherapy, stents, and photodynamic therapy. Clin Chest Med. 2002;23:241–56.
15. Chhajed PN, Baty F, Pless M, et al. Outcome of treated advanced non-small cell lung cancer with and without airway obstruction. Chest. 2006;130:1803–7.
16. Mughal MM, Gildea TR, Murthy S, et al. Short-term deployment of self-expanding metallic stents facilitates healing of bronchial dehiscence. Am J Respir Crit Care Med. 2005;172:768–71.
17. Mehta AC, Dasgupta A. Airway stents. Clin Chest Med. 1999;20:139–51.
18. Rafanan AL, Mehta AC. Stenting of the tracheobronchial tree. Radiol Clin North Am. 2000;38: 395–408.
19. Dunne JA, Sabanathan S. Use of metallic stents in relapsing polychondritis. Chest. 1994;105:864–7.
20. Collard PH, Freitag L, Reynaert MS, et al. Terminal respiratory failure from tracheobronchomalacia. Thorax. 1996;51:224–6.
21. Murgu SD, Colt HG. Complications of silicone stent insertion in patients with expiratory central airway collapse. Ann Thorac Surg. 2007;84:1870–7.

22. Colt HG, Meric B, Dumon JF. Double stents for carcinoma of the esophagus invading the tracheobronhial tree. Gastrointest Endosc. 1992;38:485–9.
23. Freitag L, Tekolf E, Steveling H, et al. Management of malignant esophago-tracheal fistulas with airway stenting and double stenting. Chest. 1996;110:1155–60.
24. Dumon J, Cavaliere S, Diaz-Jimenez JP, et al. Seven-year experience with the Dumon prosthesis. J Bronchol. 1996;3:6–10.
25. Diaz-Jimenez JP, Farrero Munoz E, et al. Silicone stents in the management of obstructive tracheobronchial lesions: 2 year experience. J Bronchol. 1994;1:15–8.
26. Noppen M, Meysman M, Claes I, et al. Screw-thread vs. Dumon endoprosthesis in the management of tracheal stenosis. Chest. 1999;115:532–5.
27. Gildea TR, Murthy SC, Sahoo D, et al. Performance of a self-expanding silicone stent in palliation of benign airway conditions. Chest. 2006;130:1419–23.
28. Slonim SM, Razavi M, Kee S, et al. Transbronchial Palmaz stent placement for tracheo-bronchial stenosis. J Vasc Interv Radiol. 1998;9:153–60.
29. Strecker EP, Liermann D, Barth KH, et al. Expandable tubular stents for treatment of arterial occlusive diseases: experimental and clinical results. Radiology. 1990;175:87–102.
30. Miyazawa T, Yamakido M, Ikeda S, et al. Implantation of Ultraflex nitinol stents in malignant tracheobronchial stenoses. Chest. 2000;118:959–65.
31. Herth F, Becker HD, LoCicero J, Thurer R, Ernst A. Successful bronchoscopic placement of tracheobronchial stents without fluoroscopy. Chest. 2001;119:1910–2.
32. Saad CP, Murthy S, Krizmanich G, et al. Self-expandable metallic airway stents and flexible bronchoscopy. Chest. 2003;124:1993–9.
33. Hoag JB, Juhas W, Morrow K, Standiford SB, Lund ME. Predeployment length modification of a self-expanding metallic stent. J Bronchol. 2008;15:185–90.
34. Trisolini R, Paioli D, Fornario V, Agli LL, Grosso D, Patelli M. Collapse of a new type of self-expanding metallic tracheal stent. Monaldi Arch Chest Dis. 2006;65:56–8.

Bronchial Thermoplasty for Severe Asthma

10

Sumita B. Khatri and Thomas R. Gildea

Abstract

Bronchial thermoplasty (BT) is a new therapeutic modality for the treatment of severe asthmatics refractory to optimal medical therapy. Individuals with uncontrolled symptoms despite treatment with high dose inhaled corticosteroids and long-acting bronchilator therapy are eligible for this procedure. BT uses radiofrequency energy to reduce the excess airway smooth muscles that can occur in asthma. Since airway smooth muscle is implicated in hyperreactivity and bronchoconstriction, BT can be adjunctive to anti-inflammatory therapy. Thermal treatment is delivered distal to mainstem bronchi to visible airways between 3 and 10 mm in diameter, excluding the right middle lobe. Treatments occur in three separate sessions with careful monitoring before and after the procedure, as the most frequent complication is exacerbation of asthma symptoms. Clinical trials have demonstrated an acceptable safety profile while improving asthma quality of life scores, symptoms, and health care utilization, resulting in FDA approval of this procedure in 2010. More recent evidence demonstrates persistence of beneficial effects up to 2 years after the procedure. Proper patient selection, optimization of confounding conditions, and ongoing asthma management are key factors in improving outcomes and minimizing adverse respiratory events. As experience with the procedure increases, better characterization of asthmatics that may benefit from this procedure will become available.

Keywords

Severe asthma • Refractory asthma • Bronchial thermoplasty • Radiofrequency ablation

S.B. Khatri, M.D., M.S. (✉)
Asthma Center, Cleveland Clinic, Respiratory Institute,
Cleveland, OH 44195, USA
e-mail: khatris@ccf.org

T.R. Gildea, M.D., M.S.
Bronchoscopy, Cleveland Clinic, Respiratory Institute,
Cleveland, OH, USA

A.C. Mehta and P. Jain (eds.), *Interventional Bronchoscopy: A Clinical Guide*, Respiratory Medicine 10,
DOI 10.1007/978-1-62703-395-4_10,

Introduction

Bronchial thermoplasty (BT) is a novel non-pharmacologic therapy for patients with severe persistent asthma who remain uncontrolled despite maximal medical therapy. Approved for use in severe asthma by the Food and Drug Administration (FDA) in 2010, BT uses radiofrequency energy in a controlled manner to provide thermal treatment to smooth muscle in visible conducting airways [1, 2]. The entire treatment is performed over 3 sessions each separated by at least 3 weeks, and is usually an outpatient procedure. Treatments occur by introducing a catheter through the channel of a flexible bronchoscope to apply thermal energy to visible airways between 3 and 10 mm in diameter. Treatments are delivered sequentially in a distal to proximal fashion. Initially the right lower lobe is treated, then the left lower lobe, and lastly bilateral upper lobes. The right middle lobe is not treated due to potential for development of atelectasis and right middle lobe syndrome. Clinical trials of feasibility and efficacy demonstrated that in appropriately selected severe asthmatics not well controlled with currently available medical therapies, bronchial thermoplasty is safe and has a positive impact on the clinical metrics of asthma including symptoms, quality of life, and healthcare utilization. The most common adverse events are respiratory complications, such as an exacerbation of asthma [2–5]. Proper patient selection and optimization of asthma management are important for the success of this procedure. The procedure is most suitable for those individuals who remain symptomatic despite maximal medical therapy but well enough to tolerate it. In this chapter, we discuss the scientific basis, clinical applications, procedure, and complications associated with this emerging technology.

Scientific Basis: Asthma Pathophysiology and Potential Mechanisms of Therapeutic Effect

Asthma is associated with chronic airway inflammation, increased airway reactivity and airflow obstruction. Various cells play a role in pathogenesis of asthma, including eosinophils, mast cells, T lymphocytes, macrophages, neutrophils, and epithelial cells [6]. Episodic shortness of breath and symptoms of bronchoconstriction are common and can be a result of mediators such as histamine, leukotrienes, and prostaglandins from allergic or nonallergic triggers. Persistent inflammation can result in airway wall remodeling causing thickening of basement membrane due to deposition of collagen, goblet cell hyperplasia with excess mucus secretion, blood vessel proliferation, and smooth muscle hypertrophy [6, 7]. These changes can lead to irreversible narrowing of the airways with persistent symptoms of airflow obstruction that may be difficult to manage, even with the best available medical therapies [6]. In patients with chronic and refractory asthma, there is excessive hyperplasia and hypertrophy of airway smooth muscles that can predispose to abnormal bronchoconstriction and airway closure in some instances. Although airway sensitivity and hyperresponsiveness can be temporarily reversed with bronchodilator and anti-inflammatory therapies, prevention of progressive airway remodeling and smooth muscle hypertrophy can be challenging. Bronchial thermoplasty targets this potential gap in asthma treatment.

The role of airway smooth muscle in asthma is not fully elucidated. Early investigations into the mechanisms of airflow obstruction and airway resistance have demonstrated that 75 % of postnasal airflow resistance occurs in the first 6–8 generations of airways, indicating that larger airways are involved [8]. In normal airways, smooth muscle has a role in providing structural support, distribution of ventilation, propulsion of mucus for clearance, cough mechanism, and in promotion of lymphatic flow. In asthma, however, airway smooth muscle is involved in bronchoconstriction and in promoting bronchial hyperresponsiveness through signaling of inflammatory mediators. Furthermore, airway smooth muscle mediates airway inflammation and remodeling through cytokine synthesis and mast cell infiltration [9–11]. Its putative nonessential role has led some to dub airway smooth muscle as "the appendix of the lung" [12]. There are no studies to demonstrate that elimination of these physiological roles of airway smooth muscle greatly inhibit the normal airway function, but there is evidence to suggest that abnormal airway smooth muscle mass contributes to asthma severity. Therefore, hypertrophied airway smooth muscle is an appropriate target for intervention in severe persistent asthma [13].

Clinical Applications: Severe Refractory Asthma and Candidates for Bronchial Thermoplasty

Asthma is a chronic inflammatory condition of the airways characterized by episodic symptoms of breathlessness, cough, and wheezing. Asthma is common, affecting approximately 8% of the population [6]. Regardless of severity at presentation, most patients with asthma are able to gain control of their symptoms with anti-inflammatory therapy, behavioral changes, and trigger management. Since the publications of National Asthma Education and Prevention Program (NAEPP) clinical practice guidelines in 1991, 1997 and 2002, there have been significant gains in the understanding of asthma pathophysiology and treatment [14–16]. The latest guidelines published in 2007 emphasize the importance of categorizing asthma severity. However assessing asthma control which involves evaluation of impairment (symptoms and limitations) and risk (exacerbations) is equally important. Severe asthma is present in about 10 % of all asthma patients and these patients experience frequent symptoms and exhibit disease-related morbidity. Patients with severe asthma also disproportionately utilize heath care resources due to frequent exacerbations, emergency room visits and hospital admissions. The burden of hospitalizations for asthma remains high, with more than 456,000 hospitalizations and 14 million missed days of work annually according to some estimates [6, 17].

In most cases, individuals with asthma are able to control their symptoms with proper adherence to anti-inflammatory therapies and avoidance of triggers. However, a subset of this population has severe asthma that becomes difficult to control despite all medical therapies available. To address the challenges in identification and management of these patients with severe and refractory asthma, the American Thoracic Society (ATS) hosted a workshop to characterize this condition (Fig. 10.1) [18]. Individuals with severe refractory asthma were defined as those who are adherent to and require treatment with continuous or near continuous (>50 % of year) oral corticosteroids or high-dose inhaled corticosteroids to control asthma symptoms. In addition, two minor criteria are needed that include persistent airway obstruction and peak expiratory flow (PEF) variability, additional daily controller medication, deterioration with reduction in inhaled/oral steroid dose, ≥3 oral steroid bursts/year, urgent care visits for asthma, or near-fatal asthma event in the past [19]. These severe asthmatics may be good candidates for bronchial thermoplasty.

Clinical Trials: Development and Evaluation of Bronchial Thermoplasty for Asthma

Radiofrequency ablation therapy has been used in a variety of medical conditions such as lung cancer and cardiac arrhythmias [20, 21]. The use of this technology to treat airway smooth muscle was initially evaluated in animal studies which showed feasibility of using radiofrequency energy to decrease airway smooth muscle mass [1]. Subsequently, clinical studies and trials in non-asthmatics, mild to moderate asthmatics, and finally moderate to severe refractory asthmatics were performed to help identify appropriate candidates, adverse events, and expected outcomes [2–5].

Early animal studies in dogs demonstrated that applying thermal energy to the airways at 65 and 75 °C attenuated methacholine responsiveness for up to 3 years after the treatment [1]. Altered airway smooth muscle, defined as degenerating or absent muscle, were seen as early as 1 week after treatments, and these changes were inversely proportional to the airway hyper-responsiveness. The post-procedure adverse effect in these animals were cough, inflammatory edema of the

REFRACTORY ASTHMA: WORKSHOP CONSENSUS FOR TYPICAL CLINICAL FEATURES*,†

Major Characteristics

In order to achieve control to a level of mild–moderate persistent asthma:

1. Treatment with continuous or near continuous (≥ 50% of year) oral corticosteroids
2. Requirement for treatment with high-dose inhaled corticosteroids:

Drug	Dose (*μg/d*)	Dose (*puffs/d*)
a. Beclomethasone dipropionate	> 1,260	> 40 puffs (42 μg/inhalation > 20 puffs (84 μg/inhalation
b. Budesonide	> 1,200	> 6 puffs
c. Flunisolide	> 2,000	> 8 puffs
d. Fluticasone propionate	> 880	> 8 puffs (110 μg), > 4 puffs (220 μg)
e. Triamcinolone acetonide	> 2,000	> 20 puffs

Minor Characteristics

1. Requirement for daily treatment with a controller medication in addition to inhaled corticosteroids, e.g., long-acting β-agonist, theophylline, or leukotriene antagonist
2. Asthma symptoms requiring short-acting β-agonist use on a daily or near daily basis
3. Persistent airway obstruction (FEV_1 < 80% predicted; diurnal PEF variability > 20%)
4. One or more urgent care visits for asthma per year
5. Three or more oral steroid "bursts" per year
6. Prompt deterioration with ≤ 25% reduction in oral or inhaled corticosteroid dose
7. Near fatal asthma event in the past

* Requires that other conditions have been excluded, exacerbating factors treated, and patient felt to be generally adherent.
† Definition of refractory asthma requires one or both major criteria and two minor criteria.

Fig. 10.1 The American Thoracic Society consensus definition of severe and refractory asthma. (Reprinted with permission of the American Thoracic Society. Copyright © 2012 American Thoracic Society. Proceedings of the ATS workshop on refractory asthma: current understanding, recommendations, and unanswered questions. American Thoracic Society. Am J Respir Crit Care Med. Dec 2000;162(6):2341–2351. Official journal of the American Thoracic Society)

airway wall, retained mucus, and blanching of airway wall at site of catheter contact. Over 3 years of this study, there was no evidence of a regenerative muscle response.

A pilot study was subsequently performed in individuals scheduled for resections for lung cancer [2]. Eight individuals (mean age 58 ± 8.3 years) underwent thermoplasty treatments to visible airways 1 cm from known tumor area and within areas to be resected. Thermoplasty with 55 and 65 °C was performed at 3–9 treatment sites in each patient 5–20 days prior to planned lung resection. At the time of resection, bronchoscopy was generally unremarkable, except for some airway narrowing or linear blanching. Histological review of the resected airways showed an average of 50 % reduction in smooth muscle mass in the airways treated at 65 °C as compared to the untreated airways. There were no significant adverse events such as hemoptysis, respiratory infections or excessive bronchial irritation.

The first prospective observational study of bronchial thermoplasty in asthmatics was performed in 16 individuals with mild to moderate disease [22]. All patients were treated with 30–50 mg prednisone the day prior and day of the procedure. Three bronchial thermoplasty treatments were spaced 3 weeks apart, and the right middle lobe was spared. Pre-bronchodilator FEV_1 improved at 12 week and 1 year but showed no significant change from baseline to 2 years post bronchial thermpoplasty. Symptom-free days increased between baseline and 12 weeks after treatment (50–73 %, $p = 0.015$) and a significant decrease in airway hyper-responsiveness as measured by methacholine was observed over the next 2 years. The most frequent side effects were cough, dyspnea, wheezing, and bronchospasm, which developed within 2–5 days after the procedure, though not severe enough for hospitalization. Chest computed tomography performed 1 and 2 years after the treatment showed no changes in parenchyma or bronchial wall structure. This pilot study demonstrated the safety and feasibility of using this technology in mild to moderate asthma.

The first large multicenter trial of bronchial thermoplasty (Asthma Intervention Research [AIR] trial) was a prospective randomized non-blinded study in moderate to severe asthmatics treated with inhaled corticosteroids (ICS) and long-acting B-agonists (LABA) [3]. Asthmatics requiring 200 μg or more of beclomethasone-equivalent ICS dose who demonstrated respiratory impairment with LABA withdrawal were randomized to receive either BT with ICS and LABA or usual care with ICS and LABA alone. One hundred twelve patients between the ages of 18 and 65 years with percent predicted FEV_1 of 60–85 %, and airway hyper-responsiveness as demonstrated by a concentration of methacholine to decrease FEV1 by 20 % (PC_{20}) of <8 mg/ml and stable asthma for 6 weeks prior to enrollment were recruited for the study. Treatments occurred in 3 sessions over 9 weeks, followed by attempts to discontinue LABA at 3, 6, and 9 months post-procedure. With BT treatment, the number of mild exacerbations and rescue medication use were significantly lower at 3 and 12 months, and changes in morning peak flow at 3, 6, and 12 months were improved from baseline in the treatment group. Symptom free days as well as asthma quality of life scores, assessed using Asthma Quality of Life Questionnaire (AQLQ) and Asthma Control Questionnaire (ACQ), also showed a significant improvement compared to the baseline. However, the study group also experienced more respiratory adverse events around the time of thermoplasty than patients in the control group. There were also more hospitalizations in the treatment group, including for asthma exacerbations, lower lobe atelectasis, and pleurisy [3]. Further, no significant change in FEV1 or methacholine reactivity was noted in BT group. Therefore, although the AIR trial demonstrated improvement in asthma symptoms and incidence of mild exacerbations, the non-blinded study design and the presence of a strong placebo effect in asthma highlighted a need for a randomized trial with a sham treatment arm [3].

To evaluate the safety and efficacy of bronchial thermoplasty in more severe asthmatics, Pavord and associates performed the Research in Severe Asthma (RISA) trial [4]. In this study, asthmatics on high dose inhaled steroids (>750 μg fluticasone-equivalent/day), on prednisone ≤30 mg/day, pre-bronchodilator FEV_1 percent predicted of ≥50 % and positive methacholine tests were randomized to receive either a bronchial thermoplasty ($n = 17$) or medical management ($n = 17$). For 16 weeks after the completion of bronchial thermoplasty, inhaled and oral steroid doses were not changed, after which a protocol driven 14-week corticosteroid wean phase was initiated (20–25 % reduction every 2–4 weeks). Adverse effects included seven hospitalizations for worsening asthma control (4 patients), lobar collapse (2 patients). After the short term increase in asthma-related morbidity in the immediate posttreatment period, there was significant reduction in rescue inhaler use, improvement in pre-bronchodilator FEV_1, as well as improved AQLQ and ACQ scores during the steroid stable phase in the BT group. Up to 1 year after treatment, there was continued decrease in rescue medication use and improvement in AQLQ/ACQ scores. Although the potential for placebo effect in asthma treatments exist, those who received treatment did have improvement in asthma [4].

The clinical trial that followed the AIR study (the AIR2 trial) addressed the placebo effect [5]. In this study, a subset of participants were randomized to a sham control arm in which bronchoscopy was performed, but no radiofrequency treatment was administered. All patients as well the investigators, except for the operators performing the bronchoscopy, were blinded to study allocation allowing it to be a true randomized double-blind clinical trial with sham controls. The primary outcome was to evaluate the changes in AQLQ scores from baseline to 6, 9, and 12 months in the treatment vs. sham group. Secondary outcomes included absolute changes in the asthma control scores, symptom scores, peak flows, rescue medication use, and FEV_1. There were 196 participants in BT group and 101 participants in the sham control group. The baseline characteristics were similar in both groups.

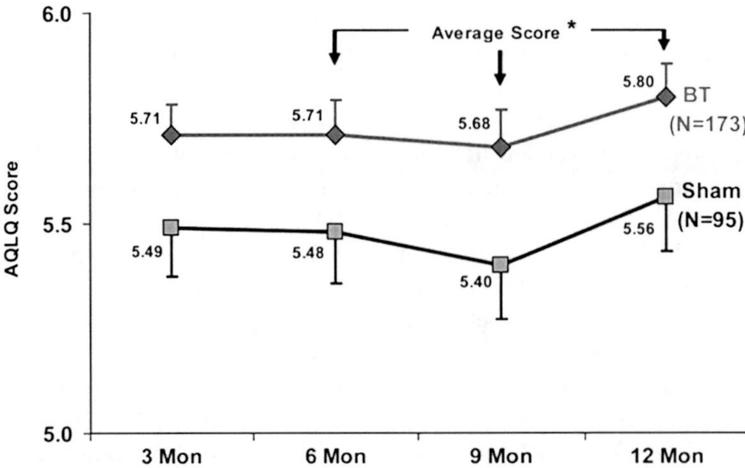

Fig. 10.2 Change in asthma quality of life by treatment group. Change in asthma quality of life questionnaire (AQLQ) score over 12 months after treatment with bronchial thermoplasty (BT) (*diamonds*) or sham control (*squares*) in the per protocol population. *Posterior probability of superiority = 97.9 % (reprinted with permission of the American Thoracic Society. Copyright © 2012 American Thoracic Society. Castro M, Rubin AS, Laviolette M, et al. Effectiveness and safety of bronchial thermoplasty in the treatment of severe asthma: a multicenter, randomized, double-blind, sham-controlled clinical trial. Am J Respir Crit Care Med. Jan 15 2010;181(2):116–124. Official Journal of the American Thoracic Society)

More than 80% participants in each arm met ATS criteria for severe refractory asthma [19]. However, patients with a history of three or more hospitalizations for asthma exacerbation, three or more lower respiratory tract infections, and four or more pulse steroid doses over the preceding year were excluded from the study. Results showed a statistically significant increase in AQLQ from baseline to the average of 6, 9, and 12 months in the BT vs. sham group (Fig. 10.2). Though, difference in the improvement in AQLQ score between two groups was lower than clinically meaningful change of 0.5 or greater. The BT group experienced reduction in severe exacerbations as compared with the sham group (0.48 vs. 0.70 exacerbations/subject/year, posterior probability of superiority of 96 %). Patients treated also had 84% risk reduction in Emergency Department (ED) visits (Fig. 10.3). Adverse events occurred in both groups; however, during the treatment phase, 16 patients in BT group needed hospitalizations for respiratory symptoms including worsening asthma, atelectasis, lower respiratory tract infections, decreased FEV_1, and an aspirated tooth. One episode of hemoptysis required bronchial artery embolization. In contrast, only 2 in the sham group needed hospitalization. Interestingly, there was a significant and clinically meaningful improvement in AQLQ in 64 % of the sham group, highlighting the relative importance of placebo effect in asthma populations [23]. However, a larger proportion (79 %) of BT treated group had a clinically meaningful improvement in AQLQ (>0.5 change) than in the sham group. Therefore, this large multicenter randomized blinded sham-controlled study demonstrated long-term improved asthma quality of life and decreased healthcare utilization in patients with severe asthma treated with bronchial thermoplasty [5]. These benefits, however, were achieved at the cost of significantly higher incidence of early complications in the BT group.

FDA Clearance and Long-Term Follow-Up

The FDA approved the Alair® system (Boston Scientific, MA) in 2010 for the treatment of severe persistent asthma in patients 18 years and older whose asthma is not well controlled with

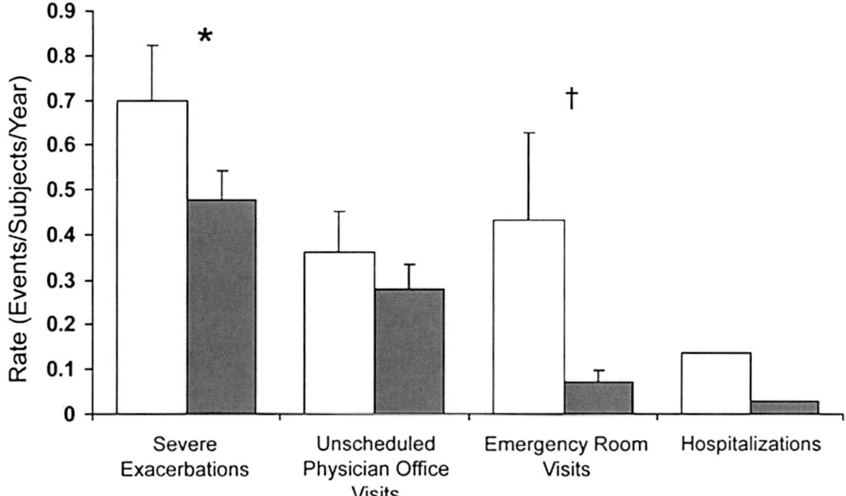

Fig. 10.3 Healthcare utilization events during the post-treatment period. Severe exacerbations (exacerbation requiring treatment with systemic corticosteroids or doubling of the inhaled corticosteroids dose), emergency department visits, and hospitalizations occurring in the posttreatment period. *Open bars*, sham; *shaded bars*, bronchial thermoplasty. All values are means ± SEM. *Posterior probability of superiority = 95.5 %. †Posterior probability of superiority = 99.9 % (reprinted with permission of the American Thoracic Society. Copyright © 2012 American Thoracic Society. Castro M, Rubin AS, Laviolette M, et al. Effectiveness and safety of bronchial thermoplasty in the treatment of severe asthma: a multicenter, randomized, double-blind, sham-controlled clinical trial. Am J Respir Crit Care Med. Jan 15 2010;181(2):116–124. Official Journal of the American Thoracic Society)

inhaled corticosteroids and long-acting beta agonists [24]. Patient selection at most institutions is based on the study populations described in the published trials. Individuals who have well-documented severe persistent asthma not well controlled on ICS and LABA can be considered for bronchial thermoplasty. As part of the final conditions of approval, the FDA has required a post approval study based on the long-term follow-up of the AIR2 trial. There is a specific need to identify the features that predict higher likelihood of desirable long-term outcomes after BT as compared to those who do not achieve any meaningful benefits from it. A 2-year follow-up study from AIR2 demonstrated that individuals who received BT continued to have sustained benefit 2 years after the procedure with persistence of lower exacerbation rates, asthma adverse events, emergency department visits, and hospitalizations. Unfortunately this could not be compared with the sham arm as patients in this group were not followed beyond 1 year post bronchial thermoplasty. Furthermore, asthma quality of life information was not collected [25]. A second post approval study will be a prospective, open label, single arm, multicenter study conducted in the USA to assess the treatment effect and short-term and long-term safety profile.

Procedural Aspects: Bronchial Thermoplasty Instruments and Protocols

Bronchial thermoplasty is performed with a Alair® system (Boston Scientific, MA) which is designed to deliver a specific amount of radiofrequency (thermal) energy through a dedicated catheter (Fig. 10.4) [26]. The catheter is deployed through a 2.0 mm working channel of an adult or pediatric sized flexible bronchoscope. Under direct vision, the electrode array is deployed treating distal airways measuring as small as 3 mm in diameter and working proximally to

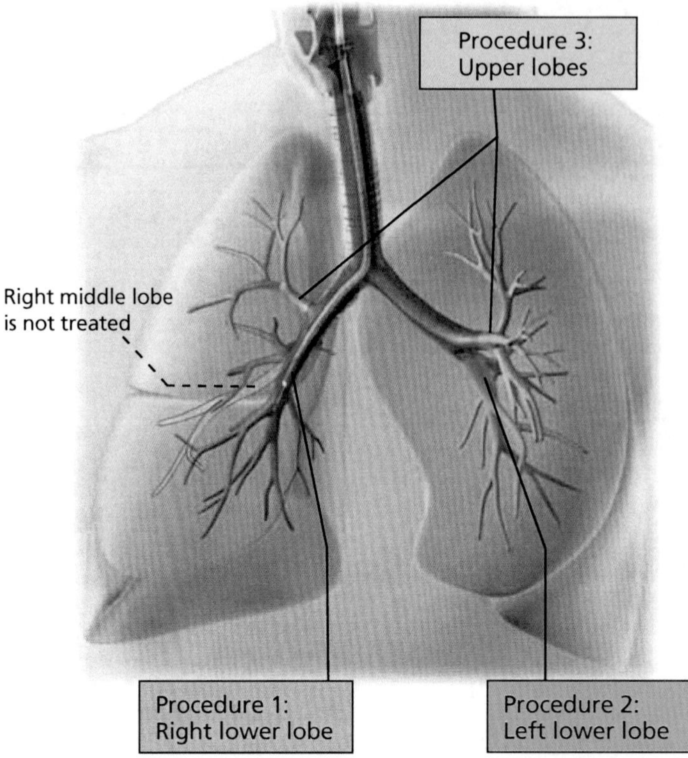

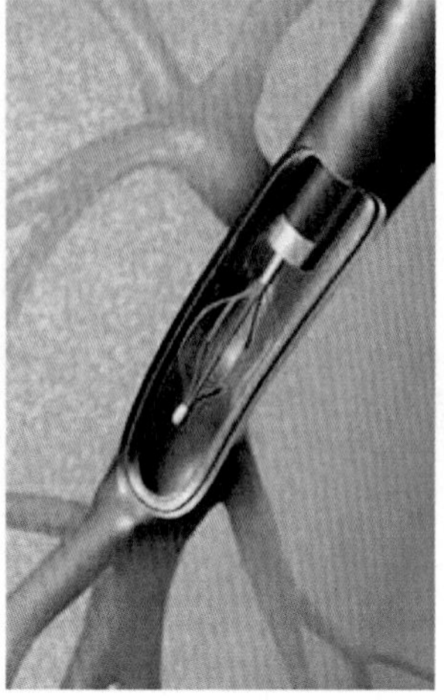

The thermoplasty device within the airway with the electrodes deployed.

Fig. 10.4 Bronchial thermoplasty involves delivery of radiofrequency energy to the airway wall, which ablates the smooth muscle layer, lessening bronchoconstriction and improving symptoms. Treatments are done in three separate procedures, with meticulous mapping of the areas treated. The right lower lobe is treated in the first procedure, the left lower lobe in the second, and the two upper lobes in the third. The right middle lobe is not treated (from: Gildea TR, Khatri SB, Castro M. Bronchial thermoplasty: A new treatment for severe refractory asthma. Cleve Clin J Med 2011; 78:477–485. Reprinted with permission. Copyright © 2011 Cleveland Clinic Foundation. All rights reserved)

sequentially treat all airways to the lobar bronchi. The electrode array is manually expanded to make contact with the airway walls and has a 5 mm treatment area of exposed electrodes on each of the four struts. As the energy is delivered via the electrodes, the control unit measures electrical resistance converted to thermal energy and will stop when an appropriate dosage is given. This thermal energy is what is responsible for altering the airway smooth muscle.

A thorough patient evaluation is essential prior to the procedure. Important aspects of pre and post-procedure care are summarized in Table 10.1. Potential candidates for bronchial thermoplasty are those with the following: (1) a confirmed diagnosis of asthma which is established to be refractory to current maximal medical therapy, (2) a current nonsmoking status (for at least 1 year), (3) no significant contraindications to bronchoscopy and radiofrequency ablation, (4) ability to temporarily suspend anticoagulation therapy, and (5) control of confounding conditions such as gastroesophageal reflux disease, sinus disease, obstructive sleep apnea, and vocal cord dysfunction. Patients with pacemakers or defibrillators are not eligible, and women of childbearing age need to undergo pregnancy test prior to the procedure.

To minimize the development of airway inflammation, patients should receive prophylactic prednisone at a dose of 50 mg per day 3 days before, on the day of and 1 day after the procedure. The procedure should be delayed if there has been an asthma exacerbation within past

Table 10.1 Overview of care of patients undergoing bronchial thermoplasty treatment

Patient selection
• Confirmed diagnosis of asthma
• Asthma refractory to maximal medical therapy
• Pre-bronchodilator FEV1 > 60 %
• Control of confounding conditions such as gastroesophageal reflux disease, obstructive sleep apnea, sinus disease
• No significant coronary artery disease or arrhythmias
• Ability to tolerate cessation of anticoagulation therapy
• Nonsmoker for 1 year or more
• No pacemaker or defibrillator
• Ability to undergo bronchoscopy
Pre-procedure measures
• Maximize asthma treatment
• Oral prednisone 50 mg/day starting 3 days prior to procedure, and day of procedure
• Rule out pregnancy. Perform pregnancy test in childbearing age group
• Administer nebulized albuterol before bronchoscopy
Delay treatment if
• Uncontrolled bronchospasm
• SpO_2<90 % on room air
• Any recent exacerbation within last 6 weeks requiring increase in dose of steroids
• Previously treated airways showing persistence of airway inflammation and erythema, or infection
• Upper respiratory infection within past 2 weeks
• Lower respiratory tract infection within past 6 weeks
During procedure
• Place grounding pad
• Keep FiO_2 less than 40 %
• Have at least two catheters available
• Control cough during bronchoscopy
Post-procedure care
• Observe for 3–4 h in recovery room
• Discharge if patient is stable and the post-procedure FEV1 is within 80 % of pre-procedure value
• Take 50 mg of prednisone on day after the procedure
• Contact patient via phone call in 24–48 h
• Office visits at 2–3 weeks to assess response and schedule subsequent BT session

6 weeks that required systemic steroids, a history of lower respiratory tract infection within the last 6 weeks, or an upper respiratory infection in the last 1–2 weeks. Individuals should be assessed prior to and on the day of the procedure to ensure asthma stability. Nebulized albuterol (2.5–5.0 mg) is given prior to the procedure and screening spirometry is performed to ensure stable pulmonary functions. Patients should be within 10–15 % of their baseline FEV_1 on the day of procedure. A full course of treatment requires three separate bronchoscopic sessions at 2–3-week intervals. Most commonly, right lower lobe is treated in the first session, followed by left lower lobe in second session, and finally both upper lobes in the third session (Fig. 10.5). The treatments are performed via a standard sized flexible bronchoscope with a minimum 2 mm working channel. Moderate sedation (e.g., fentanyl, midazolam, and topical lidocaine) is typically used; however, in certain instances of protracted coughing or difficulty obtaining adequate level of comfort, deeper sedation via general anesthesia can be used. Important safety elements of the procedure include maintaining oxygen at or less than 40 % FiO_2 and placing the appropriate gel grounding pad on the patient's torso.

Technical expertise and ability to navigate the small airways with meticulous mapping of treated areas is essential to ensure that treatment sites are not skipped or overlapped. Each procedure usually requires approximately 50–75 activations of the device and up to 40–60 min of procedure time. Recovery time of 3-4 hours post procedure and ensuring post-procedure spirometry is within 20% of pre-procedure baseline is recommended. An additional 50 mg dose of prednisone is prescribed for the day after the procedure [27].

Complications

The most common complication of the procedure is an exacerbation of asthma symptoms that usually occurs within the first to seventh day after a procedure. Adverse events were more common in the study arms of active treatment and included hospitalizations for worsening asthma, atelectasis, lower respiratory tract infections, and pleurisy [3, 6]. To ensure patient safety, proper patient selection, active monitoring throughout and after the procedure, and appropriate followup, and delaying further procedures until adequate stabilization is necessary (Table 10.1).

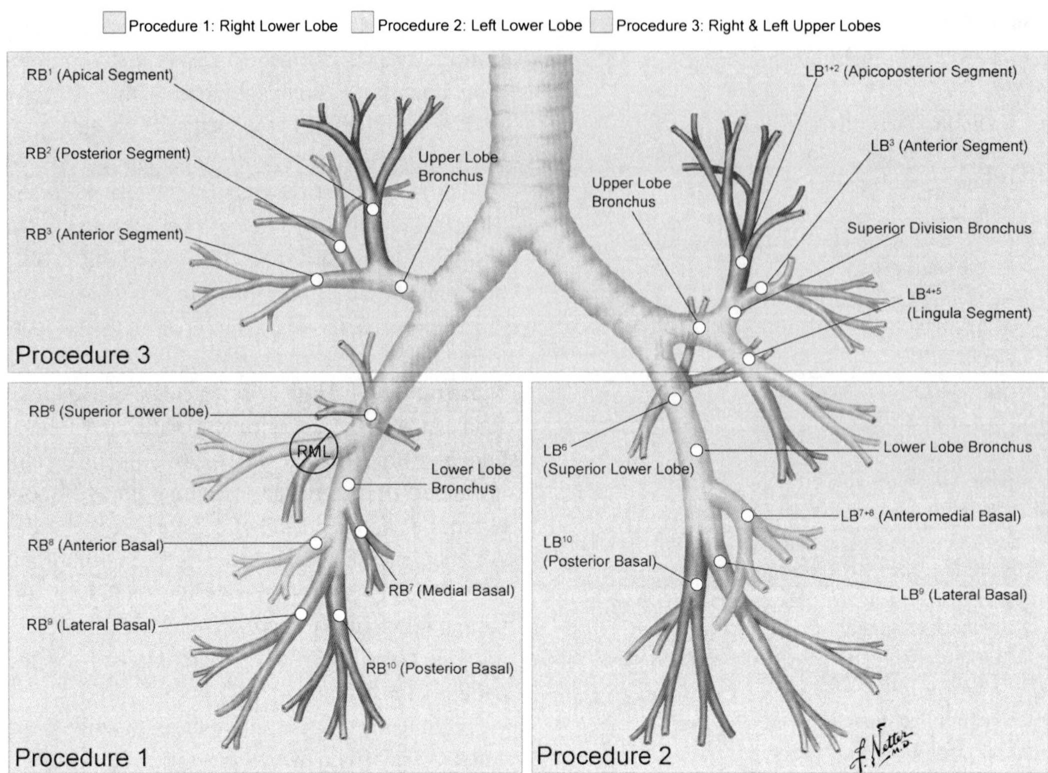

Fig. 10.5 Bronchial thermoplasty is performed in three bronchoscopic sessions as depicted. Right middle lobe is not treated. Careful mapping is needed to make sure that treated areas are not skipped or overlapped (image provided courtesy of Boston Scientific Corporation)

Limitations

Bronchial thermoplasty should be reserved for a select group of severe asthmatics as all are not eligible. In most instances, asthma can be well controlled with the available medical anti-inflammatory therapy and trigger avoidance. In those individuals with persistent symptoms despite maximal medical therapy, confounding conditions need to be considered. Patients with severely impaired lung function or current instability of symptoms are not appropriate candidates due to the known complications that can occur with the procedure.

Bronchial thermoplasty is an expensive treatment. High cost is a major impediment to the wider use of this technology. Formal cost-effective analysis is not available. High cost, unknown durability, and long-term effects of bronchial thermoplasty warrant careful patient selection for the most appropriate candidates.

It should also be noted that bronchial thermoplasty has only been evaluated in asthma, and that experience cannot be extrapolated to COPD or bronchiectasis. Current smokers are not included in clinical trials and in most instances, are not considered for this treatment. Other considerations include the need to be able to tolerate bronchoscopy, be off of anticoagulant therapy temporarily around the procedure, presence of other respiratory diseases such as interstitial lung disease, emphysema, or cystic fibrosis. People with uncontrolled hypertension, clinically significant cardiovascular disease, and internal or external pacemaker or defibrillators are not suitable candidates for this technique.

Future Directions

Since bronchial thermoplasty is a relatively new procedure in the treatment of asthma, ongoing clinical experience will help inform those performing the procedure which patients are likely to gain most benefit. Although not a cure, this mode of therapy directly affects airway smooth muscle, the vehicle of bronchospasm and hyperresponsiveness. Having trained and meticulous operators and close patient follow-up certainly will be beneficial for patients. In addition, observational studies to identify patient characteristics and biomarkers that predict successful outcome are needed so that bronchial thermoplasty may be targeted to those patients who will be helped most by this procedure.

Conclusions and Summary

To summarize, several clinical trials demonstrate the feasibility, safety, and improved clinical outcomes in patients with severe asthma who undergo bronchial thermoplasty when medical therapies do not control their symptoms. The series of trials outlined here demonstrate that although asthma is a disease of the airways, including the small airways, treatment of airways at 3 mm or larger has demonstrated improvement in asthma symptoms, quality of life and health care utilization [5].

References

1. Danek CJ, Lombard CM, Dungworth DL, et al. Reduction in airway hyperresponsiveness to methacholine by the application of RF energy in dogs. J Appl Physiol. 2004;97:1946–53.
2. Miller JD, Cox G, Vinic L, Lombard CM, Loomas BE, Danek CJ. A prospective feasibility study of bronchial thermoplasty in the human airway. Chest. 2005;127:1999–2006.
3. Cox G, Thomson NC, Rubin AS, et al. Asthma control during the year after bronchial thermoplasty. N Engl J Med. 2007;356:1327–37.
4. Pavord ID, Cox G, Thomson NC, et al. Safety and efficacy of bronchial thermoplasty in symptomatic, severe asthma. Am J Respir Crit Care Med. 2007;176: 1185–91.
5. Castro M, Rubin AS, Laviolette M, et al. Effectiveness and safety of bronchial thermoplasty in the treatment of severe asthma: a multicenter, randomized, double-blind, sham-controlled clinical trial. Am J Respir Crit Care Med. 2010;181:116–24.
6. National Asthma Education and Prevention Program, National Heart Lung and Blood Institute. Expert Panel Report 3:Guidelines for the Diagnosis and Management of Asthma, summary report 2007. J Allergy Clin Immunol. 2007;120:S94–138.
7. Akinbami L, Moorman J, Liu X. Asthma prevalence, health care use, and mortality: United States, 2005–2009. National health statistics reports, No. 32. Hyattsville, MD: National Center for Health Statistics; 2011.
8. Ingram RH, McFadden ER. Localization and mechanisms of airway responses. N Engl J Med. 1977;297: 596–600.
9. Solway J, Irvin CG. Airway smooth muscle as a target for asthma therapy. N Engl J Med. 2007;356:1367–9.
10. Berger P et al. Tryptase-stimulated human airway smooth muscle cells induce cytokine synthesis and mast cell chemotaxis. FASEB J. 2003;17:2139–41.
11. Carroll NG, Mutavdzic S, James AL. Distribution and degranulation of airway mast cells in normal and asthmatic subjects. Eur Respir J. 2002;19:879–85.
12. Mitzner W. Airway smooth muscle: the appendix of the lung. Am J Respir Crit Care Med. 2004;169: 787–90.
13. Cox PG et al. Radiofrequency ablation of airway smooth muscle for sustained treatment of asthma: preliminary investigations. Eur Respir J. 2004;24(4): 659–63.
14. NHLBI, EPR. Expert panel report: guidelines for the diagnosis and management of asthma (EPR 1991). NIH Publication No. 91-3642. Bethesda, MD: US Department of Health and Human Services; National Institutes of Health; National Heart, Lung, and Blood Institute; National Asthma Education and Prevention Program, 1991; 1991.
15. NHLBI, EPR-2. Expert panel report 2: guidelines for the diagnosis and management of asthma (EPR-2 1997). NIH Publication No. 97-4051. Bethesda, MD: US Department of Health and Human Services; National Institutes of Health; National Heart, Lung, and Blood Institute; National Asthma Education and Prevention Program, 1997; 1997.
16. NHLBI, EPR-Update 2002. Expert panel report: guidelines for the diagnosis and management of asthma. Update on selected topics 2002 (EPR–Update 2002). NIH Publication No. 02-5074. Bethesda, MD: US Department of Health and Human Services; National Institutes of Health; National Heart, Lung, and Blood Institute; National Asthma Education and Prevention Program, June 2003; 2002.
17. National Center for Health Statistics (NCHS), Centers for Disease Control and Prevention, National health interview survey (NHIS 2005). 2005.

18. American Thoracic Society. Proceedings of the ATS workshop on refractory asthma: current understanding, recommendations, and unanswered questions. Am J Respir Crit Care Med, 2000;162:2341–51.
19. Moore WC, Bleecker ER, Curran-Everett D, et al. Characterization of the severe asthma phenotype by the National Heart, Lung, and Blood Institute's Severe Asthma Research Program. J Allergy Clin Immunol. 2007;119:405–13.
20. Ambrogi MC, Fanucchi O, Lencioni R, Cioni R, Mussi A. Pulmonary radiofrequency ablation in a single lung patient. Thorax. 2006;61:828–9.
21. Benussi S, Cini R, Gaynor SL, Alfieri O, Calafiore AM. Bipolar radiofrequency maze procedure through a transseptal approach. Ann Thorac Surg. 2010;90:1025–7.
22. Cox G, Miller JD, McWilliams A, Fitzgerald JM, Lam S. Bronchial thermoplasty for asthma. Am J Respir Crit Care Med. 2006;173:965–9.
23. Wise RA, Bartlett SJ, Brown ED, et al. Randomized trial of the effect of drug presentation on asthma outcomes: the American Lung Association Asthma Clinical Research Centers. J Allergy Clin Immunol. 2009;124:436–44. 444e1-8.
24. FDA. Approval of Alair bronchial thermoplasty system: Alair catheter and Alair RF controller. 2010.
25. Castro M, Rubin A, Laviolette M, et al. Persistence of effectiveness of bronchial thermoplasty in patients with severe asthma. Ann Allergy Asthma Immunol. 2011;107:65–70.
26. Gildea TR, Khatri SB, Castro M. Bronchial thermoplasty: a new treatment for severe refractory asthma. Cleve Clin J Med. 2011;78:477–85.
27. Mayse M, Laviolette M, Rubin AS, et al. Clinical pearls for bronchial thermoplasty. J Bronchol. 2007; 14:115–23.

11 Bronchoscopic Lung Volume Reduction

Cheng He and Cliff K.C. Choong

Abstract

Chronic obstructive pulmonary disease (COPD) is one of the leading causes of respiratory morbidity and mortality worldwide. Lung volume reduction surgery has been shown to be useful in selected COPD patients with upper lobe predominance and low exercise capacity, but is associated with significant complications, prolonged hospital stay and high cost. In recent years, several bronchoscopic techniques have been tried to achieve similar benefits while aiming to reduce the complications and cost. Modest clinical benefits have been reported with placement of unidirectional bronchial valves in the airways in heterogeneous emphysema. Better functional results are achieved in patients with complete lobar occlusion and in the absence of collateral ventilation. Airway bypass using specially designed stents has been attempted in homogeneous emphysema, but stent occlusion remains a significant problem. Studies are also emerging on the use of bronchial lung volume reduction coils, endobronchial sealants and bronchoscopic thermal vapor ablation to achieve similar goals. The field of bronchoscopic lung volume reduction is rapidly evolving and more clinical studies are needed to identify the ideal patient and the most effective technique.

Keywords

Bronchoscopic lung volume reduction • Chronic obstructive pulmonary disease • Bronchial valves • Airway bypass • Bronchoscopic thermal vapor ablation • Lung volume reduction coils

Introduction

Emphysema is an irreversible, progressive, debilitating disease characterised by loss of lung tissue. Current treatment modalities for severe emphysema include medical and surgical therapy. Despite benefits from optimal medical therapy involving

C. He, M.B.B.S., B.Med.Sc., P.G.Dip.Surg.Anat.
Department of Surgery (MMC), Monash University, Monash Medical Center, Clayton, VIC, Australia

C.K.C. Choong, M.B.B.S., F.R.C.S., F.R.A.C.S. (✉)
Department of Surgery (MMC), Monash University, The Valley Hospital, Melbourne, VIC, Australia
e-mail: cliffchoong@hotmail.com

A.C. Mehta and P. Jain (eds.), *Interventional Bronchoscopy: A Clinical Guide*, Respiratory Medicine 10, DOI 10.1007/978-1-62703-395-4_11,

inhaled therapies and pulmonary rehabilitation, many patients remain significantly disabled. Surgical options include lung volume reduction surgery (LVRS) and lung transplantation. Lung transplantation is performed only in highly selected patients and is limited by a lack of donors, the requirement for lifelong immune-suppressive therapy and the permanent risk of rejection, bronchiolitis obliterans and infection. The National Emphysema Treatment Trial (NETT) demonstrated that in appropriately selected patients, with predominant heterogeneous pattern of emphysema with upper lobe predominance and low exercise capacity, LVRS significantly improved lung function, exercise tolerance, quality of life and survival [1]. However, owing to the highly strict LVRS selection criteria and the potential morbidity and mortality associated with surgery, a search for newer and safer approaches to produce lung volume reduction has been underway.

Endobronchial treatment of severe emphysema has emerged over the past 10 years. Various approaches, from bronchial valves and coils, as well as biological agents to induce reactionary scarring, in addition to bronchoscopically placed airway bypass stents, have been described [2–9]. The aims of these novel approaches are to provide a minimally invasive method of treating severe emphysema without the morbidity, mortality and costs of traditional surgical therapy. It is also hoped that these different therapies can be applied to a wider patient population, in comparison to the relatively few highly select patients considered for LVRS or lung transplantation. The choice of technique is dependent upon the emphysema subtype, either homogeneous or heterogeneous, based on computed tomography (CT) morphology. We shall provide an overview of the various bronchoscopic techniques and the current data.

Concept One: One-Way Valves Placed Within Lumen of Bronchial Airways for Heterogeneous Emphysema

The first concept is the usage of one-way valves which are placed within the lumen of airways, allowing air to flow only uni-directionally out of the airways (i.e. airflow in the direction of expiration) but does not allow air to be inspired through the valves. The aim is to place several bronchial valves to occlude all the segmental or subsegmental airways supplying a specific hyperinflated segment or lobe of the lung, thereby producing effective volume reduction. The bronchial valves are of variable sizes to allow placement within different bronchial lumen sizes. They are deployed via the working channel of a flexible bronchoscope and can be removed if necessary [10, 11].

This treatment is targeted at patients with heterogeneous emphysema, a similar population as that considered for LVRS. Two different companies, Pulmonx Inc. and Spiration Inc., produce the Zephyr® endobronchial valves (EBV) (Fig. 11.1) and the Intrabronchial Valve® (IBV), respectively (Fig. 11.2) [12, 13]. Despite the dif-

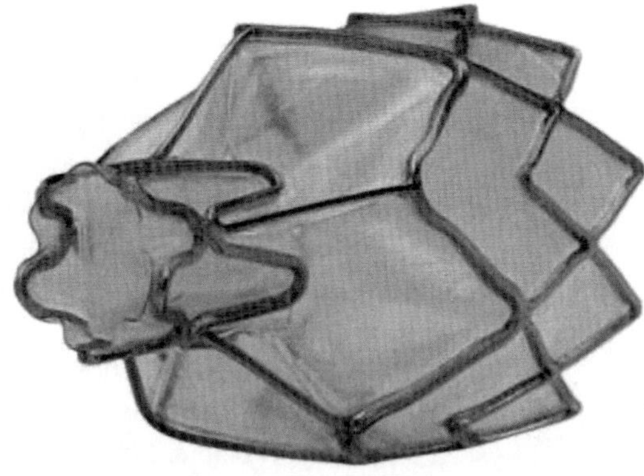

Fig. 11.1 Zephyr® endobronchial valves (EBV) [courtesy of Pulmonx Inc., California]

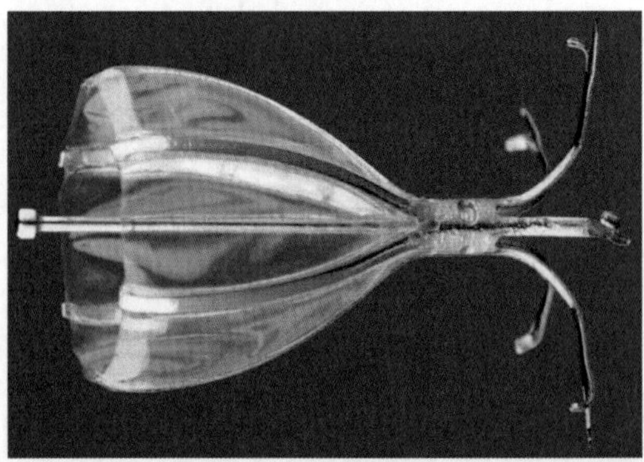

Fig. 11.2 Spiration intra-bronchial valve

ferent designs, both valves share the common features described above. The specific designs and features of the valves can be found on their respective company Websites [12, 13].

Zephyr Pulmonx Valve

The Zephyr® implant is a one-way silicone duck-bill valve mounted on a nitinol self-expanding retainer that is covered with a silicone membrane [12]. It can be deployed via a 2.8 mm instrument of a flexible bronchoscope. The purpose of this device is to isolate a diseased (hyperinflated) part of lung, allowing only venting of expired gas and secretions from that portion of lung, without air entering the blocked segment. A reduction in lung volume from the induced atelectasis of the isolated emphysematous segments would ideally be achieved, thereby shifting lung functions towards more physiological values.

Two randomised trials were conducted following promising results from several individual case series and a multicentre registry [3, 14–17]. The Endobronchial Valve for Emphysema Palliation Trial (VENT) was a randomised, prospective, multicentre study which examined the safety and efficacy of Zephyr EBV endobronchial valves (Pulmonx) in comparison to optimal medical care, in patients with advanced heterogeneous emphysema. Co-primary efficacy endpoints were percent changes (baseline to 6 months) in FEV_1 and 6-min walk test (6MWT) by multiple-imputation, intent-to-treat analysis. In the US VENT study 321 subjects were enrolled, with 220 subjects randomised to EBV and 101 to control (standard medical care). Modest improvements in FEV_1 (mean difference between groups was 6.8 %, $p=0.002$) and 6MWT (median difference was 5.8 %, $p=0.019$) in the treatment compared to control group were observed, in favor of EBV [3]. These modest improvements in lung function, exercise tolerance and symptoms came with a cost of more frequent exacerbations of chronic obstructive pulmonary disease (COPD), pneumonia and haemoptysis. Overall results were similarly observed in the European VENT study [14].

Findings from both the US and European arms of the VENT study have offered valuable insight into key patient factors influencing positive physiological and clinical outcomes. In subgroup analyses, two factors in achieving optimal lung volume reduction and clinical response were identified: (1) complete lobar occlusion and (2) the presence of greater heterogeneity and complete fissures between treated and adjacent lobes.

High-resolution CT (HRCT) was used to quantify volumetric changes in the target treatment lobe, to determine inter-lobar fissure integrity and to identify lobar occlusion following EBV therapy. In both VENT studies, patients with complete fissures who received EBV had a significantly better improvement in FEV_1 than patients with incomplete fissures (the US VENT study: 16.2 vs. 2 %, at 6 months). Optimal isolation of the target lobe from its segmental airways using EBVs would theoretically lead to the desired volume reduction effect. Indeed, of the EBV patients possessing fissure integrity on CT, those classified as having lobar occlusion (i.e. those with optimal valve placements) demonstrated even better outcomes compared with EBV patients without lobar occlusion: target lobe volume decreased by a mean 80 vs. 29 % and FEV_1 increased by 26 vs. 6 %, at 6 months (European VENT study). Not surprisingly, further analysis of the European VENT cohort found that the clinical response was directly related to the degree of lung volume reduction [18].

It is clear that some patients do not achieve significant volume reduction irrespective of optimal valve placement. This has been attributed to the phenomenon known as collateral ventilation (CV) [18, 19]. Studies on excised human lungs identified major defects in inter-lobar fissures across 21–30 % of oblique and up to 88 % of right horizontal fissures and CV can occur through these areas of incomplete fissures [20, 21]. In normal lungs, resistance in these collateral channels is high, resulting in minimal CV. In contrast, resistance across these channels in emphysema is low relative to airway resistance, allowing CV to occur between lobes. Where CV is present, atelectasis is unlikely to be achieved

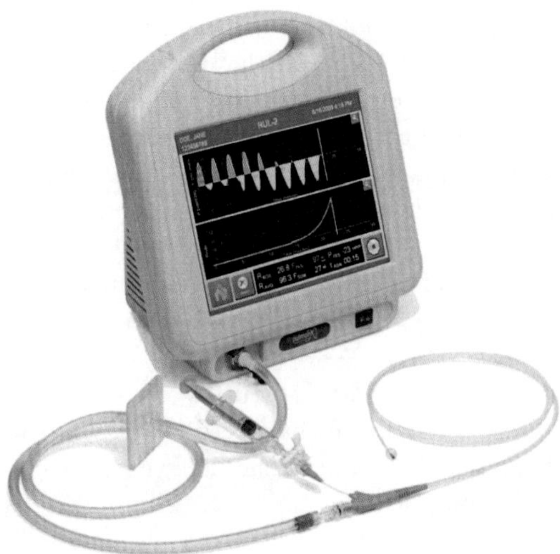

Fig. 11.3 Chartis system [courtesy of Pulmonx Inc., California]

following EBV placement due to air entering the targeted lobe via collateral channels. Thus, the ability to identify these "back-door" channels and target only lobes of lung where CV is low or absent would optimise lobar isolation, leading to markedly improved outcomes with bronchial valves [18].

In VENT study, a correlation was noted between complete inter-lobar fissure on chest CT and the magnitude of lobar volume change and improvement in FEV_1 after endobronchial valve placement. Based on this observation, it is speculated that fissure completeness on CT may be used as a marker of absence of CV while selecting patients for bronchoscopic lung volume reduction. Greater heterogeneity of emphysema on high-resolution CT is also considered as an imaging biomarker for low or absent collateral ventilation.

A bronchoscopic system for detecting CV has also been developed (Chartis), consisting of a single-patient-use catheter with a compliant balloon component at the distal tip, which upon inflation blocks the airway [12]. Air can then flow out from the target compartment into the environment only through the catheter's central lumen. By connecting to a console, airway flow and pressure can be displayed (Fig. 11.3). Airway resistance can be calculated and the presence or the absence of CV in isolated lung compartment can then be measured. A gradual reduction of measured airflow would indicate the absence of CV feeding the airways distal to the point of balloon occlusion, whilst a continuous flow reading would indicate the presence of CV in the target lobe. The effectiveness of this system in identifying those who would benefit from bronchial valve therapy was assessed in a recent study of 80 patients [18]. The HRCT was used to identify the lobe with the greatest emphysematous destruction, deemed the target lobe for bronchial valve placement, and that lobe was assessed with Chartis. Chartis was attempted prior to valve deployment but did not affect the choice of the target lobe. The primary endpoint was ≥350 ml target lobe volume reduction (TLVR), which was derived from the VENT study observation that the maximum TLVR in the control (medical therapy only) group rarely exceeded this level [3, 18]. Chartis achieved an accuracy of 75 % in predicting a significant volume reduction in response to valve placement: 36 of 51 patients classified as CV negative achieved TLVR ≥350 ml. This was equivalent to HRCT fissure analysis alone, where the accuracy was 77 % [22]. Technical issues were encountered resulting in some patients having no measurements displayed [23]. The Chartis system may be a valuable supplement to HRCT in identifying suitable target lobes where minimal CV exists, to ensure optimal response to bronchial valve therapy. However, further higher powered randomised assessments of its predictive potential would be useful.

IBV® Spiration Valve

The IBV, similar to the Zephyr valve, is also an indwelling endobronchial device, designed to obstruct airflow into targeted segments of diseased emphysematous lung. This one-way valve is built upon six nitinol struts covered by polyurethane in the shape of an umbrella to allow conformation and sealing to the airways, with minimal pressure exerted on the mucosa (Fig. 11.4) [13]. IBV are readily visible on chest radiographs (Fig. 11.5) and in many cases, a

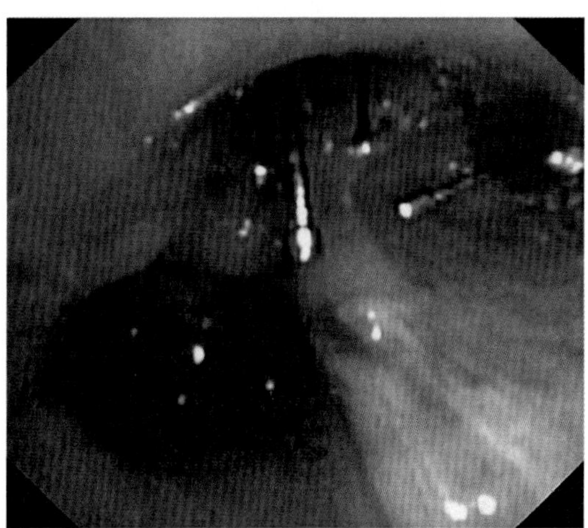

Fig. 11.4 Endoscopic appearance of spiration valve placed into segmental bronchi

follow-up radiograph reveals a significant reduction in air trapping (Fig. 11.6).

The IBV® Valve Pilot Trials Research Team published a report in 2009 on 98 patients with upper-lobe predominant heterogeneous emphysema, who were treated at 13 international sites during the 3-year single-arm series, open-label study, with EBV placed bilaterally into upper lobes [10]. 56 % of subjects had a clinically meaningful improvement in health-related quality of life, but this did not correlate to improvements in standard pulmonary function and exercise studies. TLVR were demonstrated in over 85 % of subjects on CT. A comparable proportion of patients also experienced an increase in non-targeted (i.e. non-UL) lobe volumes so that total lung volume remained unchanged. A redirection of inspired air, involving an interlobar shift of inspired volume to healthier lung tissue, corroborated by perfusion scan changes, suggested an improved ventilation and perfusion matching in non-upper (non-treated) lobe lung parenchyma as the mechanism for the improved clinical outcomes.

The most common device-related adverse effect was pneumothorax ($n = 8$), presumably due to tension on adjacent tissue, overexpansion of blebs or bullae or adhesions when lobar or segmental lung volume reduction occurred. The association between induction of lobar atelectasis and development of pneumothorax was most evident when treatment of the lingular segment was added to left upper lobe (UL) treatment, resulting in 6 of 18 subjects developing left-sided pneumothorax. Further episode of left-sided pneumothorax was not observed following discontinuation of lingular targeting. There were no procedural related deaths and the 30-day mortality was 1.1 %, which compared favorably with LVRS (16 % 30-day mortality from the NETT [24]). And with a 99.7 % technical success of stent placement, no stent migration nor erosion and a rate of associated infection <2.5 %, the authors concluded successful achievement of the primary safety outcome goal [10].

The US multicentre data, which included 91 of 98 subjects from the above study, was published in 2010, with expectantly similar findings and conclusions [4].

The first blinded, controlled evaluation of bronchial valve therapy was published in 2012 by Ninane et al. [25]. This randomised study utilised the IBV valve, using a strategy of bilateral treatment with incomplete occlusion of the target lobes. 37 patients received valves whilst 36 had a sham bronchoscopy. A positive responder was based on a composite endpoint of St George's Respiratory Questionnaire (SGRQ) change ≥4 points and lung volume changes measured by CT (volume decrease in upper lobes with a compensatory volume increase in non-treated lobes of ≥7.5 %). After 3 months, 24 % of patients in the treatment arm and none in the control arm were identified as positive responders. There was a significant shift in volume in the treated group from the upper lobes (mean ± SD, −7.3 ± 9.0 %) to the non-treated lobes (6.7 ± 14.5 %), with no significant change in control group ($p < 0.05$). However, no statistically significant differences in lung function, breathlessness and SGRQ was evident between the groups. Furthermore, owing to the presence of a control group, a significant placebo effect was demonstrated, with both arms having an ~4-point improvement in SGRQ. This raises questions about the validity of findings of clinical efficacy in the absence of functional changes

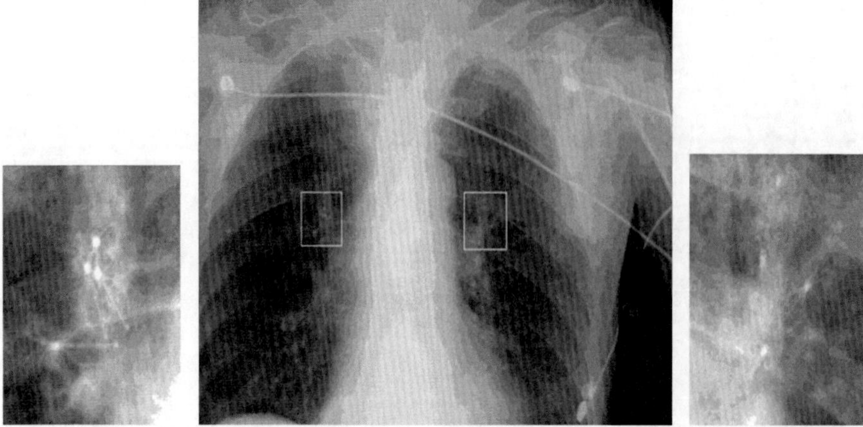

Fig. 11.5 Chest radiograph showing placement of spiration valves in both upper lobes

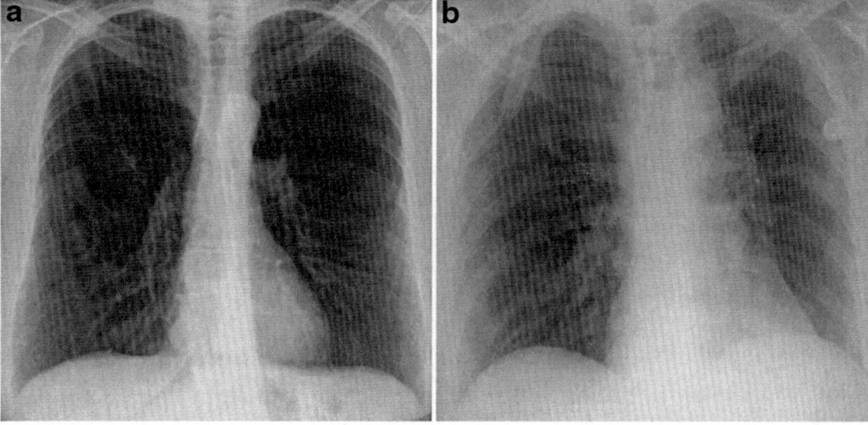

Fig. 11.6 Chest radiographs before (**a**) and after (**b**) placement of spiration valve. A significant decrease in hyperinflation and air trapping is observed in post-procedure radiograph

[10]. Importantly, this randomised-control study showed that a non-complete lobar occlusion approach was safe but not effective in the majority of patients undergoing bronchial valve treatment for heterogeneous emphysema. This is further supported by a recent small, randomised study that showed that IBV valves were indeed superior in providing both clinically and physiologically significant improvements when a single-lobe complete occlusion approach was undertaken, as compared to bilateral-partial lobe treatment [26].

Concept Two: Airway Bypass for Homogeneous Emphysema

The second concept is the usage of airway bypass stents. As previously mentioned, the ability of gas to move from one part of the lung to another part (within the lung) through nonanatomic pathways is termed "collateral ventilation", and was first observed by Van Allen and colleagues in 1930 [27]. In contrast to normal lungs, where high resistance in collateral channels abolishes any CV, in emphysematous lungs CV tends to exist and provides important channels for gas distribution. Whilst CV is a hindrance to the success of EBV therapy in preventing complete lobar occlusion, it may also be used to therapeutic advantage. Experimental and clinical work has demonstrated that creation of direct passages between emphysematous pulmonary parenchyma and bronchial airways (i.e. airway bypass) could take advantage of the extensive CV present in emphysema to provide improvement in expiratory flow and volume, which is otherwise limited by the collapse of the small, peripheral airways during expiration [6, 8].

Airway bypass involves transbronchial fenestration followed by placement of an airway bypass stent device [6, 9, 28, 29]. The stent is made of stainless steel embedded within silicone rubber, which is impregnated with paclitaxel to improve stent patency [9]. It is mounted on a delivery device and delivered endoscopically through a 2 mm working channel of a flexible bronchoscope. The stent is placed through segmental or sub-segmental airways to provide an extra-anatomic airway for trapped gas to escape, thereby reducing hyperinflation.

Airway bypass stents are targeted at patients with severe homogeneous emphysema, unlike the unidirectional bronchial valves (EBV and IBV), which are targeted at patients with heterogeneous emphysema. The airway bypass stent (Exhale Emphysema Treatment System) is manufactured by Broncus Technologies Inc., Mountain View, California, USA. Its design and features can be viewed at the company Website [30].

The EASE Trial: Exhale Airway Stents for Emphysema Trial

The findings of the Exhale Airway Stents for Emphysema (EASE) randomised trial, which aimed to evaluate the safety and clinical efficacy of bronchoscopic airway bypass in patients with severe homogeneous emphysema, were published in 2012 [5]. 315 patients with severe hyperinflation (ratio of residual volume to total lung capacity ≥0.65) secondary to homogeneous pulmonary emphysema were randomised to either airway bypass or a sham surgical control. The 6-month primary endpoint was based on a composite of lung function and clinical efficacy measure: ≥12 % in FVC and a ≥1-point decrease in the modified Medical Research Council (mMRC) dyspnoea score.

Significant improvements in lung function were observed in airway bypass patients compared to the control group at day 1 post bronchoscopy. However, these acute benefits declined by month 1, and continued to do so until the final, 12-month follow-up. Mean mMRC scores in the stent group were better than the control throughout follow-up, but in the absence of improvements in lung function parameters, these clinical measures may be of limited significance.

All primary and secondary measures, except mMRC, returned to baseline by 6 months. Loss of the initial benefits was attributed to a combination of factors, including passages that were created but not stented, stents that were expectorated and loss of stent patency. CT analyses showed that, in lobes in which stents placed were free of tissue density (a surrogate for stent patency), observed RV reduction at 6 months (−8.4 %) was comparable to results at day 1 (−10 %). Therefore, the paclitaxel–silicone polymer dose-release combination appeared inadequate at preserving stent patency, with only 21 % of stents deemed patent on CT analyses at 6 months, compared with 66 % on day 1.

Higher rates of pneumothorax, haemoptysis and COPD exacerbations were observed in patients assigned to airway bypass. However, at 12 months, rates of COPD exacerbation and pulmonary infection were similar between the two treatment groups. Mortality at 12 months was 6.7 % in the airway bypass arm and 6.5 % in the sham control, exhibiting similar Kaplan–Meier curves.

Paclitaxel did not appear as effective in maintaining stent patency as it did in animal studies [9]. Despite an acceptable safety profile, the EASE trial failed to show sustained long-term benefits in patients with severe homogeneous emphysema who underwent airway bypass stenting.

Other Concepts

Several other bronchoscopic approaches to lung volume reduction have been described.

Bronchial Lung Volume Reduction Coils

The bronchial lung volume reduction coils (LVRC) (RePneu® LVRC) are made from nitinol wires that result in parenchymal compression following bronchoscopic deployment (Fig. 11.7). The LVRC approach has no dependency upon the absence of collateral ventilation to achieve efficacy, unlike the unidirectional bronchial valves. A feasibility study evaluating LVRC performed on 11 patients observed no severe adverse effects after 3 months. Patients with either heterogeneous or homogeneous emphysema were included in the study. Despite the small cohort, patients with heterogeneous disease appeared to show better clinical efficacy post procedure than patients with homogeneous emphysema [2].

Sealant

Bronchoscopic lung volume reduction using direct application of a sealant to collapse areas of emphysematous lung has been reported. Initial tests of a synthetic polymeric foam sealant (emphysematous lung sealant, ELS, Aeriseal) were performed in 25 patients with severe (Global Initiative for Chronic Obstructive Lung Disease, GOLD stage III and IV) heterogeneous emphysema [7]. After 6 months, ELS treatment correlated with improvements in pulmonary function, exercise capacity and quality of life measures. CT analysis indicated induction of local atelectasis at sites of treatment. Interestingly, patients with GOLD stage III disease showed greater physiological gains than stage IV patients. This may reflect the greater extent of tissue destruction in stage IV patients, presumably requiring additional volume reduction to produce improvements comparable to stage III patients. Despite the encouraging early results it must be remembered that ELS therapy, in contrast to EBV, is an irreversible procedure.

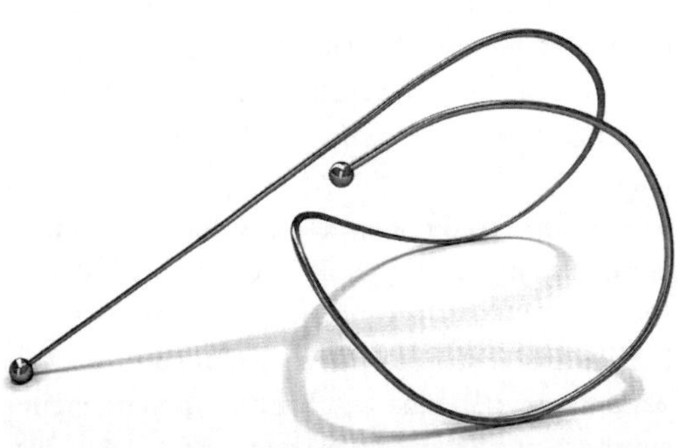

Fig. 11.7 RePneu® lung volume reduction coil [courtesy of PneumRx Inc., California]

Bronchoscopic Thermal Vapor Ablation

Bronchoscopic thermal vapor ablation (BTVA) involves delivery of precise amounts of steam water vapor directly into target lung segments via a specialised catheter. The thermal reaction leads to a localised inflammatory response, resultant permanent fibrosis, and atelectasis in order to achieve targeted, complete and permanent LVR in patients with heterogeneous emphysema. A potential advantage of BTVA is that success is independent of CV. Snell et al. [31] reported outcomes in 44 patients with upper-lobe predominant heterogeneous emphysema who underwent unilateral BTVA. Adverse events were reported in 19 patients, with COPD exacerbation being the most common. Most adverse events (62 %) occurred within the first 30 days following BTVA. An average of 48 % LVR in the target lobar and 17 % improvement in FEV_1 were achieved at 3 months, both of which were sustained at 6 months follow-up. The majority of patients (73 %) also reported a significant improvement in functional measures (SGRQ) at 6 months.

Conclusion

It is increasingly pertinent to separate emphysematous patients by their pattern of disease. Recent evidence demonstrates significant physiological and clinical benefits from the use of bronchial valves in patients with heterogeneous emphysema. Importantly, this effect appeared most marked when valve placement resulted in total lobar occlusion and was symbiotically related to the absence of collateral ventilation, of which the presence of complete fissures on CT was an indirect marker for. In practice, this highlights the need for routine utilisation of HRCT, not only to appropriately select patients for the different bronchoscopic techniques but also to more accurately identify positive responders, by targeting lobes where complete fissures exist to ensure complete lobar occlusion, thereby resulting in effective TLVR. Two recent reports also suggest a survival advantage in those patients with a good response to bronchial valve treatment [15, 16]. Additionally, as new developments such as the Chartis® system are refined, we will have tools by which the presence or the absence of collateral ventilation may be gauged, thus facilitating improvement in patient selection. Disappointingly, the EASE trial failed to report sustained benefits of airway bypasses for patients with homogeneous emphysema. However, this should not negate the positive acute-term benefits demonstrated, which suggests that it could be a worthwhile approach if the issue of stent occlusion can be mitigated.

The role of bronchoscopic LVR techniques will continue to evolve as better understanding of their effects in different emphysema phenotypes becomes more apparent and a clearer definition of patient characteristics determining successful responses emerges. Newer approaches, such as bronchoscopic coils, biological agents and thermal methods, show promise but need further investigation involving randomised control studies. A key issue will be to reach a consensus about endpoints that are clinically relevant yet physiologically practical, in order to offer a platform with which to compare the different endoscopic treatment modalities.

References

1. Fishman A, Martinez F, Naunheim K, Piantadosi S, Wise R, Ries A, et al. A randomized trial comparing lung-volume-reduction surgery with medical therapy for severe emphysema. N Engl J Med. 2003;348:2059–73.
2. Herth FJ, Eberhard R, Gompelmann D, Slebos DJ, Ernst A. Bronchoscopic lung volume reduction with a dedicated coil: a clinical pilot study. Ther Adv Respir Dis. 2010;4:225–31.
3. Sciurba FC, Ernst A, Herth FJ, Strange C, Criner GJ, Marquette CH, et al. A randomized study of endobronchial valves for advanced emphysema. N Engl J Med. 2010;363:1233–44.
4. Sterman DH, Mehta AC, Wood DE, Mathur PN, McKenna Jr RJ, Ost DE, et al. A multicenter pilot study of a bronchial valve for the treatment of severe emphysema. Respiration. 2010;79:222–33.
5. Shah PL, Slebos DJ, Cardoso PF, Cetti E, Voelker K, Levine B, et al. group Ets. Bronchoscopic lung-volume reduction with Exhale airway stents for emphysema (EASE trial): randomised, sham-controlled, multicentre trial. Lancet. 2011;378:997–1005.
6. Choong CK, Cardoso PF, Sybrecht GW, Cooper JD. Airway bypass treatment of severe homogeneous emphysema: taking advantage of collateral ventilation. Thorac Surg Clin. 2009;19:239–45.
7. Herth FJ, Gompelmann D, Stanzel F, Bonnet R, Behr J, Schmidt B, et al. Treatment of advanced emphysema with emphysematous lung sealant (AeriSeal(R)). Respiration. 2011;82:36–45.
8. Choong CK, Macklem PT, Pierce JA, Das N, Lutey BA, Martinez CO, et al. Airway bypass improves the mechanical properties of explanted emphysematous lungs. Am J Respir Crit Care Med. 2008;178:902–5.
9. Choong CK, Phan L, Massetti P, Haddad FJ, Martinez C, Roschak E, et al. Prolongation of patency of airway bypass stents with use of drug-eluting stents. J Thorac Cardiovasc Surg. 2006;131:60–4.
10. Springmeyer SC, Bolliger CT, Waddell TK, Gonzalez X, Wood DE, Teams IBVVPTR. Treatment of heterogeneous emphysema using the spiration IBV valves. Thorac Surg Clin. 2009;19:247–53. ix–x.
11. Venuta F, Rendina EA, Coloni GF. Endobronchial treatment of emphysema with one-way valves. Thorac Surg Clin. 2009;19:255–60. x.
12. Pulmonx Inc. 2012. http://www.pulmonx.com. Accessed 19 Sept 2012.
13. Spiration Inc. 2012. http://www.spiration.com. Acessed 19 Sept 2012.
14. Herth FJ, Noppen M, Valipour A, Leroy S, Vergnon JM, Ficker JH, et al. Efficacy predictors of lung volume reduction with Zephyr valves in a European cohort. Eur Respir J. 2012;39:1334–42.
15. Hopkinson NS, Kemp SV, Toma TP, Hansell DM, Geddes DM, Shah PL, et al. Atelectasis and survival after bronchoscopic lung volume reduction for COPD. Eur Respir J. 2011;37:1346–51.
16. Venuta F, Anile M, Diso D, Carillo C, De Giacomo T, D'Andrilli A, et al. Long-term follow-up after bronchoscopic lung volume reduction in patients with emphysema. Eur Respir J. 2012;39:1084–9.
17. Kotecha S, Westall GP, Holsworth L, Pham A, Williams TJ, Snell GI. Long-term outcomes from bronchoscopic lung volume reduction using a bronchial prosthesis. Respirology. 2011;16:167–73.

18. Herth FJ, Eberhardt R, Gompelmann D, Ficker JH, Wagner M, Ek L, Schmidt B, Slebos DJ. Radiological and clinical outcomes of using chartis to plan endobronchial valve treatment. Eur Respir J 2013;41: 302–8
19. Shah PL, Geddes DM. Collateral ventilation and selection of techniques for bronchoscopic lung volume reduction. Thorax. 2012;67:285–6.
20. Kent EM, Blades B. The Anatomic Approach to Pulmonary Resection. Ann Surg. 1942;116:782–94.
21. Herth FJ, Gompelmann D, Ernst A, Eberhardt R. Endoscopic lung volume reduction. Respiration. 2010;79:5–13.
22. Gompelmann D ER, Slebos DJ, et al. Study of the Use of Chartis® Pulmonary Assessment System as a Predictor of Collateral Ventilation as Compared to Computed Tomography. Pulmonx Inc.: http://www.zephyrelvr2012.com/media/28872/ers_poster_chartis_and_ct_final_14_sept_2011pdf. Accessed 19 Sept 2012.
23. Gompelmann D, Eberhardt R, Michaud G, Ernst A, Herth FJ. Predicting atelectasis by assessment of collateral ventilation prior to endobronchial lung volume reduction: a feasibility study. Respiration. 2010;80: 419–25.
24. Criner GJ, Sternberg AL. National Emphysema Treatment Trial: the major outcomes of lung volume reduction surgery in severe emphysema. Proc Am Thorac Soc. 2008;5:393–405.
25. Ninane V, Geltner C, Bezzi M, Foccoli P, Gottlieb J, Welte T, et al. Multicentre European study for the treatment of advanced emphysema with bronchial valves. Eur Respir J. 2012;39:1319–25.
26. Eberhardt R, Gompelmann D, Schuhmann M, Reinhardt H, Ernst A, Heussel CP. Herth FJ. Chest: Complete unilateral versus partial bilateral endoscopic lung volume reduction in patients with bilateral lung emphysema; 2012.
27. Van Allen CLG, Richter HG. Gaseous interchange between adjacent lung lobules. Yale J Biol Med. 1930;2:297.
28. Choong CK, Haddad FJ, Gee EY, Cooper JD. Feasibility and safety of airway bypass stent placement and influence of topical mitomycin C on stent patency. J Thorac Cardiovasc Surg. 2005;129: 632–8.
29. Lausberg HF, Chino K, Patterson GA, Meyers BF, Toeniskoetter PD, Cooper JD. Bronchial fenestration improves expiratory flow in emphysematous human lungs. Ann Thorac Surg. 2003;75:393–7. discussion 398.
30. Broncus Technologies Inc. 2012. http://www.broncus.com. Acessed 19 Sept 2012.
31. Snell G, Herth FJ, Hopkins P, Baker KM, Witt C, Gotfried MH, et al. Bronchoscopic thermal vapour ablation therapy in the management of heterogeneous emphysema. Eur Respir J. 2012;39:1326–33.

Role of Bronchoscopy in Management of Bronchopleural Fistula

12

Yaser Abu El-Sameed

Abstract

Bronchopleural fistula (BPF) refers to a direct communication between the bronchial tree and pleural space. Lung resection is the most common cause of bronchopleural fistula. Other common causes include pulmonary infections, tuberculosis, spontaneous pneumothorax, and trauma. BPF is one of the most serious complications of lung surgery, associated with high morbidity and mortality. Chest computed tomography (CT) and bronchoscopy are useful in establishing diagnosis, identifying the cause and localization of fistulous track. The management of BPF is difficult and depends on underlying cardiopulmonary reserve, nutritional status, fitness to undergo a major surgical procedure, expertise available, and the size and location of fistula. Patients with >5 mm sized centrally located fistula are most likely to benefit from surgery. Several bronchoscopic techniques have also been described for management of BPF. Bronchoscopic interventions may be considered for ≤5 mm peripheral BPF, especially in debilitated and high-surgical-risk patients. In recent years, endobronchial valves have successfully resolved BPF in many such patients.

Keywords

Bronchopleural fistula • Prolonged air leak • Pneumothorax • Endobronchial valves

Introduction

Bronchopleural fistula (BPF) is defined as a communication between the tracheobronchial tree and the pleural space [1, 2]. The incidence of BPF has decreased significantly since the availability of effective antimicrobial and antitubercular treatment, and with advances in surgical techniques. The incidence of BPF after

Y.A. El-Sameed, M.B.B.S. (✉)
Respirology Division, Medical Institute, Sheikh Khalifa Medical City, Karama Street, Abu Dhabi 51900, United Arab Emirates
e-mail: yelsameed@skmc.ae

A.C. Mehta and P. Jain (eds.), *Interventional Bronchoscopy: A Clinical Guide*, Respiratory Medicine 10, DOI 10.1007/978-1-62703-395-4_12,

pulmonary resection ranges from 1.5 to 28 % [3–7]. The incidence after lobectomy is lower (0.5 %) [6]. It is also affected by the method of the bronchus closure and the underlying disease process for which the surgery is performed [8–10]. In this chapter, the etiology, risk factors, diagnosis, and treatment of BPF are discussed. The main focus is on the emerging role of bronchoscopy in the management of BPF. A detailed discussion of surgical options and techniques is beyond the scope of this review.

Etiologies and Risk Factors

More than two-thirds of BPFs occur as a postoperative complication after pulmonary resection, including pneumonectomy [7, 11]. Other causes include pulmonary infections, spontaneous pneumothorax, chest trauma, chemotherapy or radiotherapy for lung cancer, tuberculosis (TB), and as a complication of mechanical ventilation [2, 7, 11]. In lung cancer surgeries, right pneumonectomy is associated with significantly increased risk of BPF, especially when mediastinal lymph node dissection is performed and there is residual carcinoma at the bronchial stump [12]. BPF is well described after pulmonary resections are performed due to inflammatory lung conditions, especially active TB [13]. Other risk factors include acute respiratory distress syndrome (ARDS), malnutrition, and emphysema [4, 14–18]. Radiofrequency ablation (RFA) used to treat pulmonary malignancies can be complicated by fistula formation [19]. BPFs may also occur spontaneously.

The most common location for BPF to develop in lung cancer patients after resection is the surgical stump [20]. Certain factors increase the risk to develop BPF in these patients. These factors include fever, steroid use, elevated erythrocyte sedimentation rate, leukocytosis, anemia, and bronchoscopy for mucus suctioning [20]. In one study that included 221 pneumonectomies for non-small-cell lung cancer (NSCLC), five patients (2.3 %) developed BPF [21]. Univariate analysis revealed that perioperative blood transfusion, preoperative respiratory infection, neoadjuvant therapy, right pneumonectomy, manual closure of the bronchus, days of postoperative hospitalization, and mechanical ventilation are significant risk factors for BPF development. On multivariate analysis, preoperative respiratory infection and right pneumonectomy were the only independent risk factors [21]. Local factors have been identified as risk factors for development of post-pneumonectomy BPF. These include residual carcinoma at the bronchial-stump margin, long bronchial stump, disrupted bronchial blood supply, inadequate technique of stump closure, presence of empyema, extended resection, and preoperative radiation [22–24].

The association between TB and BPF remains significant [16, 25, 26]. These fistulae can occur after pulmonary resections for TB or spontaneously from the cavitary disease [16, 26, 27]. Pomerantz et al. noted an incidence of 10.5 % after resections in 85 patients with drug-resistant mycobacterial infection [28]. Almost all BPFs occurred after right pneumonectomy in patients with multiple resistant TB.

The best bronchial closure technique to prevent BPFs has been debated. One report assessed bronchial closures in 625 consecutive patients [29]. BPF rate was 3.8 % and was more common among patients who had stapler closure than in patients who had manual closure of the bronchial stump. In one series of 209 pneumonectomies performed because of malignant disease, Hubaut et al. [30] found the incidence of BPF with manual closure of stump to be 2.4 %. Others have similarly reported a low incidence of fistula development by manual closure as well [12, 23, 31]. Still, considerable controversy continues as some experts prefer routine stapler use while others suggest manual closure [32]. The stated benefits of using staplers in pulmonary resections include minimizing contamination of operation area, reducing the time required for closure, and their safety in vascular divisions [32–34]. Due to these considerations, some authors continue to advocate the routine use of stapling in these patients [33–35].

Morbidity and Mortality

BPF is one of the most feared complications after pulmonary resection for NSCLC. It is still associated with a high mortality rate ranging from 25 to 71.2 %, with death most commonly resulting from aspiration pneumonia and subsequent ARDS [12, 16, 23, 36–38]. Pneumonia can also develop from the contamination of normal lung by empyema material via the fistula [36, 39, 40]. BPFs are also associated with high morbidity [6]. Delayed closure of the BPF may lead to empyema, need for surgical drainage, and prolonged antibiotics therapy [41]. Not unexpectedly, many patients develop significant malnutrition and low albumin levels. Factors that add to worsening outcome include impaired respiratory mechanics, contralateral lung contamination, and chronic pleural infection [42]. Apart from prolonged hospital stay, other complications include atelectasis, hospital-acquired pneumonia, and thromboembolic disease [19, 39].

Mechanical ventilation is an established risk factor for development of BPF. One study reviewed all instances of mechanical ventilation during a 4-year period and found that 39 of the 1,700 patients developed BPF [17]. The mortality rate in these 39 patients was 67 % and was higher when BPF developed late in the illness. All eight patients whose maximum air leak exceeded 500 ml per breath succumbed to the illness [17]. The management of BPF in ventilator-dependent patients is especially challenging because positive airway pressure interferes with closure of the fistulous track between the airways and pleura. According to one report, timely intervention in patients with chronic empyema and BPF with omentopexy and muscle transposition is associated with decreased morbidity and mortality [43].

Presentation

BPF patients can have either an early acute presentation or a delayed insidious onset. Acutely, BPF can be life-threatening secondary to tension pneumothorax or pulmonary flooding [2]. BPF may cause sudden entry of potentially infected material into the airways and lung parenchyma from the pleural space [1, 44]. This exudate may flood the airways of both lungs leading to acute respiratory deterioration. Other acute manifestations of BPF include subcutaneous emphysema, and decrease or disappearance of pleural effusion on the chest radiograph in postoperative cases. A persistent air leak from the chest tube postoperatively may indicate a BPF. Postoperatively, and after chest tube removal, the diagnosis of BPF can be suspected in the face of fever, cough productive of purulent sputum, and new or increasing air fluid level in the pleural space [3].

Alternatively, patients with a BPF may present with a slow deterioration associated with fever, weight loss, and cough. The pleural space in these cases is usually fibrotic and chronically infected [1, 15, 16].

Diagnosis and Localization of BPF

Chest computed tomography (CT) scan can be useful in detecting the etiology of BPF. Ricci et al. [45] reported that CT scan was useful in identifying and localizing the cause of BPF in 55 % of their patients who required surgical management of their patients with BPFs. Methylene blue has been used to localize BPF in patients with chest tube [46]. This is done by injecting the material into the bronchial stump and observing if it would be seen in the chest tube [47], but this method for localizing BPF is no longer favored.

Bronchoscopy allows not only direct visualization of central BPFs but also adequate localization of peripheral ones in many instances [48–50]. The localization of distal BPF requires passing a balloon catheter to the bronchial segment leading to the fistula using the balloon-catheter occlusion method [51–54]. In this technique, a balloon is systematically passed through the working channel of the bronchoscope and into each bronchial segment in question and then inflated for a period of 30–120 s. A reduction in air leak in the collection chamber indicates localization of a bronchial segment communicating with the BPF [51–54]. A 5-F Fogarty catheter can be used; however, other catheters have also been described [55]. If a proximal BPF cannot be visualized directly or occlusion of a distal BPF does not significantly decreases or stops the air leak, bronchoscopic methods will not be suitable to manage these fistulae.

Management

Management options of BPF include both surgical and medical therapies, in addition to different bronchoscopic interventions. The first step in the management of patients with BPF should be directed to any urgent condition like tension pneumothorax [56, 57]. Other important components of the treatment are proper drainage of the pleural space, adequate antibiotic therapy, nutritional support, and treatment of underlying disorder leading to development of BPF [58–61].

Different surgical procedures directed at closing BPFs have a success rate between 80 and 95 %; however, they are associated with high morbidity and mortality [43, 62, 63]. Surgical procedures focus on empyema drainage and reinforcement of the bronchial stump with different flaps. Chronic empyema may need thoracoplasty with removal of part of the chest wall [64, 65]. Completion of bronchial resection is usually necessary when BPF complicates lobectomy [66]. Video-assisted thoracoscopy surgery (VATS) has been increasingly used to manage prolonged BPF with a high rate of success [67]. One recent surgical technique includes debridement of the pleural space followed by suturing of the bronchial stump and reinforcement by intrathoracic transposition of omentum or muscle flaps [68, 69]. If the BPF cannot be identified, then open-window thoracotomy and daily dressing may be helpful.

In the past, the role of bronchoscopy in the management of BPF was limited to evaluation of the bronchial stump and for exclusion of different infections. More recently, bronchoscopy has gained a more prominent role in the treatment of patients with BPF. Bronchoscopic interventions now provide an option to manage those patients with BPF who are poor surgical candidates, unable to tolerate major thoracic surgeries [37, 70]. Bronchoscopy can also be used as a bridge in very sick patients until their condition improves and can undergo surgical correction of the fistula [71]. In one report, fiberoptic bronchoscopy has been also used percutaneously to visualize and investigate broncho-pleuro-cutaneous fistula [72]. Unfortunately, the overwhelming data on bronchoscopic interventions are limited to isolated case reports or short case series. The current literature does not allow adequate comparison of different bronchoscopic options available. The interventionists need to use clinical judgment in selecting the patient and the specific intervention in management of these patients.

Hartmann and Rausch [73] were the first to report closure of a postoperative peripheral BPF using methylcyanoacrylate in 1977. In the same year, Ratliff et al. [54] reported bronchoscopic control of a BPF by placement of lead shot. Since then, many reports using different devices have appeared for management of BPF via bronchoscopy. Bronchoscopic interventions are usually reserved for small fistulas or for patients with poor general condition [2, 7]. The efficacy of the bronchoscopic techniques in controlling BPF decreases as the diameter of the fistula increases [12, 74].

In a review of 96 cases describing the natural history of BPF after pneumonectomy [36], surgical procedures achieved closure of BPFs in 21 patients while bronchoscopic techniques were successful in 11 patients. Nonetheless, the overall postoperative mortality rate was 31 %. Another major review was performed to compare bronchoscopic approaches for closure of BPFs to conventional thoracotomy in post-pneumonectomy BPFs [42]. The search identified six case series with greater than two post-pneumonectomy BPF fistula patients. There were 85 patients with post-pneumonectomy BPFs who underwent bronchoscopic procedures to manage BPF. The success rate of different bronchoscopic techniques was 30 %. The mortality was 40 %, again reflecting a very high mortality rate in this patient's population.

No studies compared different bronchoscopic interventions in managing BPFs. BPF size is an important factor in predicting the outcome of the procedure as bronchoscopic options usually do not have a good success rate in fistulas larger than 5 mm [75–77]. Reports of successful treatment using bronchoscopic techniques are with BPF size not exceeding 5 mm [75–78]. Taken together, the most suitable candidate for bronchoscopic closure of a BPF is a patient who is at high surgical risk with a fistula <5 mm [79]. In cases of large BPFs, open surgery is often required [80].

Bronchoscopic management of BPF is based on the delivery of different materials and small devices into the BPF sites. Examples include using different glues, gel foam, antibiotics, ethanol injections, silicone fillers, coils, airway stents, amplatzer devices, endobronchial valves, among others [50–55, 81–100].

Synthetic Glue

Cyanoacrylate glue is a commonly used sealant to treat BPFs. Once the glue comes in contact with tissue, it forms a polymer and solidifies. Used in this manner, the glue acts like a barrier and later on induces inflammation followed by fibrous tissue formation. During bronchoscopy, after BPF is localized using aforementioned techniques, a catheter is passed through the working channel in proximity to the BPF location. The next step is to inject 0.5–1 ml of the glue into the fistula [37, 50, 101–105]. Glue treatment is considered a low-cost intervention and can be done on outpatient basis [103]. One report used methyl-2-cyanoacrylate to close post-resection BPF bronchoscopically [106]. Of the 12 patients included, the success rate was 83 %. Another series of nine cases used bronchoscopic injection of *N*-butyl-cyanoacrylate glue to close BPF [103]. In eight patients, the glue was able to successfully seal the fistulae. There were no complications in this study which made the authors recommend this approach in high-risk surgical patients. Histo-acryl glue has also been used in the form of submucosal injection to treat BPF [107]. In this report, the patient had BPF after right pneumonectomy for NSCLC. The submucosal injection of glue helped in closing the fistula by reducing the diameter of the fistula. The glue also enhanced granulation tissue formation. Despite these successful reports, Belda-Sanchís et al. [108] published a Cochrane review on the use of surgical sealants in air leaks after pulmonary resection in patients with lung cancer that did not recommend their use. The 2010 review included 16 trials that showed decrease in postoperative air leaks but no consistent reduction in the hospital length of stay [108].

Fibrin Glue

Fibrin glue has been used successfully to close small post-resection BPFs via bronchoscopy [70, 96, 109–112]. It is used in the management of proximal [70, 96, 109] and peripheral BPF [51]. The procedure involves injection of 1 ml of fibrinogen via a catheter at the desired site followed rapidly by injecting another ml of thrombin (1,000 U/ml). The resulting mixture forms a fibrin clot and seals the fistula. In an animal study, the effectiveness of fibrin glue in reducing experimental pulmonary air leak was evaluated [113]. The glue was applied to the pleural side of a BPF. Postoperative evaluations disclosed no increased adhesions in the glue-treated animals and complete resorption of the glue at 3 months.

Tissue Adhesives

One report examined the use of albumin–glutaraldehyde tissue adhesive in the management of BPFs in 38 patients who underwent thoracic surgeries [114]. The adhesive was able to close the pulmonary fistulae and prevent air leakage from surgical stumps. Another report of successful closure of complicated BPFs with the same material in two patients is also published [115].

Gel Foam

The technique for occlusion of peripheral BPFs using gel foam as a temporary endobronchial blocker has been described by Jones et al. [97]. Gel foam is readily available and easily administered. It is totally absorbed within 1 month [3].

Tissue Expander

A successful technique that uses submucosal injection of a tissue expander for bronchoscopic occlusion of BPFs has been reported. This method may be used either alone or in combination with bronchoscopic instillation of *N*-butyl-cyanoacrylate glue [74]. In one report, successful treatment of two patients with BPF was described [74]. The tissue expander used was a biocompatible agent composed of pyrolytic carbon-coated beads suspended in a water-based carrier gel containing beta-glucan. The carbon-coated beads acted as physical filler which kept the fistula closed. Another report on using a tissue expander for management of persistent alveolar fistula after lobectomy had a successful outcome [116]. In that report, the patient developed a thoracic empyema after right bi-lobectomy for lung cancer. After draining the empyema, a muscle flap was used to close the fistula. However, a residual space remained, and air leak persisted. Implanting a tissue expander was able to tightly fix the flap and solve the air leak.

Antibiotics

Doxycycline has been used successfully as a pleural sclerosing agent when given through a chest tube for persistent BPFs [117]. In one case report, doxycycline was used for management of BPF in a patient with severe pneumonia resulting in chronic fistula formation and respiratory failure [90]. Intrabronchial instillation of tetracycline caused the fistula to close and improvement in the patient condition. Similar case reports have been published [52].

Ethanol

Initially, alcohol was used for the treatment of protuberant lesions of the stomach by intramural injection under direct vision [118]. There are reports of intra-tumoral ethanol injection to manage malignant tracheobronchial lesions via bronchoscopy [95]. Local injection of absolute alcohol has also been used for bronchoscopic closure of BP fistula. The swelling of the mucosa caused by the injection is responsible for the initial control of the BPF. At a later date, granulation tissue develops which keeps the fistula closed [118, 119]. One report included five patients with central BPFs who were successfully treated by injecting absolute ethanol directly into the submucosal layer of the fistula under bronchoscopy [89]. No complications occurred as a result of this treatment. This intervention allowed reduction in the cost and duration of hospitalization and improved the patients' quality of life.

Argon Plasma Coagulation and Nd:YAG Laser

One report presented a case that used argon plasma coagulation (APC) for the management of BPF developed secondary to tracheobronchial anastomosis failure [120]. It aimed at providing an alternative treatment for small uncomplicated fistulae that develop after pneumonectomy. In this report, a 56-year-old patient underwent a sleeve pneumonectomy for NSCLC. The patient developed cough and productive sputum 3 months after surgery. He was found to have two small fistulae at the anastomosis junction with no evidence of tumor recurrence. APC was applied using bronchoscopy under local anesthesia with no complications. The patient was followed up for 18 months without any symptoms. The healing of the fistula can be attributed to mechanical trauma and wound healing resulting in fibrosis. Kiriyama et al. reported the use of endobronchial neodymium:yttrium–aluminum–garnet (Nd:YAG) laser for noninvasive closure of small proximal BPF after lung resection [121].

Silicone Fillers

Silicone fillers have been used successfully in the management of BPF caused by intractable pneumothorax. Watanabe et al. [93] reported their experience in using bronchial occlusion with endobronchial spigots (Fig. 12.1) in patients with prolonged BPFs. The air leak either stopped or was markedly reduced in 77.6 % of all patients (Fig. 12.2). Endoscopic bronchial occlusion with

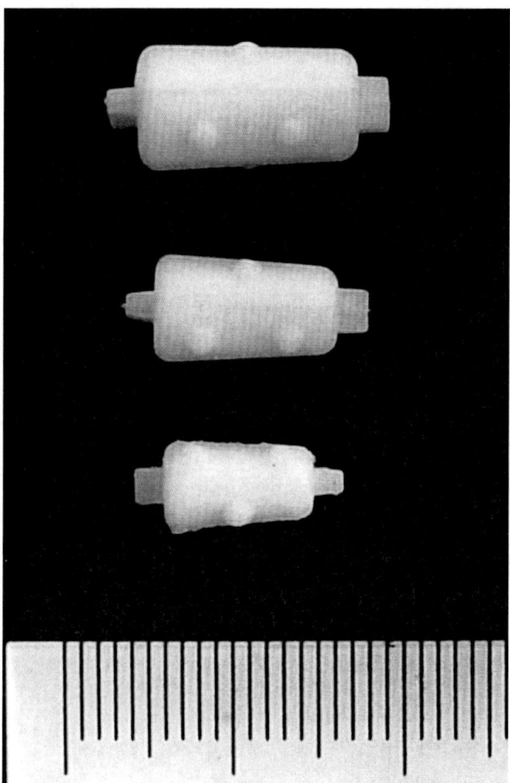

Fig. 12.1 Endobronchial Watanabe spigots (courtesy of Dr. Sukagawa and Dr. Watanabe)

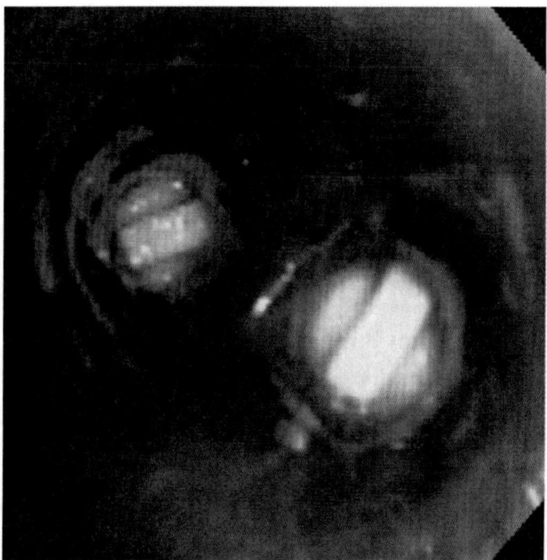

Fig. 12.2 Endobronchial Watanabe spigot placed via flexible bronchoscope (courtesy of Dr. Sukagawa and Dr. Watanabe)

silicone embolic material has also been used to control an intractable BPF caused by RFA [122]. In this report, a 58-year-old man with NSCLC underwent RFA that was complicated by a pneumothorax. Air leak continued despite prolonged chest drainage. Bronchial occlusion was performed with a silicone embolus, causing cessation of the air leakage.

Coils

There are several published reports on using coils to control BPFs [99, 100, 123]. In one such report, bronchoscopy was used to place angiographic occlusion coils over large bronchopleural fistula with good control of the leak [99]. Another case series reported a method of permanently blocking small peripheral airways using vascular occlusion coils placed endobronchially by modified angiographic techniques [100]. The procedure was applied in five cases of complicated parenchymal air leaks. Complete or substantial partial control was achieved in all cases with no complications. The technique for endobronchial occlusion of BPF with metallic coils and glue applied using bronchoscopy under local anesthesia has been described [91]. In this technique, after anchoring the vascular embolization coils at the fistula bronchus, cyanoacrylate glue was sprayed. The sprayed glue obliterates gaps between the coils and stabilizes them. The procedure was successful in all patients except one case with large fistula [91]. Another report of a woman with BPFs treated with the endobronchial placement of vascular embolization coils was published by Uchida et al. [124]. She developed multiple BPFs after surgical treatment for empyema. These fistulae were occluded endobronchially by the placement of vascular embolization coils. Soon after the procedure, air leak from the fistulas stopped and the drainage tube was removed 2 days later.

Airway Stents

Airway stents are commonly used to manage tracheal or bronchial fistulae communicating with the esophagus [125–128]. Their use has been extended to management of BPFs after pulmonary resections [129–133]. Watanabe et al. [129] described successful management of a BPF with bronchial stent placement combined with irrigation of the empyema cavity. The BPF developed in a 67-year-old man after lobectomy for lung cancer. Re-suturing of the bronchial stump and using different flaps were not effective. Placement of a Dumon stent in the bronchus to close the stump was able to control the fistula. Another report by Tayama et al. [130] described a similar case where a BPF developed after pneumonectomy for lung cancer. It involved placement of modified Dumon which effectively closed the stump. The high incidence of silicone stent migration causing recurrence of the BPF may make a case to use the fully covered self-expandable metallic stents (SEMSs) in order to provide better control over the fistula. Takahashi et al. [134] reported using the Ultraflex expandable stent in the management of large post-pneumonectomy BPF [134]. The patient developed postoperative empyema and aspergillosis. A covered Ultraflex expandable stent was implanted to block a major air leak from the BPF. The patient's general condition improved and he was discharged 1 month after stenting. Recently, the efficacy and outcome of using customized conical tracheobronchial SEMSs were evaluated in the multidisciplinary management of large post-pneumonectomy fistulae [132]. These stents were used in seven patients with post-pneumonectomy BPFs that are larger than 6 mm in diameter. Air leak was stopped in all patients after the procedure but mortality remained high at 57 %, mainly secondary due to sepsis. Another recent study aimed at assessing the feasibility, efficacy, and safety of conical SEMSs in the treatment of post-pneumonectomy BPFs had positive results [80]. Six patients underwent the procedure with the aim of excluding the bronchial dehiscence from the airflow. Five patients presented with a BPF larger than 5 mm following pneumonectomy. One patient had an anastomotic dehiscence after tracheal sleeve pneumonectomy. The prosthesis was secured to tracheal mucosa with titanium helical fastener tacks. Immediate resolution of the bronchial air leak was obtained in all patients. Permanent closure of the bronchial dehiscence was achieved in all the patients followed by successful removal without complications.

Amplatzer Devices

Amplatzer devices (ADs) are usually used to treat congenital heart defects [135–138].

One report described three patients who underwent bronchoscopic control of their fistulae by inserting atrial septal defect occluders [139]. Two of the fistulae were larger than 10 mm in diameter. The procedure was minimally invasive and resulted in resolution of BPFs. Another case report described successful closure of the BPF using bronchoscopic implantation of an AD in a patient with a right main stem BPF following pneumonectomy [140]. Similarly, an atrial septal defect occluder was used to close a bronchial fistula that developed after lobectomy for aspergilloma with immediate reduction in the air leak [141]. On follow-up bronchoscopy examination, the device was almost covered by granulation tissue. This endobronchial technique seems to be safe and effective to manage large BPFs. Passera et al. [142] presented a case of lower bi-lobectomy complicated by a large BPF and empyema 1 month after primary surgery. The patient was immediately treated with an open-window thoracostomy. After surgical debridement, an AD was positioned to close the fistula. Thereafter, the thoracostomy was rapidly closed with vacuum-assisted closure therapy. The combined approach led to a successful outcome.

A recent series describing the management of 10 patients with 11 BPFs using ADs was published by Fruchter et al. [86]. Procedures were done under conscious sedation. A nitinol double-disk occluder device was delivered under direct bronchoscopic guidance over a guide-wire causing occlusion of the fistula. The procedure was successful in nine patients and symptoms related to the BPF disappeared. It was well tolerated by patients with no side effects or complications. The results were maintained over a median follow-up of 9 months. Compared to SEMSs, the

ADs leave the airway free from foreign material which avoids the issue of mucous impaction. The AD does not need to be removed as usually required for a metallic stent.

Endobronchial Valves

Endobronchial valves (EBVs) are one of the recent additions to different devices for the management of BPF. They were initially designed to perform bronchoscopic lung volume reduction in selected emphysema patients [143]. The EBV functions as a unidirectional valve allowing both expiratory air and secretions to flow but stopping inspiratory flow. It is anchored within the airway creating an airtight seal against the bronchial wall, hence preventing any air leak around the device itself. Early case reports described the use of EBVs to control intractable pulmonary-pleural fistulas [55, 66, 144]. These reports included patients who developed empyema but surgical treatment could not close the BPF. Other patients were too sick to undergo surgery [19, 145–150]. A large group of cases was published by Travaline et al. that included 40 patients with prolonged air leak [151]. Patients underwent EBV insertion as the primary method to manage their BPFs. The rates of complete and partial resolution of air leak were 47.5 and 45 %, respectively. Chest tubes remained for a mean time of 21 days (median 7.5; interquartile range [IQR] 3–29 days) after EBV insertion. The mean time from valve procedure to hospital discharge was 19 ± 28 days (median 11; IQR 4–27 days). Another report presented the results of seven consecutive patients who had complex BPFs and were managed successfully with EBVs [152]. El-Sameed et al. [153] reported their successful experience in managing persistent BPFs with EBVs and included a review of the literature. They treated four patients who presented with varying forms of prolonged air leak (Figs. 12.3 and 12.4). Two of their patients had TB as a cause of the BPF. All patients had improvement after the procedure and all valves were removed successfully with no complications. These reports show that EBVs can be placed easily using flexible bronchoscopy and under conscious sedation. Currently, Emphasys bronchial valves (EBV) and Spiration intrabronchial valve (IBV) are available for use. The Food and Drug Administration (FDA) has granted Spiration IBV humanitarian use designation since 2006 under the Humanitarian Device Exemption Program that allows it to be used for any patient who has undergone lung resection surgery or

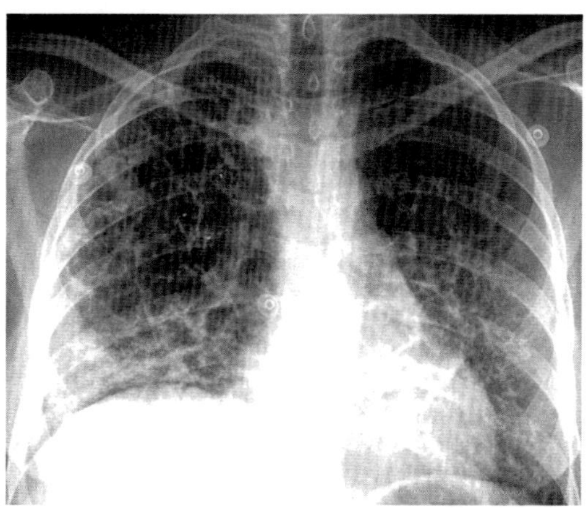

Fig. 12.3 Chest radiograph showing three endobronchial valves in the right upper lobe in a patient who had prolonged bronchopleural fistula from advanced bronchiectasis (reprinted from [153] with permission from Springer Science + Business Media)

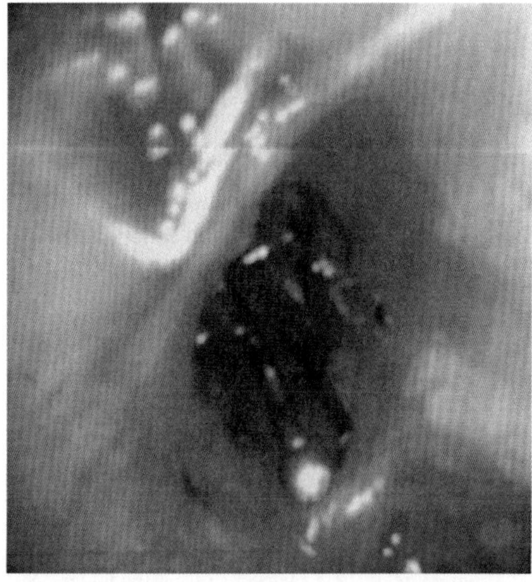

Fig. 12.4 A bronchoscopic image showing an endobronchial valve placed in a disrupted bronchial stump

lung volume reduction operation with a prolonged air leak present 7 or more days after the surgery [154]. While this is an attractive option for some of these patients, larger studies are needed to define the exact role of EBVs in the management of BPF.

Summary

There are multiple bronchoscopic interventions that can be offered to manage BPF. However, most publications are case series or limited case reports with no definite guidelines on the best approach to manage difficult BPFs. Bronchoscopic procedures seem beneficial in high-risk surgical patients. The size and the ability to localize the fistula can help in determining the choice between surgical and bronchoscopic options. There are no comparative studies to support any particular bronchoscopic intervention over the other. Along with the patient's condition and the BPF assessment, availability of resources and the bronchoscopist expertise remain important factors in choosing a particular technique. Future research is definitely necessary in this field to help guide the management of such challenging condition.

References

1. Baumann MH, Sahn SA. Medical management and therapy of bronchopleural fistulas in the mechanically ventilated patient. Chest. 1990;97:721–8.
2. Lois M, Noppen M. Bronchopleural fistulas: an overview of the problem with special focus on endoscopic management. Chest. 2005;128:3955–65.
3. McManigle JE, Fletcher GL, Tenholder MF. Bronchoscopy in the management of bronchopleural fistula. Chest. 1990;97:1235–8.
4. Sonobe M, Nakagawa M, Ichinose M, et al. Analysis of risk factors in bronchopleural fistula after pulmonary resection for primary lung cancer. Eur J Cardiothorac Surg. 2000;18:519–23.
5. Turk AE, Karanas YL, Cannon W, Chang J. Staged closure of complicated bronchopleural fistulas. Ann Plast Surg. 2000;45:560–4.
6. Cerfolio RJ. The incidence, etiology, and prevention of postresectional bronchopleural fistula. Semin Thorac Cardiovasc Surg. 2001;13:3–7.
7. Sirbu H, Busch T, Aleksic I, et al. Bronchopleural fistula in the surgery of non-small cell lung cancer: incidence, risk factors, and management. Ann Thorac Cardiovasc Surg. 2001;7:330–6.
8. Sato M, Saito Y, Nagamoto N, et al. An improved method of bronchial stump closure for prevention of bronchopleural fistula in pulmonary resection. Tohoku J Exp Med. 1992;168(3):507–13.
9. Al-Kattan K, Cattelani L, Goldstraw P. Bronchopleural fistula after pneumonectomy for lung cancer. Eur J Cardiothorac Surg. 1995;9:479–82.
10. Conlan AA, Lukanich JM, Shutz J, Hurwitz SS. Elective pneumonectomy for benign lung disease: modern-day mortality and morbidity. J Thorac Cardiovasc Surg. 1995;110(4 Pt 1):1118–24.
11. Algar FJ, Alvarez A, Aranda JL, et al. Prediction of early bronchopleural fistula after pneumonectomy: a multivariate analysis. Ann Thorac Surg. 2001;72: 1662–7.
12. Asamura H, Naruke T, Tsuchiya R, et al. Bronchopleural fistulas associated with lung cancer operations. Univariate and multivariate analysis of risk factors, management, and outcome. J Thorac Cardiovasc Surg. 1992;104:1456–64.
13. Shields TW, Ponn RB. Complications of pulmonary resection. In: Shields TW, LoCicero J, Ponn RB, editors. General thoracic surgery. 5th ed. Philadelphia: Williams and Wilkins; 2000. p. 1113–22.
14. Malave G, Foster ED, Wilson JA, Munro DD. Bronchopleural fistula—present-day study of an old problem. A review of 52 cases. Ann Thorac Surg. 1971;11:1–10.
15. Hankins JR, Miller JE, Attar S, Satterfield JR, McLaughlin JS. Bronchopleural fistula. Thirteen-year experience with 77 cases. J Thorac Cardiovasc Surg. 1978;76:755–62.
16. Steiger Z, Wilson RF. Management of bronchopleural fistulas. Surg Gynecol Obstet. 1984;158:267–71.
17. Pierson DJ, Horton CA, Bates PW. Persistent bronchopleural air leak during mechanical ventilation. A review of 39 cases. Chest. 1986;90:321–3.
18. Frytak S, Lee RE, Pairolero PC, Arnold PG, Shaw JN. Necrotic lung and bronchopleural fistula as complications of therapy in lung cancer. Cancer Invest. 1988;6:139–43.
19. Abu-Hijleh M, Blundin M. Emergency use of an endobronchial one-way valve in the management of severe air leak and massive subcutaneous emphysema. Lung. 2010;188:253–7.
20. Sato M, Saito Y, Fujimura S, et al. Study of postoperative bronchopleural fistulas—analysis of factors related to bronchopleural fistulas. Nihon Kyobu Geka Gakkai Zasshi. 1989;37:498–503.
21. Panagopoulos ND, Apostolakis E, Koletsis E, et al. Low incidence of bronchopleural fistula after pneumonectomy for lung cancer. Interact Cardiovasc Thorac Surg. 2009;9:571–5.
22. Ferguson MK. Assessment of operative risk for pneumonectomy. Chest Surg Clin N Am. 1999;9: 339–51.
23. Wright CD, Wain JC, Mathisen DJ, Grillo HC. Postpneumonectomy bronchopleural fistula after

sutured bronchial closure: incidence, risk factors, and management. J Thorac Cardiovasc Surg. 1996;112:1367–71.
24. Klepetko W, Taghavi S, Pereszlenyi A, et al. Impact of different coverage techniques on incidence of postpneumonectomy stump fistula. Eur J Cardiothorac Surg. 1999;15:758–63.
25. Ellis JH, Sequeira FW, Weber TR, Eigen H, Fitzgerald JF. Balloon catheter occlusion of bronchopleural fistulae. AJR Am J Roentgenol. 1982; 138:157–9.
26. Donath J, Khan FA. Tuberculous and posttuberculous bronchopleural fistula. Ten year clinical experience. Chest. 1984;86:697–703.
27. Johnson TM, McCann W, Davey WN. Tuberculous bronchopleural fistula. Am Rev Respir Dis. 1973; 107:30–41.
28. Pomerantz M, Madsen L, Goble M, Iseman M. Surgical management of resistant mycobacterial tuberculosis and other mycobacterial pulmonary infections. Ann Thorac Surg. 1991;52:1108–11; discussion 1112.
29. Uçvet A, Gursoy S, Sirzai S, et al. Bronchial closure methods and risks for bronchopleural fistula in pulmonary resections: how a surgeon may choose the optimum method? Interact Cardiovasc Thorac Surg. 2011;12:558–62.
30. Hubaut JJ, Baron O, Al Habash O, et al. Closure of the bronchial stump by manual suture and incidence of bronchopleural fistula in a series of 209 pneumonectomies for lung cancer. Eur J Cardiothorac Surg. 1999;16:418–23.
31. Péterffy A, Calabrese E. Mechanical and conventional manual sutures of the bronchial stump. A comparative study of 298 surgical patients. Scand J Thorac Cardiovasc Surg. 1979;13:87–91.
32. Asamura H, Kondo H, Tsuchiya R. Management of the bronchial stump in pulmonary resections: a review of 533 consecutive recent bronchial closures. Eur J Cardiothorac Surg. 2000;17:106–10.
33. Weissberg D, Kaufman M. Suture closure versus stapling of bronchial stump in 304 lung cancer operations. Scand J Thorac Cardiovasc Surg. 1992;26: 125–7.
34. Vester SR, Faber LP, Kittle CF, Warren WH, Jensik RJ. Bronchopleural fistula after stapled closure of bronchus. Ann Thorac Surg. 1991;52:1253–7; discussion 1257-8.
35. Takaro T. Use of staplers in bronchial closure. In: Grillo HC, Eschapasse H, editors. International trends in general thoracic surgery. Philadelphia: W.B. Saunders; 1987. p. 452–7.
36. Hollaus PH, Lax F, El-Nashef BB, et al. Natural history of bronchopleural fistula after pneumonectomy: a review of 96 cases. Ann Thorac Surg. 1997;63:1391–6; discussion 1396-7.
37. Torre M, Chiesa G, Ravini M, Vercelloni M, Belloni PA. Endoscopic gluing of bronchopleural fistula. Ann Thorac Surg. 1987;43:295–7.
38. Uramoto H, Hanagiri T. The development of bronchopleural fistula in lung cancer patients after major surgery: 31 years of experience with 19 cases. Anticancer Res. 2011;31:619–24.
39. Sarkar P, Chandak T, Shah R, Talwar A. Diagnosis and management bronchopleural fistula. Indian J Chest Dis Allied Sci. 2010;52:97–104.
40. Darling GE, Abdurahman A, Yi Q-L, et al. Risk of a right pneumonectomy: role of bronchopleural fistula. Ann Thorac Surg. 2005;79:433–7.
41. Fernández-Díaz JA, García-Gallo C, Goicolea-Ruigómez J, Varela-de UA. Use of amplatzer® device for closure of bronchopleural fistulas, a hybrid procedure using bronchoscopy and radiology. Rev Esp Cardiol. 2011;64:1065–6.
42. West D, Togo A, Kirk AJB. Are bronchoscopic approaches to post-pneumonectomy bronchopleural fistula an effective alternative to repeat thoracotomy? Interact Cardiovasc Thorac Surg. 2007;6:547–50.
43. Stamatis G, Freitag L, Wencker M, Greschuchna D. Omentopexy and muscle transposition: two alternative methods in the treatment of pleural empyema and mediastinitis. Thorac Cardiovasc Surg. 1994;42: 225–32.
44. Høier-Madsen K, Schulze S, Møller Pedersen V, Halkier E. Management of bronchopleural fistula following pneumonectomy. Scand J Thorac Cardiovasc Surg. 1984;18:263–6.
45. Ricci ZJ, Haramati LB, Rosenbaum AT, Liebling MS. Role of computed tomography in guiding the management of peripheral bronchopleural fistula. J Thorac Imaging. 2002;17:214–8.
46. Hsu JT, Bennett GM, Wolff E. Radiologic assessment of bronchopleural fistula with empyema. Radiology. 1972;103:41–5.
47. Alifano M, Sepulveda S, Mulot A, Schussler O, Regnard J-F. A new method for detection of postpneumonectomy broncho-pleural fistulas. Ann Thorac Surg. 2003;75:1662–4.
48. Kim EA, Lee KS, Shim YM, et al. Radiographic and CT findings in complications following pulmonary resection. Radiographics. 2002;22:67–86.
49. Misthos P, Konstantinou M, Kokotsakis J, Skottis I, Lioulias A. Early detection of occult bronchopleural fistula after routine standard pneumonectomy. Thorac Cardiovasc Surg. 2006;54:264–7.
50. Roksvaag H, Skalleberg L, Nordberg C, Solheim K, Høivik B. Endoscopic closure of bronchial fistula. Thorax. 1983;38:696–7.
51. Regel G, Sturm JA, Neumann C, Schueler S, Tscherne H. Occlusion of bronchopleural fistula after lung injury—a new treatment by bronchoscopy. J Trauma. 1989;29:223–6.
52. Lan RS, Lee CH, Tsai YH, Wang WJ, Chang CH. Fiberoptic bronchial blockade in a small bronchopleural fistula. Chest. 1987;92:944–6.
53. Pace R, Rankin RN, Finley RJ. Detachable balloon occlusion of bronchopleural fistulae in dogs. Invest Radiol. 1983;18:504–6.

54. Ratliff JL, Hill JD, Tucker H, Fallat R. Endobronchial control of bronchopleural fistulae. Chest. 1977;71: 98–9.
55. Ferguson JS, Sprenger K, Van Natta T. Closure of a bronchopleural fistula using bronchoscopic placement of an endobronchial valve designed for the treatment of emphysema. Chest. 2006;129:479–81.
56. Cooper WA, Miller JI. Management of bronchopleural fistula after lobectomy. Semin Thorac Cardiovasc Surg. 2001;13:8–12.
57. Baldwin JC, Mark JB. Treatment of bronchopleural fistula after pneumonectomy. J Thorac Cardiovasc Surg. 1985;90:813–7.
58. Phillips YY, Lonigan RM, Joyner LR. A simple technique for managing a bronchopleural fistula while maintaining positive pressure ventilation. Crit Care Med. 1979;7:351–3.
59. Powner DJ, Grenvik A. Ventilatory management of life-threatening bronchopleural fistulae. A summary. Crit Care Med. 1981;9:54–8.
60. Hazerian TE, Berrezueta R, Pittokopitis K, Buckle FG, Robinson L. Technical consideration of synchronized chest tube occlusion in bronchopleural fistula. Crit Care Med. 1983;11:484.
61. Bishop MJ, Benson MS, Sato P, Pierson DJ. Comparison of high-frequency jet ventilation with conventional mechanical ventilation for bronchopleural fistula. Anesth Analg. 1987;66:833–8.
62. Sabanathan S, Richardson J. Management of postpneumonectomy bronchopleural fistulae. A review. J Cardiovasc Surg. 1994;35:449–57.
63. Hollaus PH, Huber M, Lax F, et al. Closure of bronchopleural fistula after pneumonectomy with a pedicled intercostal muscle flap. Eur J Cardiothorac Surg. 1999;16:181–6.
64. Stefani A, Jouni R, Alifano M, et al. Thoracoplasty in the current practice of thoracic surgery: a single-institution 10-year experience. Ann Thorac Surg. 2011;91:263–8.
65. Walsh MD, Bruno AD, Onaitis MW, et al. The role of intrathoracic free flaps for chronic empyema. Ann Thorac Surg. 2011;91:865–8.
66. Snell GI, Holsworth L, Fowler S, et al. Occlusion of a broncho-cutaneous fistula with endobronchial one-way valves. Ann Thorac Surg. 2005;80:1930–2.
67. Sedrakyan A, van der Meulen J, Lewsey J, Treasure T. Video assisted thoracic surgery for treatment of pneumothorax and lung resections: systematic review of randomised clinical trials. BMJ (Clinical research ed). 2004;329(7473):1008.
68. Nosotti M, Cioffi U, De Simone M, et al. Omentoplasty and thoracoplasty for treating postpneumonectomy bronchopleural fistula in a patient previously submitted to aortic prosthesis implantation. J Cardiothorac Surg. 2009;4:38.
69. Molnar TF. Current surgical treatment of thoracic empyema in adults. Eur J Cardiothorac Surg. 2007; 32:422–30.
70. Glover W, Chavis TV, Daniel TM, Kron IL, Spotnitz WD. Fibrin glue application through the flexible fiberoptic bronchoscope: closure of bronchopleural fistulas. J Thorac Cardiovasc Surg. 1987;93:470–2.
71. Hollaus PH, Lax F, Janakiev D, et al. Endoscopic treatment of postoperative bronchopleural fistula: experience with 45 cases. Ann Thorac Surg. 1998; 66:923–7.
72. Chowdhury JK. Percutaneous use of fiberoptic bronchoscope to investigate bronchopleurocutaneous fistula. Chest. 1979;75:203–4.
73. Hartmann W, Rausch V. New therapeutic application of the fiberoptic bronchoscope. Chest. 1977;71:237.
74. García-Polo C, León-Jiménez A, López-Campos JL, et al. Endoscopic sealing of bronchopleural fistulas with submucosal injection of a tissue expander: a novel technique. Can Respir J. 2010;17:e23–4.
75. Baumann WR, Ulmer JL, Ambrose PG, Garvey MJ, Jones DT. Closure of a bronchopleural fistula using decalcified human spongiosa and a fibrin sealant. Ann Thorac Surg. 1997;64:230–3.
76. Sivrikoz CM, Kaya T, Tulay CM, et al. Effective approach for the treatment of bronchopleural fistula: application of endovascular metallic ring-shaped coil in combination with fibrin glue. Ann Thorac Surg. 2007;83:2199–201.
77. Keckler SJ, Spilde TL, St Peter SD, Tsao K, Ostlie DJ. Treatment of bronchopleural fistula with small intestinal mucosa and fibrin glue sealant. Ann Thorac Surg. 2007;84:1383–6.
78. Andreetti C, D'Andrilli A, Ibrahim M, et al. Submucosal injection of the silver-human albumin complex for the treatment of bronchopleural fistula. Eur J Cardiothorac Surg. 2010;37:40–3.
79. Varoli F, Roviaro G, Grignani F, et al. Endoscopic treatment of bronchopleural fistulas. Ann Thorac Surg. 1998;65:807–9.
80. Andreetti C, D'Andrilli A, Ibrahim M, et al. Effective treatment of post-pneumonectomy bronchopleural fistula by conical fully covered self-expandable stent. Interact Cardiovasc Thorac Surg. 2012;14: 420–3.
81. Paul S, Talbot SG, Carty M, Orgill DP, Zellos L. Bronchopleural fistula repair during Clagett closure utilizing a collagen matrix plug. Ann Thorac Surg. 2007;83:1519–21.
82. Tao H, Araki M, Sato T, et al. Bronchoscopic treatment of postpneumonectomy bronchopleural fistula with a collagen screw plug. J Thorac Cardiovasc Surg. 2006;132:99–104.
83. Ranu H, Gatheral T, Sheth A, Smith EEJ, Madden BP. Successful endobronchial seal of surgical bronchopleural fistulas using BioGlue. Ann Thorac Surg. 2009;88:1691–2.
84. Bellato V, Ferraroli GM, De Caria D, et al. Management of postoperative bronchopleural fistula with a tracheobronchial stent in a patient requiring mechanical ventilation. Intensive Care Med. 2010; 36:721–2.
85. Chae EY, Shin JH, Song H-Y, et al. Bronchopleural fistula treated with a silicone-covered bronchial occlusion stent. Ann Thorac Surg. 2010;89:293–6.

86. Fruchter O, Kramer MR, Dagan T, et al. Endobronchial closure of bronchopleural fistulae using amplatzer devices: our experience and literature review. Chest. 2011;139:682–7.
87. Eckersberger F, Moritz E, Klepetko W, Müller MR, Wolner E. Treatment of postpneumonectomy empyema. Thorac Cardiovasc Surg. 1990;38:352–4.
88. Matthew TL, Spotnitz WD, Kron IL, et al. Four years' experience with fibrin sealant in thoracic and cardiovascular surgery. Ann Thorac Surg. 1990;50:40–3; discussion 43-4.
89. Takaoka K, Inoue S, Ohira S. Central bronchopleural fistulas closed by bronchoscopic injection of absolute ethanol. Chest. 2002;122:374–8.
90. Martin WR, Siefkin AD, Allen R. Closure of a bronchopleural fistula with bronchoscopic instillation of tetracycline. Chest. 1991;99:1040–2.
91. Watanabe S, Watanabe T, Urayama H. Endobronchial occlusion method of bronchopleural fistula with metallic coils and glue. Thorac Cardiovasc Surg. 2003;51:106–8.
92. Kanno R, Suzuki H, Fujiu K, Ohishi A, Gotoh M. Endoscopic closure of bronchopleural fistula after pneumonectomy by submucosal injection of polidocanol. Jpn J Thorac Cardiovasc Surg. 2002;50: 30–3.
93. Watanabe Y, Matsuo K, Tamaoki A, Komoto R, Hiraki S. Bronchial occlusion with endobronchial Watanabe spigot. J Bronchol. 2003;10:264–7.
94. Roukema JA, Verpalen MC, Lobach HJ, Palmen FM. Bronchopleural fistula: the use of tissue glue. J Thorac Cardiovasc Surg. 1992;103:167.
95. Fujisawa T, Hongo H, Yamaguchi Y, et al. Intratumoral ethanol injection for malignant tracheobronchial lesions: a new bronchofiberscopic procedure. Endoscopy. 1986;18:188–91.
96. Jessen C, Sharma P. Use of fibrin glue in thoracic surgery. Ann Thorac Surg. 1985;39:521–4.
97. Jones DP, David I. Gelfoam occlusion of peripheral bronchopleural fistulas. Ann Thorac Surg. 1986;42:334–5.
98. Mathisen DJ, Grillo HC, Vlahakes GJ, Daggett WM. The omentum in the management of complicated cardiothoracic problems. J Thorac Cardiovasc Surg. 1988;95:677–84.
99. Salmon CJ, Ponn RB, Westcott JL. Endobronchial vascular occlusion coils for control of a large parenchymal bronchopleural fistula. Chest. 1990;98: 233–4.
100. Ponn RB, D'Agostino RS, Stern H, Westcott JL. Treatment of peripheral bronchopleural fistulas with endobronchial occlusion coils. Ann Thorac Surg. 1993;56:1343–7.
101. Menard JW, Prejean CA, Tucker WY. Endoscopic closure of bronchopleural fistulas using a tissue adhesive. Am J Surg. 1988;155:415–6.
102. Wood RE, Lacey SR, Azizkhan RG. Endoscopic management of large, postresection bronchopleural fistulae with methacrylate adhesive (Super Glue). J Pediatr Surg. 1992;27(2):201–2.
103. Chawla RK, Madan A, Bhardwaj PK, Chawla K. Bronchoscopic management of bronchopleural fistula with intrabronchial instillation of glue (N-butyl cyanoacrylate). Lung India. 2012;29:11–4.
104. Chang C-C, Hsu H-H, Kuo S-W, Lee Y-C. Bronchoscopic gluing for post-lung-transplant bronchopleural fistula. Eur J Cardiothorac Surg. 2007;31:328–30.
105. Keller FS, Rösch J, Barker AF, Dotter CT. Percutaneous interventional catheter therapy for lesions of the chest and lungs. Chest. 1982;81: 407–12.
106. Scappaticci E, Ardissone F, Ruffini E, Baldi S, Mancuso M. Postoperative bronchopleural fistula: endoscopic closure in 12 patients. Ann Thorac Surg. 1994;57:119–22.
107. Hamid UI, Jones JM. Closure of a bronchopleural fistula using glue. Interact Cardiovasc Thorac Surg. 2011;13:117–8.
108. Belda-Sanchís J, Serra-Mitjans M, Iglesias Sentis M, Rami R. Surgical sealant for preventing air leaks after pulmonary resections in patients with lung cancer. Cochrane Database Syst Rev (Online). 2010;(1): CD003051.
109. Onotera RT, Unruh HW. Closure of a post-pneumonectomy bronchopleural fistula with fibrin sealant (Tisseel). Thorax. 1988;43:1015–6.
110. York EL, Lewall DB, Hirji M, Gelfand ET, Modry DL. Endoscopic diagnosis and treatment of postoperative bronchopleural fistula. Chest. 1990;97: 1390–2.
111. Kinoshita T, Miyoshi S, Katoh M, et al. Intrapleural administration of a large amount of diluted fibrin glue for intractable pneumothorax. Chest. 2000;117: 790–5.
112. Vietri F, Tosato F, Passaro U, et al. The use of human fibrin glue in fistulous pathology of the lung. G Chir. 1991;12(6):399–402.
113. McCarthy PM, Trastek VF, Bell DG, et al. The effectiveness of fibrin glue sealant for reducing experimental pulmonary air leak. Ann Thorac Surg. 1988; 45:203–5.
114. Potaris K, Mihos P, Gakidis I. Preliminary results with the use of an albumin-glutaraldehyde tissue adhesive in lung surgery. Med Sci Mon Int Med J Exp Clin Res. 2003;9:PI79–83.
115. Lin J, Iannettoni MD. Closure of bronchopleural fistulas using albumin-glutaraldehyde tissue adhesive. Ann Thorac Surg. 2004;77:326–8.
116. Sakamaki Y, Kido T, Fujiwara T, Kuwae K, Maeda M. A novel procedure using a tissue expander for management of persistent alveolar fistula after lobectomy. Ann Thorac Surg. 2005;79:2130–2.
117. Heffner JE, Standerfer RJ, Torstveit J, Unruh L. Clinical efficacy of doxycycline for pleurodesis. Chest. 1994;105:1743–7.
118. Asaki S. Tissue solidification in coping with digestive tract bleeding: hemostatic effect of local injection of 99.5 % ethanol. Tohoku J Exp Med. 1981; 134:223–7.

119. Otani T, Tatsuka T, Kanamaru K, Okuda S. Intramural injection of ethanol under direct vision for the treatment of protuberant lesions of the stomach. Gastroenterology. 1975;69:123–9.
120. Aynaci E, Kocatürk CI, Yildiz P, Bedirhan MA. Argon plasma coagulation as an alternative treatment for bronchopleural fistulas developed after sleeve pneumonectomy. Interact Cardiovasc Thorac Surg. 2012;14:912–4.
121. Kiriyama M, Fujii Y, Yamakawa Y, et al. Endobronchial neodymium:yttrium-aluminum garnet laser for noninvasive closure of small proximal bronchopleural fistula after lung resection. Ann Thorac Surg. 2002;73:945–8; discussion 948-9.
122. Kodama H, Yamakado K, Murashima S, et al. Intractable bronchopleural fistula caused by radiofrequency ablation: endoscopic bronchial occlusion with silicone embolic material. Br J Radiol. 2009; 82:e225–7.
123. Shen H-N, Lu FL, Wu H-D, Yu C-J, Yang P-C. Management of tension pneumatocele with high-frequency oscillatory ventilation. Chest. 2002; 121:284–6.
124. Uchida T, Wada M, Sakamoto J, Arai Y. Treatment for empyema with bronchopleural fistulas using endobronchial occlusion coils: report of a case. Surg Today. 1999;29:186–9.
125. Albes JM, Schäfers HJ, Gebel M, Ross UH. Tracheal stenting for malignant tracheoesophageal fistula. Ann Thorac Surg. 1994;57:1263–6.
126. Witt C, Ortner M, Ewert R, et al. Multiple fistulas and tracheobronchial stenoses require extensive stenting of the central airways and esophagus in squamous-cell carcinoma. Endoscopy. 1996;28: 381–5.
127. Colt HG, Meric B, Dumon JF. Double stents for carcinoma of the esophagus invading the tracheo-bronchial tree. Gastrointest Endosc. 1992;38(4):485–9.
128. Freitag L, Tekolf E, Steveling H, Donovan TJ, Stamatis G. Management of malignant esophagotracheal fistulas with airway stenting and double stenting. Chest. 1996;110:1155–60.
129. Watanabe S, Shimokawa S, Yotsumoto G, Sakasegawa K. The use of a Dumon stent for the treatment of a bronchopleural fistula. Ann Thorac Surg. 2001;72:276–8.
130. Tayama K, Eriguchi N, Futamata Y, et al. Modified Dumon stent for the treatment of a bronchopleural fistula after pneumonectomy. Ann Thorac Surg. 2003;75:290–2.
131. Tsukada H, Osada H. Use of a modified Dumon stent for postoperative bronchopleural fistula. Ann Thorac Surg. 2005;80:1928–30.
132. Dutau H, Breen DP, Gomez C, Thomas PA, Vergnon J-M. The integrated place of tracheobronchial stents in the multidisciplinary management of large post-pneumonectomy fistulas: our experience using a novel customised conical self-expandable metallic stent. Eur J Cardiothorac Surg. 2011;39:185–9.
133. Ferraroli GM, Testori A, Cioffi U, et al. Healing of bronchopleural fistula using a modified Dumon stent: a case report. J Cardiothorac Surg. 2006;1:16.
134. Takahashi M, Takahashi H, Itoh T, et al. Ultraflex expandable stents for the management of air leaks. Ann Thorac Cardiovasc Surg. 2006;12:50–2.
135. Dua J, Chessa M, Piazza L, et al. Initial experience with the new Amplatzer Duct Occluder II. J Invasive Cardiol. 2009;21:401–5.
136. Thanopoulos BD, Laskari CV, Tsaousis GS, et al. Closure of atrial septal defects with the Amplatzer occlusion device: preliminary results. J Am Coll Cardiol. 1998;31:1110–6.
137. Butera G, Chessa M, Carminati M. Percutaneous closure of ventricular septal defects. Cardiol Young. 2007;17(3):243–53.
138. Han YM, Gu X, Titus JL, et al. New self-expanding patent foramen ovale occlusion device. Catheter Cardiovasc Interv. 1999;47:370–6.
139. Scordamaglio PR, Tedde ML, Minamoto H, Pedra CAC, Jatene FB. Endoscopic treatment of tracheobronchial tree fistulas using atrial septal defect occluders: preliminary results. J Bras Pneumol. 2009;35:1156–60.
140. Gulkarov I, Paul S, Altorki NK, Lee PC. Use of Amplatzer device for endobronchial closure of bronchopleural fistulas. Interact Cardiovasc Thorac Surg. 2009;9:901–2.
141. Tedde ML, Scordamaglio PR, Minamoto H, et al. Endobronchial closure of total bronchopleural fistula with Occlutech Figulla ASD N device. Ann Thorac Surg. 2009;88:e25–6.
142. Passera E, Guanella G, Meroni A, et al. Amplatzer device and vacuum-assisted closure therapy to treat a thoracic empyema with bronchopleural fistula. Ann Thorac Surg. 2011;92:e23–5.
143. Sciurba FC, Ernst A, Herth FJF, et al. A randomized study of endobronchial valves for advanced emphysema. N Engl J Med. 2010;363:1233–44.
144. Feller-Kopman D, Bechara R, Garland R, Ernst A, Ashiku S. Use of a removable endobronchial valve for the treatment of bronchopleural fistula. Chest. 2006;130:273–5.
145. Levin AV, Tseĭmakh EV, Saĭmulenkov AM, et al. Use of endobronchial valve in postresection empyema and residual cavities with bronchopleural fistulas. Probl Tuberk Bolezn Legk. 2007;6:46–9.
146. Toma TP, Kon OM, Oldfield W, et al. Reduction of persistent air leak with endoscopic valve implants. Thorax. 2007;62:830–3.
147. Yu WC, Yeung YC, Chang Y, et al. Use of endobronchial one-way valves reveals questions on etiology of spontaneous pneumothorax: report of three cases. J Cardiothorac Surg. 2009;4:63.
148. Conforti S, Torre M, Fieschi S, Lomonaco A, Ravini M. Successful treatment of persistent postoperative air leaks following the placement of an endobronchial one-way valve. Monaldi Arch Chest Dis. 2010;73:88–91.

149. Schweigert M, Kraus D, Ficker JH, Stein HJ. Closure of persisting air leaks in patients with severe pleural empyema—use of endoscopic one-way endobronchial valve. Eur J Cardiothorac Surg. 2011;39:401–3.
150. Rosell A, López-Lisbona R, Cubero N, et al. Endoscopic treatment of persistent alveolar-pleural air leaks with a unidirectional endobronchial valve. Arch Bronconeumol. 2011;47:371–3.
151. Travaline JM, McKenna RJ, De Giacomo T, et al. Treatment of persistent pulmonary air leaks using endobronchial valves. Chest. 2009;136:355–60.
152. Gillespie CT, Sterman DH, Cerfolio RJ, et al. Endobronchial valve treatment for prolonged air leaks of the lung: a case series. Ann Thorac Surg. 2011;91:270–3.
153. El-Sameed Y, Waness A, Al Shamsi I, Mehta AC. Endobronchial valves in the management of broncho-pleural and alveolo-pleural fistulae. Lung. 2012;190:347–51.
154. FDA approves lung valve to control some air leaks after surgery. www.fda.gov/newsEvents/newsroom/…2008/ucm116970.hmt. Accessed 15 Jul 2012.

13 Bronchoscopy for Foreign Body Removal

Erik Folch and Adnan Majid

Abstract

Suspected airway foreign body aspiration is an important indication for bronchoscopy. The clinical presentation of airway foreign body aspiration varies from asymptomatic and incidental finding to acute and life-threatening central airway obstruction. Most cases of foreign body aspiration are encountered in children and elderly patients. Several comorbid conditions such as alcohol intoxication, dementia, and other chronic neurological disorders increase the risk of foreign body aspiration. A high index of suspicion is essential in order to avoid delay in diagnosis. Bronchoscopy is the gold standard for diagnosis and management of patients with suspected aspiration of foreign bodies. Rigid bronchoscope is superior to flexible bronchoscope in removal of large airway foreign bodies, especially in pediatric patients. However, due to lack of training and expertise in rigid bronchoscopy, it is usual to employ flexible bronchoscope for airway foreign body removal, especially in adult patients. Several accessory instruments are available to facilitate removal of foreign objects from the airways using flexible bronchoscope. In recent years, the cryoprobe has become a useful adjunct for removal of organic foreign bodies. Experienced and skillful operators are able to remove the majority of airway foreign bodies using the flexible scope. In this chapter, we discuss the clinical presentation, accessory instruments, and technical aspects of airway foreign body removal using flexible bronchoscope.

E. Folch, M.D., M.Sc. • A. Majid, M.D., F.C.C.P. (✉)
Division of Thoracic Surgery and Interventional Pulmonology, Beth Israel Deaconess Medical Center, Harvard Medical School, 185 Pilgrim Road, Deaconess 201, Boston, MA 02215, USA
e-mail: efolch@bidmc.harvard.edu; amajid@bidmc.harvard.edu

A.C. Mehta and P. Jain (eds.), *Interventional Bronchoscopy: A Clinical Guide*, Respiratory Medicine 10, DOI 10.1007/978-1-62703-395-4_13,

Keywords
Airway foreign body • Foreign body aspiration • Rigid bronchoscopy • Pediatric airway foreign body

Introduction

The use of bronchoscopy in its rigid and flexible forms has become the standard for the diagnosis and treatment of patients with foreign body aspiration [1]. The debate whether to use flexible or rigid bronchoscope frequently depends on local resources and expertise. The advantages of rigid bronchoscopy include better protection of the airway and ability to use tools that allow removal of large foreign bodies (FB), thus making it the safer technique for FB removal. In children, rigid bronchoscope with or without adjuvant flexible bronchoscope is often needed for successful removal of airway foreign bodies. However, in the United States the availability of operators trained in rigid bronchoscopy is highly variable [2–4] and for this reason in adult patients, flexible bronchoscopy with moderate sedation is frequently employed for FB removal from airways [5], as it is more widely available. Unfortunately, even the expertise, skill, and the facilities for flexible bronchoscopy and the accessory instruments needed for foreign body retrieval may not be available in smaller institutions or in many centers in the developing world. In this situation, an early referral to tertiary care centers is recommended for timely removal of aspirated foreign body.

Aspiration of foreign bodies occurs most commonly in the young and the elderly. Several risk factors for foreign body aspiration have been identified (Table 13.1). Although it is not uncommon for patients to present with nonspecific symptoms, a detailed history and physical examination, as well as chest imaging, are invaluable (Table 13.2). Occasionally, the patient will not recall the event and a high index of suspicion is needed to establish diagnosis in a timely fashion. Not surprisingly, in a significant number of patients the diagnosis can only be made through direct visualization with a bronchoscope. In the majority of these cases, the removal can be accomplished during the initial bronchoscopic procedure.

It is important to realize that each case of foreign body aspiration follows a different clinical course. The variables include the type of object and its location in the airway, time interval from aspiration to removal, and host's reaction to the

Table 13.1 Risk factors for foreign body aspiration in adults

Alcohol intoxication
Sedative or hypnotic drug use
Poor dentition
Senility
Mental retardation
Parkinson's disease
Primary neurologic disorders with impairment of swallowing or mental status
Trauma with loss of consciousness
Seizure
General anesthesia
Zenker's diverticulum

Table 13.2 Signs and symptoms of foreign body aspiration

History of choking episode
Chronic cough
Unilateral decrease in breath sounds
Atelectasis
Unilateral hyperinflation
Recurrent pneumonia
Unilateral or bilateral wheezing
Hemoptysis
Pneumothorax
Pneumomediastinum
Subcutaneous emphysema
Bronchiectasis
Lung abscess
Pleuritic chest pain

foreign body. The physical characteristics of the object, the clinical presentation, and the expertise of the bronchoscopist will also determine the ultimate outcome. For both patient and bronchoscopist, foreign body removal can be a very rewarding procedure, as the success rate is high and the complication rate is low.

Still, the removal of airway foreign body using bronchoscope remains a challenging task. In this chapter, we discuss the principles of diagnosis and removal of airway FB and provide a pathway that can be adapted to the specific setting, available local expertise, and technology.

Clinical Presentation

In adults, the swallowing reflex protects the airway from aspiration of foreign bodies. Whenever this protective mechanism fails, the cough reflex, which is reliably forceful, will likely be responsible for the self-resolution of most episodes of airway foreign body aspiration.

The clinical presentation of foreign body aspiration is highly variable, from trivial to life threatening, depending on the location and size of the object (Table 13.2). For example, even a small object will cause significant irritation and cough if it is located in the vicinity of the vocal cords, whereas a moderate size or occlusive object in the distal airway of the adult may cause only cough and obstructive pneumonitis. Therefore, a high degree of suspicion is critical in identifying patients at risk and when in doubt, a proactive approach will prevent serious future complications [6]. Approximately one-third of all objects are located proximal to the glottis after an episode of choking. These are usually large and can easily occlude the larynx. Patients, if alert, will present with severe cough, choking, hoarseness, and gagging.

In children, a witnessed or a reported episode of choking is the most common presentation. In some instances, children with foreign body aspiration present in extremis, and are found to have a radio-opaque object or unilateral hyperinflation on radiograph. On the other hand, in adults, aspiration of foreign bodies usually presents with chronic cough in the absence of a history of choking [7]. In acute episodes, Baharloo et al. described a "penetration syndrome" in which the patients present with sudden onset of choking and intractable cough with or without vomiting with less common symptoms being cough, fever, dyspnea, and wheezing [8]. It is important to remember that 39 % of patients with a foreign body aspiration will have no physical findings [9], and chest radiograph may be normal in 6–38 % of patients [9–15]. A significant, but unknown, number of patients expectorate the foreign body before presenting to the hospital, and some objects are even swallowed.

In the presence of a suggestive clinical scenario of aspiration, approximately 50 % of children with a history of choking have no foreign body in their airways. In these cases, it is difficult to determine whether the FB was ever aspirated or whether it is the result of spontaneous coughing out or swallowing of the foreign body.

Location

The majority of aspirated FB in adults tends to lodge in the right lower lobe. This is not seen in children as the size of the left main bronchus, and the angle of branching, is not acute, as is the case in adults [8, 16].

Mechanism

It is proposed that an inspiratory suction force frequently used while eating with chopsticks, drinking soup, or sucking on plant material may be responsible for propelling the food towards the epiglottis and predisposing to aspiration [17–19]. In the case of children, the use of incisors can propel the object into the retro-pharynx. Their natural curiosity during the oral phase as well as the habit of crying, laughing, and playing during meals are responsible for the increased incidence of FB aspiration among young children [5, 18].

Timeline

The time interval from aspiration to medical evaluation is variable among patients. Several authors describe a longer lag time for adults when compared to children. The average delay in presentation and diagnosis is also shorter for inorganic as compared with the organic foreign body aspiration [8]. Clearly, the timeliness of diagnosis also depends on the experience and clinical acumen of the clinician.

Radiologic Evaluation

The chest radiograph is often the initial diagnostic test whenever FB aspiration is suspected.

Most aspirated objects are radiolucent, thus limiting the role of standard X-rays for diagnosis. However, the use of inspiratory and expiratory films may show subtle signs such as air trapping, atelectasis, mediastinal shift, or pulmonary infiltrates that may suggest airway FB aspiration. In published studies, chest radiograph has a sensitivity of 70–82 %, specificity of 44–74 %, positive predictive value of 72–83 %, and negative predictive value of 41–73 % for detection of airway foreign bodies [11, 12]. Therefore, the presence of a radiopaque object on chest radiograph is diagnostic, but the normal or the subtle chest X-ray findings do not exclude the diagnosis and should be interpreted with caution in the context of the clinical history. In fact, whenever the possibility of foreign body aspiration is considered in the differential diagnosis, the clinician should have low threshold to advise the bronchoscopic examination, which is the cornerstone of the diagnostic workup in such patients.

In children, the presence of pneumomediastinum or subcutaneous emphysema should also alert the clinicians to consider the possibility of a foreign body aspiration [20, 21]. Lateral neck films revealing a subglottic density or swelling may suggest the presence of laryngotracheal foreign body [22]. The presence of a calcified foreign body on X-rays suggests the possibility of a previously missed airway foreign body or a broncholith, as vegetable materials in the airways can calcify over time [23].

In chronic obstruction, the computed tomography (CT) of the chest can show the late complications of FB aspiration, which include bronchial stenosis, bronchiectasis, endobronchial masses, or granulation tissue. The use of MRI to identify peanut aspiration has been described [24–26]. The presence of fat within the peanut produces a high signal on T1-weighted imaging. Sometimes the presence of mucus in the airway mimics the clinical and radiological features of airway foreign body. However, mucus on computed tomography appears to have a low-attenuation, bubbly appearance, in the dependent airways, and frequently can be mobilized by forceful coughing [27].

Recently, the use of virtual bronchoscopy (VB) in the diagnosis of suspected foreign body aspiration in 60 children was investigated [28]. The multidetector CT generated virtual bronchoscopy and demonstrated a lesion suggestive of foreign body in 40 cases and 33 objects were identified and removed with bronchoscopy. The authors suggest that VB can be used to determine the presence and localization of an FB, which can help with pre-procedural planning. In this series, foreign body was not detected on rigid bronchoscopy in any of the seven patients who had a negative VB, suggesting a high negative predictive value of VB in evaluation of airway FB. Unfortunately, virtual bronchoscopy is not therapeutic and is not available in most hospitals. It may also delay necessary interventions. A report from Sudan highlights the reach of computed tomography airway reconstruction as a diagnostic tool in centers that lack bronchoscopic equipment [29].

It is important to remember that both in children and adults, aspirated foreign bodies are frequently misdiagnosed as croup, recurrent laryngitis, asthma, recurrent pneumonia, or primary airway tumors, leading to unnecessary and inappropriate diagnostic and therapeutic interventions [30, 31].

Aspiration in Children

When compared to adults, children have a significantly higher rate of aspiration events, and life-threatening complications. The incidence of aspiration is highest from 1 to 3 years of age as curiosity and independent exploration expose infants to small objects in the prime of the oral phase [8]. This is coupled with poor airway protection mechanisms and forceful propulsion of the object to the retro-pharynx after biting with the incisors. Furthermore, children may cry, laugh, and play while attempting to swallow. The most common aspirated objects among children are peanuts, seeds, small foods, or toys.

Aspiration in Adults

The type of foreign bodies aspirated by adults vary widely and in many instances reflect cultural and lifestyle variations. The most common cause of aspiration in adults is meat [32]. However, a significant number of cases have retention of the foreign particle at the level of the glottis, which is coughed or amenable to postural drainage. Other common food particles aspirated by adults include nuts, pumpkin seeds [33], melon seeds [34, 35], watermelon seeds [35], dental fixtures, dental fillings, coins, safety pins, ear plugs, glass, fragments of tracheostomy tubes [36], and medication tablets [37] among others (Fig. 13.1). In the United States, the aspiration of nails and pins is seen in healthy young adult males [38, 39]. In Middle Eastern countries, the aspiration of prayer beads, worry beads, and pins are relatively common [35, 40, 41]. Notably, aspiration of foreign bodies in adults is seen in all age groups, but is most common in elderly patients with dental problems, swallowing difficulties, and altered mental status or dementia (Table 13.1). Some case series show a significant number of cases of aspiration of bones contained in food [42]. Aspiration of foreign bodies has also been described during medical or dental procedures such as esophagogastroduodenoscopy with band ligation [43].

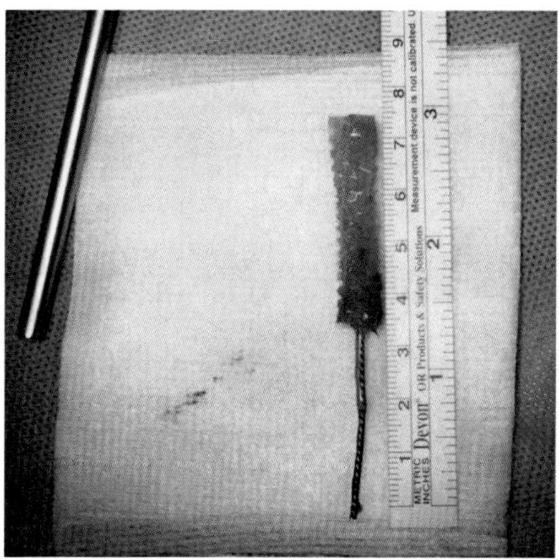

Fig. 13.1 Successful removal of tracheostomy brush accidentally aspirated during cleaning

Success Rates

Bronchoscopy is the frontline procedure for retrieval of airway foreign bodies. Several studies suggest high rates of success, 97–99 %, particularly when using a combination of rigid and flexible bronchoscope. Table 13.3 summarizes several studies of flexible and rigid bronchoscopy use for removal of foreign bodies. This list is not exhaustive and is just a representative sample of the published evidence.

All airway foreign bodies cannot be retrieved with rigid or flexible bronchoscopy. Failure to remove foreign bodies in some instances is related to deep impaction of FB in the airway that is not amenable to balloon dislodgement. Other cause is an externally impaled object, such as metal debris after an explosion [42]. Interestingly, several reports include failed initial bronchoscopies at outside institutions or by less experienced bronchoscopists that were later successful [8, 42], which attests to the importance of experience and proper training in this procedure.

Table 13.3 Case series of airway foreign body removal by flexible and rigid bronchoscopy

Author	Flexible(F), rigid(R), or both(B)	Total number of patients (*N*)	Successful removal	% of Success
Hiller [91]	F	7	6	86
Cunanan [92]	F	300	267	89
Clark [93]	F	3	3	100
Nunez [94]	F	17	12	71
Lan [95]	F	33	32	97
Limper [50]	F	23	14	61
Chen [18]	F	43	32	74
Moura e sa [96]	F	2[a]	2[a]	100
Ali Ali [41]	F	16	9	57
Gencer [40]	F	23	21	91
Debeljak [42]	B	63	61	97
Donado Uña [97]	F	56	53	95
Baharloo [8]	R	112	103	92
Kalyanappagol [98]	R	206	206	100
Lima [99]	?	83	83	100
Blanco-Ramos [100]	B	32	24	75
Saki [87]	R	967	967	100
Oguzkaya [101]	R	500	498	99
Rahbarimanesh [102]	R	44	44	100
Metrangelo [103]	R	70	70	100
Martinot [11]	R	40	40	100
Chik [104]	R	27	27[b]	100
Yetim [105]	R	38	37	97
Tang [106]	F	1027	938	91
Boyd [107]	F	20	18	90
Weissberg [108]	R	66	55	83
Zhijun [109]	R	1428	1424	99
Paşaoğlu	R	639	639	100
Skoulakis [110]	R	130	130	100
Maddali [111]	R	140	140	100
Kiyan [112]	R	153	153	100

[a]Two cases of a series of 77 patients in which the FB could not be removed with RB
[b]Four patients required repeated bronchoscopy for residual fragments

Therapeutic Approach to the Patient with Foreign Body Aspiration

All patients with suspected foreign body aspiration should remain in close observation until the diagnosis has been confirmed or excluded, and the foreign material has been removed. Even clinically stable patients can have a sudden change in their condition as a result of migration of the object, or occurrence of complications such as bleeding, or pneumothorax [44, 45].

The likelihood and extent of tissue reaction increase the longer a foreign body remains in the airway [13, 46, 47]. The delay in starting the procedure can only be justified in order to coordinate the necessary personnel and equipment, or to facilitate prompt transfer to another institution with capabilities to deal with foreign body aspiration. It is important to remember that during the first 24 h, the endobronchial mucosa suffers mild inflammation, erythema, and granulation tissue formation [13]. However, the degree of inflammatory response depends on the content of

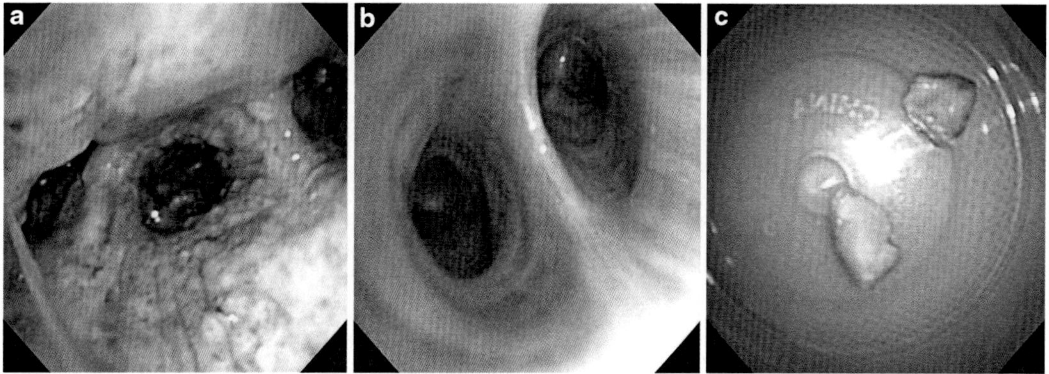

Fig. 13.2 (**a**) Localized endobronchial inflammation as a result of peanut aspiration (**b**) shows normal unaffected airways on the same patient. (**c**) Successful removal of two peanuts from the bronchi showing inflammatory changes

the FB aspirated. Nuts, peanuts, and grass are particularly irritating. Our group has removed peanuts and other nuts with various degrees of granulation tissue formation (Fig. 13.2). Unfortunately, the humid environment of the airways increases the probability of the peanuts to fragment and occlude the airways distally.

The overall management can be broken down into postural drainage, rigid bronchoscopy, and flexible bronchoscopy. Many accessory instruments specifically designed to facilitate retrieval of airway foreign body are available. In recent years, cryoprobe has emerged as the most suitable method for removal of organic material as discussed below.

Non-endoscopic Therapies

Bronchodilator inhalation and postural drainage are not recommended in the initial management of foreign body aspiration as proximal migration of the object may lead to cardiopulmonary arrest in a small percentage of patients [48]. A delay in proceeding to bronchoscopy increases the risk of complications such as pneumonia, atelectasis, and cardiopulmonary arrest while decreasing the likelihood of successful bronchoscopic removal. At least one clinical trial of bronchodilator inhalation and postural drainage for the treatment of FB aspiration has described cardiopulmonary arrest, while others have pointed out the potential for extended hospital stay and more complications with the use of such protocols [46, 48, 49].

Another technique seldom employed is the use of therapeutic percussion while the patient coughs. Nevertheless, despite anecdotal reports of success, these efforts should never delay a clearly safer and more effective therapeutic maneuver such as rigid or flexible bronchoscopy.

In patients with foreign bodies located in the oropharynx, it is important to have access to a Magill forceps since it facilitates extraction [5].

Rigid Bronchoscopy

In the most recent series, the reported success rate using rigid bronchoscopy for removal of aspirated foreign bodies is between 95 and 99 % [33–35, 44, 47, 50, 51]. The rigid bronchoscope offers several advantages. These include ability to maintain adequate ventilation, better visualization, and superior suctioning capabilities. With appropriate technique and under general anesthesia, rigid bronchoscopy is safe and effective while providing maximal comfort to the patient. A wide variety of instruments such as optical forceps, alligator forceps, four-prong hooks, baskets, cryotherapy probes, and several types of balloons are available for FB retrieval using rigid bronchoscope. The type and location of FB should dictate the type of instrument employed. In some instances more than one

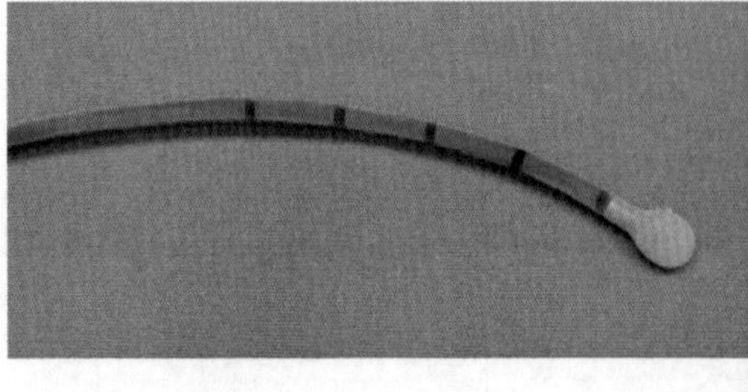

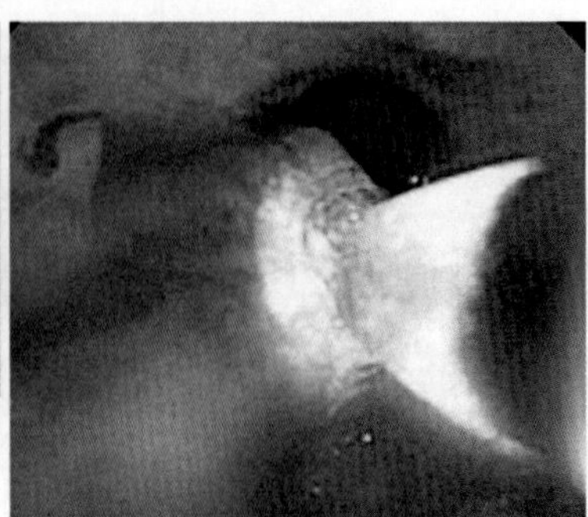

Fig. 13.3 Cryoprobe and application in benign airway disease

instrument may be needed for successful removal of airway foreign body. The rigid bronchoscope is particularly useful in the removal of sharp objects. However, several series describe successful removal of pins with the flexible bronchoscope [40, 41].

Unfortunately, rigid bronchoscopy is not widely available and only practiced by 4–8 % of pulmonologists in the United States [2–4].

Flexible Bronchoscopy

In the evaluation of foreign body aspiration in adults, the flexible bronchoscope is the usual initial diagnostic tool. Whenever foreign body is suspected, flexible bronchoscope should be introduced via oral route. A comprehensive examination is essential in every case because sometimes the foreign object is not immediately obvious to the examiner. This difficulty arises in some cases because the FB is covered by blood or granulation tissue. Less frequently, the foreign object is fragmented and is located in more than one distal airway.

Once the object type, size, and location have been identified, removal can be attempted. Whenever removal is attempted, several instruments should be readily available, ideally including a rigid bronchoscope. Instruments that have been developed for removal of FB through flexible bronchoscope include flexible forceps, ragged-tooth forceps, snares, Dormia basket, fishnet basket, cryotherapy probes (Fig. 13.3), balloon catheters (Fogarty), and magnet extractor.

A successful removal with the flexible bronchoscope spares the patient of a subsequent rigid bronchoscopy and its associated cost. Several reports attest to the successful application of the flexible bronchoscope to remove foreign bodies. These reports show a success rate of >90 % in experienced hands [42, 52, 53]. The list of FB removed is extensive and includes teeth, windscreen glass, earplugs, pins, nails, fish bone, peanuts, coins, and endodontic needles [40, 41, 54–59].

Some authors recommend the use of an endotracheal tube when removing some objects with flexible bronchoscope in order to minimize the injury risk to the upper airway [42].

Intense debate surrounds the use of flexible or rigid bronchoscope for removal of foreign bodies in the literature, partly fueled by the personal preference and individual expertise, and partly from the available instruments and technology at the time of such debate. It is the opinion of the authors that flexible bronchoscopy has acquired paramount importance in the diagnosis and removal of foreign bodies in adults. Rigid bronchoscope has an important complementary role and should be readily available whenever an FB removal is planned [2, 42, 60]. It is essential for all operators who use flexible bronchoscope to retrieve airway FB to understand the potential consequences of a failed procedure. Not every pulmonologist who performs flexible bronchoscopy is comfortable managing the potential consequences of a failed procedure. When in doubt, it is best to stabilize the patient and refer to an institution that has expertise in both flexible and rigid bronchoscopy.

Anesthesia and Analgesia

The flexible bronchoscope allows removal of the foreign body with local anesthesia under moderate sedation, unlike the rigid bronchoscope, which is performed under general anesthesia. An advantage of performing foreign body removal with moderate sedation is that it preserves the cough reflex, which can further facilitate the removal. An object brought forward to the trachea by bronchoscopic techniques can often be coughed out on command given to the patient.

The fact that foreign body removal by flexible bronchoscopy is done with moderate sedation and without a secure airway has led to much criticism. There has been some concern about the possibility of losing the object in a narrow subglottic area leading to potential asphyxiation. To our knowledge, no incident of this kind has been reported in the medical literature. Notwithstanding, in the rare event of this occurring, immediate intubation—either with bronchoscopic guidance or with a direct laryngoscope—can always be performed to secure the airway. Varying sizes of endotracheal tubes (ETT) and laryngoscopes should be readily available in most bronchoscopy suites for the rare happenstance of this complication occurring with bronchoscopy. Extraction can then proceed via ETT. Another approach (aside from emergent intubation) would be to reintroduce the flexible bronchoscope and push the foreign body into the distal airways, thus clearing up the upper-airway obstruction.

In difficult cases, when moderate sedation cannot be achieved adequately, proceeding with rigid bronchoscopy under general anesthesia is the best option. In those instances where the object is too distal and inaccessible to removal with the rigid bronchoscope, the foreign body can be removed with a flexible bronchoscope introduced via the ETT or the rigid barrel. When the object is larger than the diameter of the tube, the ETT or the rigid barrel may need to be withdrawn in conjunction with the bronchoscope and the secured foreign body [61, 62]. This should be followed by prompt reintubation and repeat inspection of the airway. An alternative to the use of ETT with general anesthesia is the laryngeal mask airway [63]. Flexible bronchoscopy can be performed with reasonable airway control even with deeper sedation [64, 65]. Recent experience with fospropofol, a prodrug of propofol, has proven it to be safe and effective during flexible bronchoscopy [66]. Interestingly, fospropofol is not a general anesthetic, and has distinct pharmacokinetic and pharmacodynamic characteristics and should not require anesthesia monitoring [67]. However, its use in therapeutic bronchoscopic procedures is yet to be described.

In children, there is no consensus on anesthesia. However, a very large review of 12,979 patients found that induction with maintenance of spontaneous ventilation is commonly practiced to minimize the risk of converting a partial proximal obstruction to a complete obstruction. Adequate ventilation combined with intravenous drugs and paralysis allows for appropriate rigid bronchoscopy conditions and a desired level of anesthesia [68].

Accessories for the Flexible Bronchoscope

Multiple instruments for the removal of foreign bodies with the flexible bronchoscope are available. The instrument of choice is largely dictated by the location, type of foreign body, and the accompanying host tissue reaction.

Grasping Forceps

The forceps is the most widely available and used instrument. These have different designs including a wide range of cup sizes and shapes, rotation mechanisms, presence or absence of teeth, and accessories such as central fenestrations or needles. Among the grasping forceps are the w-shaped, alligator jaw, rat-tooth, shark-tooth, and covered-tip forceps.

The selected forceps should have a jaw size large enough to enclose the full diameter of the foreign body. In cases where a firm grip is needed to prevent a hard object from slipping the alligator jaws, rat-tooth or shark-tooth

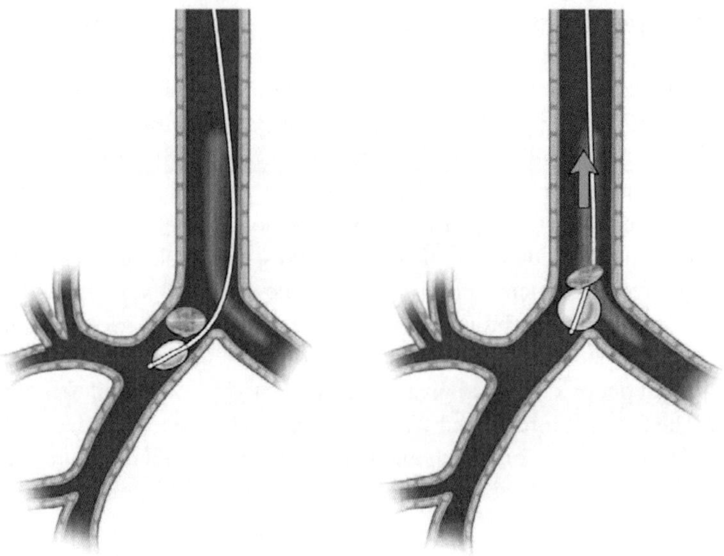

Fig. 13.4 Fogarty balloon catheter used as an aid to move foreign bodies to proximal airways

forceps are recommended. For more delicate manipulations, a w-shaped or a covered-tip forceps may be used. In general, grasping forceps are only used for the removal of flat or thin inorganic (e.g., coins, pins, screws, clips) or hard organic objects (e.g., bone), as attempted removal of friable organic foreign body will cause it to fracture, disintegrate, and disperse into the distal airways.

Balloon Catheters

Inflatable balloon catheters are probably the most useful but clearly underutilized tool available for removal of foreign objects (Fig. 13.4). Although there are a few commercially available, the Fogarty catheter remains the most frequently used. It has different sizes (4–7 F) and can be passed through the working channel of the flexible bronchoscope. The catheter is advanced distal to the object, then the balloon is inflated with 1–3 cc of saline, and the catheter is pulled until the object is dislodged proximally to facilitate removal.

Dormia Basket

A modified version of the Dormia basket used by gastroenterologists and urologists for the removal of calculi from the common bile duct and bladder is also available for the bronchoscopic removal of foreign bodies in the airway. The wings of the basket are normally retracted within a 1.6 mm diameter Teflon catheter. The basket is opened in the airway and maneuvered to allow its "wings" to surround and entrap the foreign body. The basket is most useful in the removal of large and bulky objects.

Fishnet Basket

The fishnet basket is a modified version of a polypectomy snare, in which a mesh of thin thread is attached to the snare wire for easy folding and unfolding (Fig. 13.5). The net is normally retracted within the catheter for easy passage through the channel of the flexible bronchoscope. When the snare is advanced, the fishnet is slowly released to surround the object. The snare is then

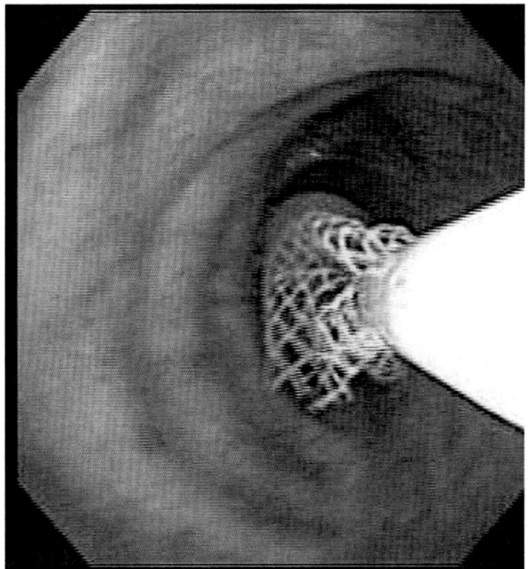

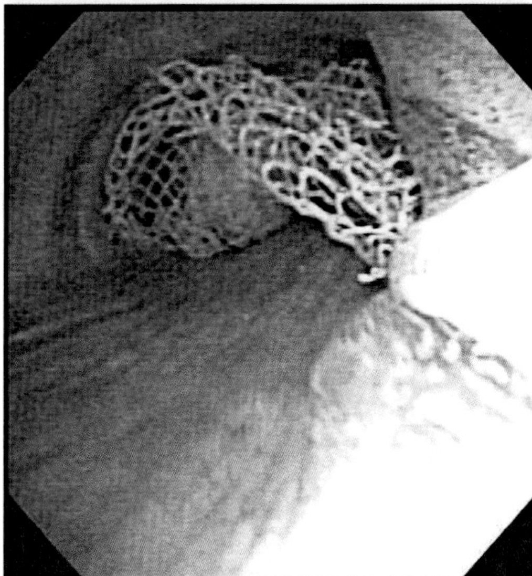

Fig. 13.5 Endoscopic use of fishnet basket to remove foreign body

slowly retracted to enclose the foreign object within the fishnet. Once this is accomplished, the basket, the captured object, and the bronchoscope are then removed as a unit. This fishnet basket is also most useful in the removal of bulky objects.

Three- or Four-Prong Snares

The snares are usually squeezed together inside the catheter. Whenever they are deployed, the snares are released surrounding the foreign object. When the operator squeezes the handle of the device, the prong's distal ends come together capturing the object. Once secured, the foreign body, snare, and flexible bronchoscope are withdrawn carefully as a single unit. Because the prongs are very flimsy, it is not advisable to use this accessory in the removal of hard, solid objects.

Magnet Extractor

A magnetic extractor consists of a flexible probe with a magnetic cylinder at its tip. This accessory is specially designed for passage through the working channel of the flexible bronchoscope. Small and mobile metallic foreign bodies, such as broken forceps or cytology brushes, can be removed easily with this instrument [69, 70].

Cryotherapy Catheter

The adhesive properties of the cryoprobe make it an ideal instrument for the removal of foreign bodies rich in water content. The system has a cryogen tank (e.g., nitrous oxide or nitrogen) that by rapid gas-decompression or principle of Joule–Thomson generates an extremely low temperature (−15 to −40 °C) at the tip of the specially designed cryoprobe (Fig. 13.3). When the cryoprobe is placed in direct contact with the object, the two become attached and the operator then removes the flexible bronchoscope along with the cryoprobe and the foreign body. This technique is extremely useful for the removal of blood clots, mucus balls, organic materials, and small inorganic objects [71].

In our experience, this is one of the most useful instruments for the removal of organic materials. We recently removed a fragmented peanut from the airway of a 2-year-old through the combined use of rigid bronchoscope, pediatric flexible bronchoscope, and pediatric cryoprobe.

The bronchoscopist should be careful to keep a clear field of view in order to prevent contact with the surrounding mucosa, and to inadvertently remove attached normal tissue.

Removal with the Flexible Bronchoscope

Whenever foreign body aspiration is suspected, the flexible bronchoscopy is performed through the oral route, in order to avoid the narrow nasal passage [72]. Initially, a thorough airway exam should be done, starting with the unaffected lung. The suspicious area of aspiration is examined last. This thorough and careful exam is done to assure that there is only one foreign object, or that fragments have not been dispersed to other airways. When the object is visualized, the shape and structure of the foreign body in relation to the surrounding areas are carefully examined before an extraction attempt is made. The entire foreign body may not be visible bronchoscopically and a review of radiologic films may be necessary during the procedure to determine the position of the unseen portion. The appropriate bronchoscopic accessory is then determined based on the size, shape, position, and density of the object.

Whenever the flexible bronchoscope is used, utmost care should be taken not to push the object farther down the airway. In general, we use the Fogarty balloon to dislodge the foreign body and to bring it proximally to the trachea, before attempting removal [54]. The Fogarty balloon catheter is positioned distal to the object. The balloon is then inflated and the foreign body is pulled out from the segmental or the lobar airways to the trachea (Fig. 13.4). Once in the trachea, the object is easily amenable to removal. We have often asked the patient to sit up and cough up the foreign body once it has been dislodged to the upper trachea. We usually employ this technique for small and soft objects and have had successful results in approximately 90 % of our cases.

The key to successfully removing a foreign body lies in being able to adequately secure the object by either grasping or enclosing it with the bronchoscopic accessory. Once the object is snared or trapped, all three (bronchoscope, grasping instrument, and object) are removed simultaneously from the patient as a unit. During removal, the bronchoscopist must make every attempt to continuously visualize the object and keep it in the center of the airway. Removal of a sharp object is a challenging task. The key to removing this type of object is to locate the sharp end and to attempt its dislodgement. Once the sharp end is freed, the object can be grabbed and removed. Grasping the shaft or the other end of a pointed instrument increases the difficulty of removal because this will most likely be caught in the mucosa.

Similarly, difficulty is also encountered when the tissue reaction surrounding the foreign body interferes with the removal process. Sometimes the surrounding granulation tissue has to be cleared prior to removal of the object. In some of these cases, bronchoscopic removal under general anesthesia may be necessary. Sometimes ablative therapies such as laser photoresection may help vaporize the surrounding granulation tissue. Laser may also be used to break a larger FB into smaller and more manageable pieces that can be easily removed with the bronchoscopic techniques [73–75]. Other modalities, such as bronchoscopic electrocautery, can also be used to similarly vaporize surrounding granulation tissue. Some authors suggest the use of a short course of steroids prior to removal of airway foreign bodies although the efficacy of this practice remains untested [14, 76].

Massive hemoptysis is a rare complication of foreign body removal and is better controlled with rigid bronchoscopy [74]. Whenever hemoptysis does occur, our practice is to instill an epinephrine solution (1:10,000 to 1:20,000) through the bronchoscope to achieve topical vasoconstriction with decrease in blood flow and eventual thrombosis of the bleeding vessels. We also find cold saline (4 °C) instillation to be effective in bleeding cessation. Cold saline causes hypothermic vasoconstriction and eventual thrombosis of the bleeding vessel.

Elusive Foreign Body Aspirations

Almost everyone who has significant experience with foreign body removal can describe a case in which the foreign body was not found, lost during the removal at the mouth, or seems to have disappeared after it was seen on radiologic imaging. The most common cause is spontaneous expectoration of the foreign body without patient's knowledge. However, it is very important to do a thorough airway examination for small fragments of the original object, or for missing objects. Whenever removed, the object should preferably be sent for pathologic analysis as some have described the presence of concomitant malignancy as an incidental finding on pathologic samples [18]. And then there is the case of the dissolved aspirated pill. Lee et al. have described a case of iron pill aspiration that was not found on bronchoscopy 2 months after the aspiration event, but endobronchial biopsies confirmed the residue of iron being responsible for severe granulation tissue [37]. A recent report by Parray et al. also describes the migration of a foreign body from the right to the left [77].

About Multidisciplinary Teams

It has been our experience as well as that of others [11, 42] that an excellent working relationship with specialists from pulmonary, otolaryngology, and thoracic surgery is an asset that expedites and improves favorable outcomes in the management of airway foreign bodies.

Rare Cases Where the Object is Left Behind

The medical literature has a few case reports where the foreign object was left behind due to the inability to be removed or the clinical deterioration of the patient that prompted the interruption of the foreign body removal [78]. Although these situations may happen, we would like to emphasize that the long-term complications of foreign objects in the airway warrant that every effort should be made to guarantee its removal, including referral to a specialized center. In extraordinarily rare cases, the patient would expectorate the foreign body left behind [79]. Also, in rare cases, the unsuccessful endoscopic removal is followed by a surgical approach [80].

Respiratory Equipment Malfunction Causing Foreign Body Aspiration

Unfortunately, the progress of respiratory therapy and mechanical ventilation has been accompanied by an increase in the number of cases of aspiration of foreign bodies. Examples of this include aspiration of intubation stylets [81], suction catheters [81, 82], and tracheostomy brushes (Fig. 13.1).

Aspiration of Medication Tablets

A relatively more common occurrence is the aspiration of pills in the airway. The consequences of such events can be dramatic, and due to the quick expansion of the tablet when humidification occurs, it can cause acute airway obstruction as has been described with sucralfate [83]. In other cases, the medication can quickly dissolve and have long-term consequences due to inflammation and fibrosis as those described with iron tablet aspiration [37]. Our group recently reported experience with two cases, with metformin and pomegranate tablets [84].

Complications of Foreign Body Aspiration

The aspiration of foreign bodies carries a high risk of short- and long-term complications. All of these have been extensively described in the literature and include acute respiratory failure and asphyxia

[72], pneumonia, empyema [85], atelectasis, cardiopulmonary arrest, hemoptysis, granulation tissue formation, laryngeal edema, pneumothorax, pneumomediastinum, tracheobronchial rupture, trachea-esophageal fistula, bronchial stricture, localized bronchiectasis [86], mediastinitis, lung torsion [18], and anoxic brain injury [87]. An interesting report by Aziz [85] demonstrated the potential cascade of events leading from a foreign body aspiration including airway obstruction, post-obstructive pneumonia, and empyema.

The Case for ECMO and Foreign Body Aspiration

Treatment of near-fatal foreign body aspiration treated with ECMO has been reported in the medical literature [88, 89]. Recently, a complicated bronchoscopic removal of a foreign body required ECMO support due to worsening respiratory failure in the setting of purulent secretion aspiration and overwhelming sepsis [90]. Although rarely used, these cases support the advantages of rapid referral to specialized airway centers, whenever it is clinically feasible.

Conclusions

The clinical presentation of aspirated foreign bodies may vary from an asymptomatic and incidental finding to an acute and life-threatening airway obstruction. Regardless, removal of foreign bodies from tracheobronchial tree should always be attempted in order to relieve the current symptoms and to prevent future complications. Bronchoscopy remains the premier diagnostic as well as therapeutic option in these patients. Most experts would agree that rigid bronchoscopy is more effective than flexible bronchoscopy in removing large airway foreign bodies. In pediatric population, rigid bronchoscope is clearly preferred over flexible bronchoscope. Unfortunately, the facilities for rigid bronchoscopy are seldom available due to lack of training and expertise. Therefore, in practical terms, flexible bronchoscope is the most commonly employed tool for retrieval of airway foreign bodies in adults. In the hands of experienced and skillful operators, the majority of airway foreign bodies can be retrieved using flexible bronchoscopy techniques. It is essential for the operators to be familiar with a variety of accessory instruments that are available to facilitate removal of airway foreign bodies. Failure to remove foreign body with the flexible bronchoscope should be promptly followed by rigid bronchoscopy. Early referral to a tertiary care center is indicated if such facility is not locally available.

References

1. Rafanan AL, Mehta AC. Adult airway foreign body removal. What's new? Clin Chest Med. 2001;22:319–30.
2. Prakash UB, Offord KP, Stubbs SE. Bronchoscopy in North America: the ACCP survey. Chest. 1991;100:1668–75.
3. Tape TG, Blank LL, Wigton RS. Procedural skills of practicing pulmonologists. A national survey of 1,000 members of the American College of Physicians. Am J Respir Crit Care Med. 1995;151:282–7.
4. Colt HG, Prakash UBS, Offord KP. Bronchoscopy in North America: survey by the American Association for Bronchology, 1999. J Bronchol. 2000;7:8–25.
5. Marquette CH, Martinot A. Interventional bronchoscopy. Basel: Karger; 2000.
6. Paksu S, Paksu MS, Kilic M, et al. Foreign body aspiration in childhood: evaluation of diagnostic parameters. Pediatr Emerg Care. 2012;28:259–64.
7. al-Majed SA, Ashour M, al-Mobeireek AF, al-Hajjaj MS, Alzeer AH, al-Kattan K. Overlooked inhaled foreign bodies: late sequelae and the likelihood of recovery. Respir Med. 1997;91:293–6.
8. Baharloo F, Veyckemans F, Francis C, Biettlot MP, Rodenstein DO. Tracheobronchial foreign bodies: presentation and management in children and adults. Chest. 1999;115:1357–62.
9. McGuirt WF, Holmes KD, Feehs R, Browne JD. Tracheobronchial foreign bodies. Laryngoscope. 1988;98:615–8.
10. Mantor PC, Tuggle DW, Tunell WP. An appropriate negative bronchoscopy rate in suspected foreign body aspiration. Am J Surg. 1989;158:622–4.
11. Martinot A, Closset M, Marquette CH, et al. Indications for flexible versus rigid bronchoscopy in children with suspected foreign-body aspiration. Am J Respir Crit Care Med. 1997;155:1676–9.
12. Hoeve LJ, Rombout J, Pot DJ. Foreign body aspiration in children. The diagnostic value of signs, symptoms and pre-operative examination. Clin Otolaryngol Allied Sci. 1993;18:55–7.

13. Wiseman NE. The diagnosis of foreign body aspiration in childhood. J Pediatr Surg. 1984;19:531–5.
14. Banerjee A, Rao KS, Khanna SK, et al. Laryngo-tracheo-bronchial foreign bodies in children. J Laryngol Otol. 1988;102:1029–32.
15. Pasaoglu I, Dogan R, Demircin M, Hatipoglu A, Bozer AY. Bronchoscopic removal of foreign bodies in children: retrospective analysis of 822 cases. Thorac Cardiovasc Surg. 1991;39:95–8.
16. Cleveland RH. Symmetry of bronchial angles in children. Radiology. 1979;133:89–93.
17. Casson AG, Guy JR. Foreign-body aspiration in adults. Can J Surg. 1987;30:193–4.
18. Chen CH, Lai CL, Tsai TT, Lee YC, Perng RP. Foreign body aspiration into the lower airway in Chinese adults. Chest. 1997;112:129–33.
19. Case records of the Massachusetts General Hospital. Weekly clinicopathological exercises. Case 33-1997. A 75-year-old man with chest pain, hemoptysis, and a pulmonary lesion. N Engl J Med. 1997;337:1220–6.
20. Burton EM, Riggs Jr W, Kaufman RA, Houston CS. Pneumomediastinum caused by foreign body aspiration in children. Pediatr Radiol. 1989;20:45–7.
21. Nimrey-Atrash N, Bentur L, Elias N. Subcutaneous emphysema and pneumomediastinum due to foreign body aspiration in children with asthma. Pediatr Pulmonol. 2012;47:88–90.
22. Esclamado RM, Richardson MA. Laryngotracheal foreign bodies in children. A comparison with bronchial foreign bodies. Am J Dis Child. 1987;141: 259–62.
23. Shepard JA. The bronchi: an imaging perspective. J Thorac Imaging. 1995;10:236–54.
24. Imaizumi H, Kaneko M, Nara S, Saito H, Asakura K, Akiba H. Definitive diagnosis and location of peanuts in the airways using magnetic resonance imaging techniques. Ann Emerg Med. 1994;23:1379–82.
25. Kitanaka S, Mikami I, Tokumaru A, O'Uchi T. Diagnosis of peanut inhalation by MRI. Pediatr Radiol. 1992;22:300–1.
26. O'Uchi T, Tokumaru A, Mikami I, Yamasoba T, Kikuchi S. Value of MR imaging in detecting a peanut causing bronchial obstruction. AJR Am J Roentgenol. 1992;159:481–2.
27. Marom EM, Goodman PC, McAdams HP. Focal abnormalities of the trachea and main bronchi. AJR Am J Roentgenol. 2001;176:707–11.
28. Cevizci N, Dokucu AI, Baskin D, et al. Virtual bronchoscopy as a dynamic modality in the diagnosis and treatment of suspected foreign body aspiration. Eur J Pediatr Surg. 2008;18:398–401.
29. Salah MT, Hamza S, Murtada M, Salma M. Delayed diagnosis of foreign body aspiration in children. Sudanese J of Public Health. 2007;2:48–50.
30. Atmaca S, Unal R, Sesen T, Kilicarslan H, Unal A. Laryngeal foreign body mistreated as recurrent laryngitis and croup for one year. Turk J Pediatr. 2009;51:65–6.
31. Barben J, Berkowitz RG, Kemp A, Massie J. Bronchial granuloma—where's the foreign body? Int J Pediatr Otorhinolaryngol. 2000;53:215–9.
32. Mittleman RE, Wetli CV. The fatal cafe coronary. Foreign-body airway obstruction. JAMA. 1982;247: 1285–8.
33. Daniilidis J, Symeonidis B, Triaridis K, Kouloulas A. Foreign body in the airways: a review of 90 cases. Arch Otolaryngol. 1977;103:570–3.
34. Abdulmajid OA, Ebeid AM, Motaweh MM, Kleibo IS. Aspirated foreign bodies in the tracheobronchial tree: report of 250 cases. Thorax. 1976;31: 635–40.
35. Elhassani NB. Tracheobronchial foreign bodies in the Middle East. A Baghdad study. J Thorac Cardiovasc Surg. 1988;96:621–5.
36. Yapici D, Atici S, Birbicer H, Oral U. Manufacturing defect in an endotracheal tube connector: risk of foreign body aspiration. J Anesth. 2008;22:333–4.
37. Lee P, Culver DA, Farver C, Mehta AC. Syndrome of iron pill aspiration. Chest. 2002;121:1355–7.
38. Clancy MJ. Bronchoscopic removal of an inhaled, sharp, foreign body: an unusual complication. J Laryngol Otol. 1999;113:849–50.
39. Vander Salm TJ, Ellis N. Blowgun dart aspiration. J Thorac Cardiovasc Surg. 1986;91:930–2.
40. Gencer M, Ceylan E, Koksal N. Extraction of pins from the airway with flexible bronchoscopy. Respiration. 2007;74:674–9.
41. Al-Ali MA, Khassawneh B, Alzoubi F. Utility of fiberoptic bronchoscopy for retrieval of aspirated headscarf pins. Respiration. 2007;74:309–13.
42. Debeljak A, Sorli J, Music E, Kecelj P. Bronchoscopic removal of foreign bodies in adults: experience with 62 patients from 1974–1998. Eur Respir J. 1999;14:792–5.
43. Betancourt M, Bekteshi E, Toth J, Alam S. Foreign body aspiration during esophagogastroduodenoscopy with band ligation. J Bronchol Intervento Pulmonol. 2008;15:204–5.
44. Kosloske AM. Bronchoscopic extraction of aspirated foreign bodies in children. Am J Dis Child. 1982;136:924–7.
45. Kosloske AM. Tracheobronchial foreign bodies in children: back to the bronchoscope and a balloon. Pediatrics. 1980;66:321–3.
46. Law D, Kosloske AM. Management of tracheobronchial foreign bodies in children: a reevaluation of postural drainage and bronchoscopy. Pediatrics. 1976; 58:362–7.
47. Steen KH, Zimmermann T. Tracheobronchial aspiration of foreign bodies in children: a study of 94 cases. Laryngoscope. 1990;100:525–30.
48. Bose P, El Mikatti N. Foreign bodies in the respiratory tract. A review of forty-one cases. Ann R Coll Surg Engl. 1981;63:129–31.
49. Cotton EK, Abrams G, Vanhoutte J, Burrington J. Removal of aspirated foreign bodies by inhalation

and postural drainage. A survey of 24 cases. Clin Pediatr (Phila). 1973;12:270–6.
50. Limper AH, Prakash UB. Tracheobronchial foreign bodies in adults. Ann Intern Med. 1990;112:604–9.
51. Hsu W, Sheen T, Lin C, Tan C, Yeh T, Lee S. Clinical experiences of removing foreign bodies in the airway and esophagus with a rigid endoscope: a series of 3217 cases from 1970 to 1996. Otolaryngol Head Neck Surg. 2000;122:450–4.
52. Surka AE, Chin R, Conforti J. Bronchoscopic myths and legends: airway foreign bodies. Clin Pulm Med. 2006;13:209–11.
53. Swanson KL, Prakash UB, MdCougall JC, Midthun DE, Edell ES, Brutinel MW, et al. Airway foreign bodies in adults. J Bronchol. 2003;10:107–11.
54. Heinz 3rd GJ, Richardson RH, Zavala DC. Endobronchial foreign body removal using the bronchofiberscope. Ann Otol Rhinol Laryngol. 1978;87:50–2.
55. Mehta AC, Grimm M. Breakage of Nd-YAG laser sapphire contact probe inside the endobronchial tree. Chest. 1988;93:1119.
56. Fieselmann JF, Zavala DC, Keim LW. Removal of foreign bodies (two teeth) by fiberoptic bronchoscopy. Chest. 1977;72:241–3.
57. Klayton RJ, Donlan CJ, O'Neil TJ, Foreman DR. Letter: foreign body removal via fiberoptic bronchoscopy. JAMA. 1975;234:806.
58. Lee M, Fernandez NA, Berger HW, Givre H. Wire basket removal of a tack via flexible fiberoptic bronchoscopy. Chest. 1982;82:515.
59. Rohde FC, Celis ME, Fernandez S. The removal of an endobronchial foreign body with the fiberoptic bronchoscope and image intensifier. Chest. 1977; 72:265.
60. Prakash UB, Midthun DE, Edell ES. Indications for flexible versus rigid bronchoscopy in children with suspected foreign-body aspiration. Am J Respir Crit Care Med. 1997;156:1017–9.
61. Downey RJ, Libutti SK, Gorenstein L, Mercer S. Airway management during retrieval of the very large aspirated foreign body: a method for the flexible bronchoscope. Anesth Analg. 1995;81: 186–7.
62. Verea-Hernando H, Garcia-Quijada RC, Ruiz de Galarreta AA. Extraction of foreign bodies with fiberoptic bronchoscopy in mechanically ventilated patients. Am Rev Respir Dis. 1990;142:258.
63. Rodrigues AJ, Scussiatto EA, Jacomelli M, et al. Bronchoscopic techniques for removal of foreign bodies in children's airways. Pediatr Pulmonol. 2012;47:59–62.
64. Hirai T, Yamanaka A, Fujimoto T, Shiraishi M, Fukuoka T. Bronchoscopic removal of bronchial foreign bodies through the laryngeal mask airway in pediatric patients. Jpn J Thorac Cardiovasc Surg. 1999;47:190–2.
65. McGrath G, Das-Gupta M, Clarke G. Bronchoscopy via continuous positive airway pressure for patients with respiratory failure. Chest. 2001;119:670–1.
66. Silvestri GA, Vincent BD, Wahidi MM, Robinette E, Hansbrough JR, Downie GH. A phase 3, randomized, double-blind study to assess the efficacy and safety of fospropofol disodium injection for moderate sedation in patients undergoing flexible bronchoscopy. Chest. 2009;135:41–7.
67. Jantz MA. The old and the new of sedation for bronchoscopy. Chest. 2009;135:4–6.
68. Fidkowski CW, Zheng H, Firth PG. The anesthetic considerations of tracheobronchial foreign bodies in children: a literature review of 12,979 cases. Anesth Analg. 2010;111:1016–25.
69. Saito H, Saka H, Sakai S, Shimokata K. Removal of broken fragment of biopsy forceps with magnetic extractor. Chest. 1989;95:700–1.
70. Mayr J, Dittrich S, Triebl K. A new method for removal of metallic-ferromagnetic foreign bodies from the tracheobronchial tree. Pediatr Surg Int. 1997;12:461–2.
71. De Weerdt S, Noppen M, Remels L, Vanherreweghe R, Meysman M, Vincken W. Successful removal of a massive endobronchial blood clot by means of cryotherapy. J Bronchol. 2005;12:23–4.
72. Mehta AC. Nasal versus oral insertion of the flexible bronchoscope. J Bronchol. 1996;3:224–8.
73. Boelcskei PL, Wagner M, Lessnau KK. Laser-assisted removal of a foreign body in the bronchial system of an infant. Lasers Surg Med. 1995;17:375–7.
74. Rees JR. Massive hemoptysis associated with foreign body removal. Chest. 1985;88:475–6.
75. Hayashi AH, Gillis DA, Bethune D, Hughes D, O'Neil M. Management of foreign-body bronchial obstruction using endoscopic laser therapy. J Pediatr Surg. 1990;25:1174–6.
76. Bolliger CT, Mathur PN. Interventional bronchoscopy. Basel: Karger; 2000.
77. Parray T, Abraham E, Apuya JS, Ghafoor AU, Saif Siddiqui M. Migration of a foreign body from right to left lung. Internet J Anesthesiol. 2010;24.
78. Mohnssen SR, Greggs D. Iatrogenic aspiration of components of respiratory care equipment. Chest. 1993;103:964–5.
79. Pinals M, Pinals D, Tracy JD, Brandstetter RD. Expectoration of an occult foreign body six asymptomatic years after aspiration. Chest. 1993;103: 1930–1.
80. Karapolat S. Foreign-body aspiration in an adult. Can J Surg. 2008;51:411; author reply -2.
81. Mohnssen SR. Iatrogenic aspiration. Follow-up. Chest. 1994;105:976.
82. Iannuzzi M, De Robertis E, Rispoli F, Piazza O, Tufano R. A complication of a closed-tube endotracheal suction catheter. Eur J Anaesthesiol. 2009;26:974–5.
83. Overdahl MC, Wewers MD. Acute occlusion of a mainstem bronchus by a rapidly expanding foreign body. Chest. 1994;105:1600–2.
84. Kinsey CM, Folch E, Majid A, Channick C. Evaluation and management of pill aspiration: case discussion. In: 17th World Congress for bronchol-

ogy and interventional pulmonology. Cleveland, OH; 2012.

85. Aziz F. Natural history of an aspirated foreign body. J Bronchol. 2006;13:161–2.
86. James P, Christopher DJ, Balamugesh T, Thomas R. Multiple foreign body aspiration and bronchiectasis. J Bronchol. 2006;13:218–20.
87. Saki N, Nikakhlagh S, Rahim F, Abshirini H. Foreign body aspirations in infancy: a 20-year experience. Int J Med Sci. 2009;6:322–8.
88. Brown KL, Shefler A, Cohen G, DeMunter C, Pigott N, Goldman AP. Near-fatal grape aspiration with complicating acute lung injury successfully treated with extracorporeal membrane oxygenation. Pediatr Crit Care Med. 2003;4:243–5.
89. Ignacio Jr RC, Falcone Jr RA, Brown RL. A case report of severe tracheal obstruction requiring extracorporeal membrane oxygenation. J Pediatr Surg. 2006;41:E1–4.
90. Isherwood J, Firmin R. Late presentation of foreign body aspiration requiring extracorporeal membrane oxygenation support for surgical management. Interact Cardiovasc Thorac Surg. 2011;12:631–2.
91. Hiller C, Lerner S, Varnum R, et al. Foreign body removal with the flexible fiberoptic bronchoscope. Endoscopy. 1977;9:216–22.
92. Cunanan OS. The flexible fiberoptic bronchoscope in foreign body removal. Experience in 300 cases. Chest. 1978;73:725–6.
93. Clark PT, Williams TJ, Teichtahl H, Bowes G, Tuxen DV. Removal of proximal and peripheral endobronchial foreign bodies with the flexible fibreoptic bronchoscope. Anaesth Intensive Care. 1989;17:205–8.
94. Nunez H, Perez Rodriguez E, Alvarado C, et al. Foreign body aspirate extraction. Chest. 1989;96:698.
95. Lan RS, Lee CH, Chiang YC, Wang WJ. Use of fiberoptic bronchoscopy to retrieve bronchial foreign bodies in adults. Am Rev Respir Dis. 1989; 140:1734–7.
96. Moura e Sa J, Oliveira A, Caiado A, et al. Tracheobronchial foreign bodies in adults—experience of the Bronchology Unit of Centro Hospitalar de Vila Nova de Gaia. Rev Port Pneumol. 2006;12:31–43.
97. Donado Una JR, de Miguel Poch E, Casado Lopez ME, Alfaro Abreu JJ. Fiber optic bronchoscopy in extraction of tracheo-bronchial foreign bodies in adults. Arch Bronconeumol. 1998;34:76–81.
98. Kalyanappagol VT, Kulkarni NH, Bidri LH. Management of tracheobronchial foreign body aspirations in paediatric age group—a 10 year retrospective analysis. Indian J Anaesth. 2007;51:20–3.
99. Lima AG, Santos NA, Rocha ER, Toro IF. Bronchoscopy for foreign body removal: where is the delay? Jornal Brasileiro de Pneumologia: Publicacao Oficial da Sociedade Brasileira de Pneumologia e Tisilogia. 2008;34:956–8.
100. Ramos MB, Fernandez-Villar A, Rivo JE, et al. Extraction of airway foreign bodies in adults: experience from 1987–2008. Interact Cardiovasc Thorac Surg. 2009;9:402–5.
101. Oguzkaya F, Akcali Y, Kahraman C, Bilgin M, Sahin A. Tracheobronchial foreign body aspirations in childhood: a 10-year experience. Eur J Cardiothorac Surg. 1998;14:388–92.
102. Rahbarimanesh A, Noroozi E, Molaian M, Salamati P. Foreign body aspiration: a five-year report in a children's hospital. Iran J Pediatr. 2008;18:191–2.
103. Metrangelo S, Monetti C, Meneghini L, Zadra N, Giusti F. Eight years' experience with foreign-body aspiration in children: what is really important for a timely diagnosis? J Pediatr Surg. 1999;34: 1229–31.
104. Chik KK, Miu TY, Chan CW. Foreign body aspiration in Hong Kong Chinese children. Hong Kong Med J. 2009;15:6–11.
105. Yetim DT, Bayarogullari H, Arica V, Akcora B, Arica SG, Tutanc M. Foreign body aspiration in children; analysis of 42 cases. J Pulmon Resp Med. 2012;2:121–5.
106. Tang LF, Xu YC, Wang YS, et al. Airway foreign body removal by flexible bronchoscopy: experience with 1027 children during 2000–2008. World J Pediatr. 2009;5:191–5.
107. Boyd M, Watkins F, Singh S, et al. Prevalence of flexible bronchoscopic removal of foreign bodies in the advanced elderly. Age Ageing. 2009;38: 396–400.
108. Weissberg D, Schwartz I. Foreign bodies in the tracheobronchial tree. Chest. 1987;91:730–3.
109. Zhijun C, Fugao Z, Niankai Z, Jingjing C. Therapeutic experience from 1428 patients with pediatric tracheobronchial foreign body. J Pediatr Surg. 2008;43: 718–21.
110. Skoulakis CE, Doxas PG, Papadakis CE, et al. Bronchoscopy for foreign body removal in children. A review and analysis of 210 cases. Int J Pediatr Otorhinolaryngol. 2000;53:143–8.
111. Maddali MM, Mathew M, Chandwani J, Alsajwani MJ, Ganguly SS. Outcomes after rigid bronchoscopy in children with suspected or confirmed foreign body aspiration: a retrospective study. J Cardiothorac Vasc Anesth. 2011;25:1005–8.
112. Kiyan G, Gocmen B, Tugtepe H, Karakoc F, Dagli E, Dagli TE. Foreign body aspiration in children: the value of diagnostic criteria. Int J Pediatr Otorhinolaryngol. 2009;73:963–7.

Role of Bronchoscopy in Hemoptysis

14

Santhakumar Subramanian, Arvind H. Kate, and Prashant N. Chhajed

Abstract

Hemoptysis is a common and alarming symptom. There are no accepted volume-based definitions of non-massive or massive hemoptysis. For practical purposes, massive hemoptysis is better defined on the basis of magnitude of effect rather than the amount of expectorated blood. Acute bronchitis is the most common cause of non-massive hemoptysis. The common causes of massive hemoptysis include bronchiectasis, tuberculosis, lung cancer, and mycetoma. Bronchoscopy plays a central role in the evaluation and management of hemoptysis. Direct inspection allows localization of the bleeding site and isolation of bleeding segment to prevent flooding of non-bleeding lung and asphyxiation. Rigid bronchoscope is preferred over flexible bronchoscope for management of massive hemoptysis but its utility is limited by lack of trained personnel in majority of medical centers. In the absence of facilities for rigid bronchoscopy, it is prudent to secure airway with a large endotracheal tube, perform early flexible bronchoscopy, and initiate aggressive resuscitative measures. Several bronchoscopic techniques such as balloon tamponade, topical application of cold saline, vasoconstrictors, and pro-coagulant substances may be applied for temporary control of bleeding. Interventional

S. Subramanian, M.D., F.C.C.P., I.D.C.C. (✉)
KG Hospital, Arts College Road, Coimbatore,
Tamil Nadu 642018, India
e-mail: drskumar.chest@gmail.com

A.H. Kate, M.D., F.C.C.P.
Lung Care and Sleep Centre, Fortis Hiranandani Hospital,
Navi Mumbai, Maharashtra, India

P.N. Chhajed, M.D., D.N.B., D.E.T.R.D., F.C.C.P.
Lung Care and Sleep Centre, Fortis Hiranandani
Hospital, Navi Mumbai, Maharashtra, India
e-mail: pchhajed@gmail.com

A.C. Mehta and P. Jain (eds.), *Interventional Bronchoscopy: A Clinical Guide*, Respiratory Medicine 10,
DOI 10.1007/978-1-62703-395-4_14, © Springer Science+Business Media New York 2013

techniques such as laser photoresection and argon plasma coagulation may be helpful in selected cases. Temporary control of bleeding may facilitate institution of definitive therapies such as bronchial artery embolization and surgery in selected patients.

Keywords

Hemoptysis • Bronchoscopy • Rigid bronchoscopy • Massive hemoptysis • Bronchial artery embolization

Introduction

Hemoptysis is one of the alarming symptoms of an underlying pulmonary problem. It may present as minimal blood-streaked sputum or a moderate to massive hemoptysis compromising the airway and hemodynamic status, endangering life. It is estimated that 6.8 % of chest clinic visits and 11 % of thoracic surgical admissions are due to hemoptysis [1]. Although mortality rate may be as high as 80 % in a massive hemoptysis, usually mortality ranges from 7 to 30 % [2–4]. Asphyxia rather than exsanguination is usually the cause of death [5], and it is commonly accompanied by cardiovascular collapse. Like any other life-threatening condition, initial management in hemoptysis would be aiming at a patent airway and resuscitation of the patient to obtain stable hemodynamic status. Once the airway patency is obtained, bronchoscopy plays a pivotal role with regard to localization of the anatomic site of bleeding, isolation of the involved airway, control of hemorrhage, and treatment of the underlying cause of hemoptysis in case of visible endoluminal lesions [6]. In this chapter we focus on role of bronchoscopy in the management of hemoptysis and review the definition, blood supply, etiology, assessment, and management of hemoptysis.

Definition

Hemoptysis may be classified as non-massive and massive hemoptysis. There is no consensus definition made so far on massive hemoptysis even though various volumetric and magnitude-related definitions have been quoted in different studies. The volumetric definitions mainly focus on the amount of expectorated blood ranging from 100 to 1,000 ml in 24 h accounting for a massive hemoptysis whereas expectoration of less than 100 ml in 24 h has been accepted as non-massive hemoptysis [6]. A widely accepted definition of massive hemoptysis is witnessing ≥600 ml of expectorated blood in 24 h, based on a study by Crocco et al. [7] in which >600 ml of blood expectorated in 4 h led to 71 % mortality whereas less than 600 ml of expectorated blood in 24–48 h was associated with a mortality rate of only up to 5 %. It is estimated that more than 400 ml of blood in the alveolar space is sufficient to cause impairment of oxygenation [8]. As the above definitions lack a consensus cutoff volume and do not consider other major determinants like rate of bleeding, patient's cardiopulmonary reserve, and ability to protect airway, a more reliable definition could be based on magnitude of effect on the patient due to hemoptysis in which the following parameters are included: need for transfusion, hospitalization, intubation, or causing aspiration and airway obstruction, hypoxemia (PaO_2 <8 kPa or 60 mmHg), or death.

Blood Supply

The respiratory system receives blood supply from two different sources: a high-pressure (systemic) bronchial circulation which supplies the airway down to the terminal bronchioles and a low-pressure pulmonary circulation which supplies the alveolar ducts and sacs [9]. Bronchial arteries originate from the descending aorta, most often at the T5, T6 level and the most common pattern is single artery on right side and two bronchial arteries on left side. In about 20 % of cases, bronchial arteries have an aberrant origin from other systemic arteries. In 5 % of patients, a spinal artery originates from a bronchial artery [10].

Etiology

It is important to establish that lung is the source of bleeding as bleeding arising from nasopharyngeal and gastrointestinal sources may mimic hemoptysis. Most important causes of hemoptysis are listed in Table 14.1. Chronic inflammatory conditions such as bronchiectasis, tuberculosis, and lung abscess, and lung malignancies, are the most common causes of massive hemoptysis [11]. Bleeding may also occur from mycetoma forming in patients with a preexisting cavitating lung disease [12].

In older studies tuberculosis accounted for 73 % of all causes of hemoptysis [7]. These included both new and inactive cases. In tuberculosis various underlying pathophysiological mechanisms account for hemoptysis such as (1) direct extension of infection and inflammation into the bronchial arterioles; (2) bronchiectasis due to chronic inflammation leading to dilated, tortuous, and fragile blood vessels that bleed spontaneously; (3) mycetomas formed inside

Table 14.1 Causes of hemoptysis

Infections • Mycobacteria, particularly tuberculosis • Fungal infections (mycetoma) • Lung abscess • Necrotising pneumonia (Klebsiella, Staphylococcus, Legionella)	Vascular • Pulmonary embolism and infarction • Mitral stenosis • Arteriobronchial fistula • Arteriovenous malformations • Bronchial telangiectasia • Left ventricular failure
Iatrogenic • Bronchoscopy • Swan–Ganz catheterization • Transbronchial biopsy • Transtracheal aspirate	Coagulopathy • Von Willebrand's disease • Hemophilia • Anticoagulant therapy • Thrombocytopenia • Platelet dysfunction • Disseminated intravascular coagulation • Vasculitis • Behcet's disease • Wegener's granulomatosis
Parasitic • Hydatid cyst • Paragonimiasis	
Trauma • Blunt/penetrating injury • Suction ulcers • Tracheoarterial fistula	
Neoplasm • Bronchogenic carcinoma • Bronchial adenoma • Pulmonary metastases • Sarcoma	Pulmonary • Bronchiectasis (including cystic fibrosis) • Chronic bronchitis • Emphysematous bullae
Hemoptysis in children • Foreign body aspiration • Bronchial adenoma • Vascular anomalies	Miscellaneous • Lymphangioleiomyometosis • Catamenial (endometriosis) • Pneumoconiosis • Broncholith • Idiopathic
	Spurious • Epistaxis • Hematemesis

large parenchymal cavities forming granulation tissue and neovascularization (Rasmussen's aneurysms); and (4) extension of tuberculous infection into pulmonary artery leading to rupture of the vessel.

Bronchiectasis resulting from various causes such as chronic inflammation, cystic fibrosis, and immotile cilia syndrome and immunoglobulin deficiency may account for a significant percentage of hemoptysis [13]. The underlying pathophysiological mechanism in these patients is enlarged, dilated, tortuous bronchial arteries forming collaterals. Pulmonary malignancies including both primary as well as metastatic disease with endobronchial involvement are usually highly vascular and bleed spontaneously and may give rise to massive hemoptysis. Although the bronchial circulation accounts for most cases of massive hemoptysis, pulmonary arteries (PA) remain the source of bleeding in a substantial number of patients. Several etiologies such as necrotizing pulmonary infections, malignancies, vasculitis, trauma from Swan–Ganz catheterization, and pulmonary A-V malformations cause bleeding to originate from the pulmonary circulation. Although alveolar hemorrhage is a well-recognized cause of hemoptysis, it rarely presents with massive bleeding since the alveoli can accommodate a large amount of blood. Curiously, despite extensive diagnostic workup, cryptogenic massive hemoptysis has been reported in 11–19 % of cases in the recent literature [14]. Pulmonary veno-occlusive disease, pulmonary endometriosis, pulmonary arteriovenous malformations, and broncho-vascular fistula are other rare sources for massive hemoptysis.

Diagnosis

After achieving airway protection and hemodynamic stabilization, diagnostic workup may be initiated in massive hemoptysis where as in mild to moderate hemoptysis a conservative approach might be sufficient initially. A thorough history and clinical examination may be useful in differentiating hemoptysis from hematemesis and upper airway bleed. There is no consensus on diagnostic approach of hemoptysis. However chest imaging including radiography and computed tomography scan (CT scan) combined with a diagnostic bronchoscopy is usually needed to reach a definitive diagnosis in majority of cases. Coagulation and vasculitis profile should be obtained in appropriate situations. Chest radiography can identify the site of bleeding in 33–82 % of cases of massive hemoptysis [15], and may reveal the underlying cause in 35 % of patients. CT scan is superior to radiography in localizing pathology and identifying the etiology as well as guiding the future definitive therapy. The yield for localization of bleeding site with CT is up to 88 % [16]. It has been a long debate whether CT should be done first before bronchoscopy or the reverse. While some authors suggest that CT can replace bronchoscopy as a first-line investigational approach in patients with massive hemoptysis because of its higher diagnostic yield [17], others advocate it as complementary to flexible bronchoscopy for bleeding site identification [18]. Recently multidetector CT has been proven to be more precise in delineation of bronchial and pulmonary vessels [19, 20]. However imaging techniques may also have limitations in certain scenarios. For example, in patient with bilateral lung disease, bronchoscopy is more likely to reveal and localize the site of bleeding than chest CT. Bronchoscopy can also be useful in hemodynamically unstable patients who cannot be moved to the CT scan department.

Flexible bronchoscopy is more useful in large or massive hemoptysis for localization (diagnostic yield: 73–93 %) where as in mild to moderate hemoptysis the diagnostic yield is lower [21, 22]. While optimal timing of bronchoscopy (early vs. late) remains a controversial issue, there is no difference in outcome and therapeutic decisions whether an early or a late bronchoscopy is performed in a case of non-massive hemoptysis [23, 24]. But it is essential to understand that flexible bronchoscopy may not be a right choice in massive life-threatening hemoptysis due to its limitations in obtaining airway control and ventilation while rigid bronchoscopy is more efficient at safeguarding airway patency, preserving ventilation, and allowing better clearance of the airways, therefore improving visualization [25].

Management of Hemoptysis

Non-massive hemoptysis

The overall goals of management of the patient with hemoptysis are threefold: cessation of bleeding, prevention of aspiration, and treatment of the underlying cause. Acute bronchitis remains the most common cause of acute, mild hemoptysis. In majority of cases, hemoptysis is transient and self-limiting in these patients. Low-risk patients with normal chest radiographs can be treated on an outpatient basis with close monitoring and appropriate oral antibiotics, if clinically indicated. An abnormal mass on a chest radiograph warrants an outpatient bronchoscopic examination. For patients with a normal chest radiograph and risk factors for lung cancer or recurrent hemoptysis, high-resolution computed tomography is indicated prior to bronchoscopy, except in urgent situations when immediate bronchoscopy is needed.

Management of Massive Hemoptysis

It may not be possible to follow a stepwise approach in a patient with massive hemoptysis because multiple interventions need to be done simultaneously to achieve cardiopulmonary stability. However airway protection and hemodynamic resuscitation are the top priorities. If the bleeding side is known patient should be kept in lateral decubitus position with the bleeding side down. The patient should be transferred to intensive care unit as soon as possible. Urgent fluid resuscitation and blood transfusion should be done as required. Coagulopathy if identified should be corrected. Rigid bronchoscopy is the most effective means of clearing the airways from secretions and blood clots, ensuring effective tamponade of airways and isolation of the non-affected lung and thereby preventing asphyxia and preserving ventilation. However rigid bronchoscopy is not feasible always, as the skilled rigid bronchoscopist may not be available at the time of massive hemoptysis or operating room may not be in a state of readiness to receive a collapsing patient for immediate management. In such cases urgent endotracheal intubation and airway stabilization could prevent imminent death from asphyxia.

Airway Protection and Resuscitation

If immediate rigid bronchoscopy cannot be done, urgent endotracheal (ET) intubation with a large-size tube (preferably eight or more) should be done and flexible bronchoscopic suctioning and clearance should be attempted through the endotracheal tube. Selective unilateral intubation of non-bleeding bronchus may be considered under flexible bronchoscopy guidance (Fig. 14.1); however selective right main bronchial intubation should be avoided as it can cause occlusion of right upper lobe bronchus and further compromise ventilation. In such circumstances, tracheal intubation can be done initially and a balloon catheter may be passed beside the ET tube via the

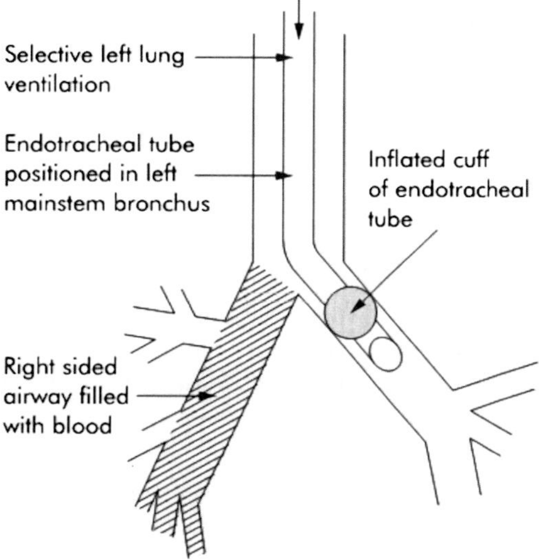

Fig. 14.1 Selective intubation of left main bronchus for management of bleeding arising from right lung (reprinted from Lordan JL, Gascoigne A, Corris PA. The pulmonary physician in critical care—illustrative case 7: assessment and management of massive haemoptysis. Thorax. 2003;58(9):814–9. With permission from BMJ Publishing Group Ltd.)

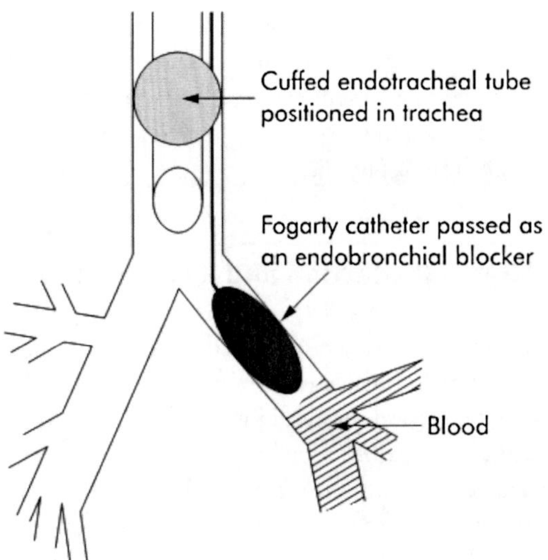

Fig. 14.2 Placement and inflation of a balloon catheter in bleeding left main bronchus (reprinted from Lordan JL, Gascoigne A, Corris PA. The pulmonary physician in critical care—illustrative case 7: assessment and management of massive haemoptysis. Thorax. 2003;58(9):814–9. With permission from BMJ Publishing Group Ltd.)

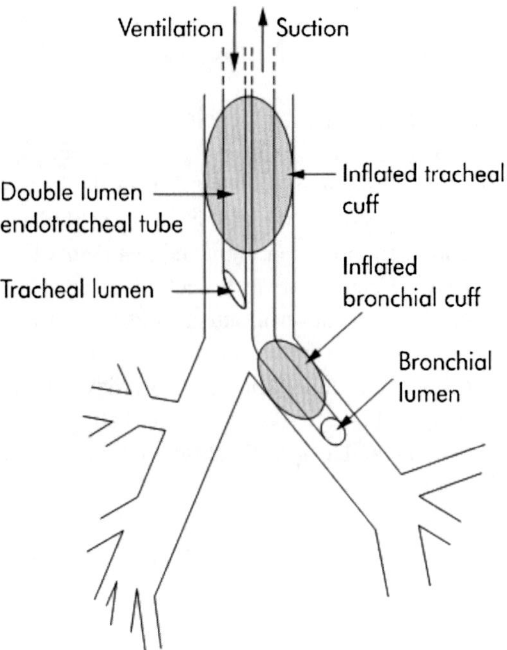

Fig. 14.3 Double-lumen endotracheal tube with inflated tracheal and bronchial cuffs (reprinted from Lordan JL, Gascoigne A, Corris PA. The pulmonary physician in critical care—illustrative case 7: assessment and management of massive haemoptysis. Thorax. 2003;58(9):814–9. With permission from BMJ Publishing Group Ltd.)

vocal cords or through ET tube itself and directed into the left main bronchus followed by balloon inflation (Fig. 14.2). In rare instances, double-lumen endotracheal tube may be placed which isolates the bleeding lung and simultaneously ventilates the normal lung (Fig. 14.3). Standard resuscitative techniques should go hand in hand with the above-mentioned bronchoscopic measures. Fluid resuscitation, vasopressor medications, and blood products should be administered as indicated. Appropriate laboratory and serologic studies are performed. Disease-specific therapies such as immunosuppressive therapy for vasculitis, connective tissue disorders, and Wegener's granulomatosis may be initiated, depending on the underlying diagnosis. Corticosteroids and plasmapheresis may be useful in the setting of Goodpasture syndrome. Once hemodynamic and respiratory conditions are stabilized, urgent endovascular therapy should be considered. In the setting of massive hemoptysis from a local source, early thoracic surgical consultation should be sought in case urgent surgical lung resection is needed to control the hemorrhage.

Bronchoscopic Interventions

Utilization of bronchoscopy in appropriate situations may either stabilize the patient temporarily by achieving hemostasis or in certain circumstances provide a long-lasting control of hemoptysis. Although it has been a long debate whether to use flexible bronchoscopy or rigid bronchoscopy there is no randomized control trial to support either of them. But it is clear that choice of the bronchoscopy depends on availability, operator's preference and technical skills, and available facilities. Both flexible and rigid bronchoscopes have their merits and limitations (Table 14.2). However rigid bronchoscopy is more efficient and safer when performed by a skilled bronchoscopist. Moreover it has several advantages over flexible bronchoscope which must be highlighted. The rigid bronchoscope has tracheobronchial ventilating ports which allow ventilation of normal lung

Table 14.2 Merits and demerits of flexible and rigid bronchoscope in management of hemoptysis

	Flexible bronchoscopy	Rigid bronchoscopy
Advantage	Technically easy to perform Ability to navigate smaller segments Can be done at bedside in ICU	Airway protection Better ventilation Better blood suctioning More therapeutic options
Disadvantage	Poor ability to suction blood Less interventions	Needs operating room Needs more skills

simultaneous with a therapeutic procedure. Rigid scope is attached with separate suction and therapeutic channels for clearing airways and passage of electrocautry or laser fiber, respectively. An important component is the ventilating side port that allows the administration of general anesthesia. The light source and telescope allow for both direct and video-assisted visualization. Through the wide bore channel, a number of endoscopic devices and therapeutic agents could be introduced. Therefore rigid bronchoscope allows stabilization of patient's hemodynamic and respiratory conditions before proceeding with further diagnostic or therapeutic interventions. However visibility through rigid bronchoscope is limited to central airways only. This limitation is easily overcome by placing a flexible bronchoscope through the lumen of the rigid bronchoscope for the inspection of distal airways. Various endoluminal bronchoscopic methods have been described in literature.

Topical Agents

Endoscopically applied topical vasoconstrictive or procoagulant agents can secure a temporary hemostasis until a definitive procedure is undertaken. These agents include cold saline, epinephrine, vasopressin and its analogues, for their vasoconstrictive effect, as well as thrombin–fibrinogen and tranexamic acid, for their procoagulant action.

Cold Saline

Topically applied ice-cold saline induces hypothermia and thus vasoconstriction leading to reduction in active bleeding. First study on cold saline was reported in 1980 by Conlan et al. in which cold saline irrigation stopped bleeding in 23 patients with massive hemoptysis temporarily until patients were taken for definitive surgical procedure [25]. Rigid bronchoscope was used and 50 ml aliquots of 4 °C saline up to maximum of 500 ml were applied to the tracheobronchial tree to achieve hemostasis. Utilization of rigid bronchoscope improved visualization and airway clearing. There were no significant complications except for transient bradycardia in one patient.

Epinephrine and Vasopressin

Topical irrigation with diluted epinephrine (1:10,000–1:20,000) may prove to be a temporary measure in cases of mild to moderate bleed following biopsy or brushing procedures [26]. However endobronchial irrigation of epinephrine may complicate with high plasma epinephrine levels leading to cardiac arrhythmias and tachycardia in a few patients [27, 28]. Alternatively some investigators have found the vasopressin analogues such as terlipressin and ornipressin to be as efficacious as epinephrine in obtaining hemostasis but without much cardiovascular adverse effects. However no randomized reports are available to support the use of these agents [29–31].

Topically Applied Procoagulants

Use of the antifibrinolytic agent tranexamic acid is well known for long time in achieving hemostasis in patients with mucosal bleeding, postsurgical bleeding, and bleeding disorders.

Systemic (intravenous and oral) administration of tranexamic acid showed good efficacy for control of hemoptysis in patients with cystic fibrosis and recurrent hemoptysis in patients with multiple aberrant bronchial arteries [32–34]. Recently topical irrigation with tranexamic acid (500–1,000 mg) has been reported to be efficient in bleeding that occurs following endobronchial procedures [35].

Topical application of fibrin–thrombin combination seems to be a promising method in moderate to massive hemoptysis in circumstances where immediate endovascular procedures are not feasible or contraindicated. Even though a few case reports [36, 37] established encouraging effects of these agents in the recent past, further large studies are needed to support their clinical use on a routine basis.

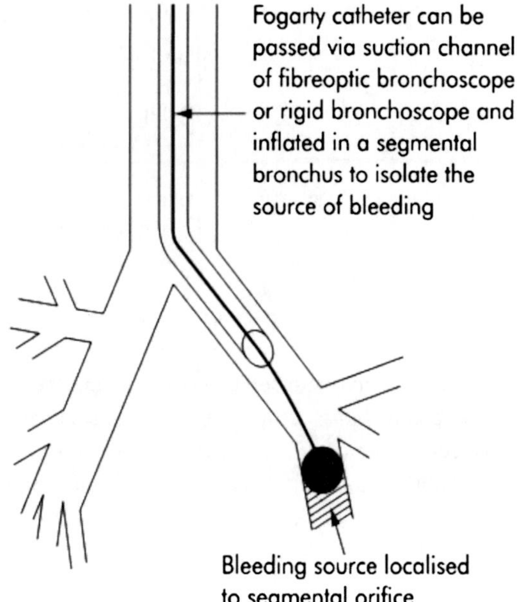

Fig. 14.4 Bronchoscopically guided placement of balloon catheter in a segmental bronchus (reprinted from Lordan JL, Gascoigne A, Corris PA. The pulmonary physician in critical care—illustrative case 7: assessment and management of massive haemoptysis. Thorax. 2003;58(9):814–9. With permission from BMJ Publishing Group Ltd.)

Bronchial Blocking Devices

In a circumstance of moderate to massive hemoptysis not responding to the above topical agents, blockade of the segmental or subsegmental bronchus at a level proximal to the bleeding site would give a tamponade effect and may stop bleeding completely (Fig. 14.4). In some instances, balloon tamponade stabilizes the patients prior to bronchial artery embolization. Tamponade or blockade effect might be created by using various techniques mentioned below.

Various types of balloon devices have proven to be effective in achieving temporary hemostasis until a definitive procedure is undertaken. These devices could be left in place for a period of up to 48–72 h before a definitive procedure. On the other hand, if left for a period more than 5 days, patients may develop postobstruction pneumonia of the occluded segment or lobe, vocal cord granulomas due to continuous contact with catheter, and recurrent bleeding due to dislocation of device from the original site. Frietag et al. have developed a double-lumen balloon catheter introduced through the working channel of flexible bronchoscope with the second lumen being utilized for administration of topical agents. Tamponade was successful in 26/27 patients with moderate hemoptysis using this catheter [38]. Dutau et al. developed a silicone spigot which is placed endobronchially with the use of rigid and flexible bronchoscope under direct vision and left in place at the bleeding segment for a few hours until bronchial artery embolization is undertaken [39]. Recently, Valipour and his colleagues placed oxidized regenerated cellulose mesh in the endobronchial segments using flexible bronchoscope and achieved immediate arrest of hemoptysis in 56/58 patients [40].

Endobronchial Sealing with Biocompatible Glue

Endobronchial sealing with *N*-acetyl cyanoacrylate, a bioadhesive material that solidifies on contact with humidity, is an efficient, safe, and simple method, described recently. Bhattacharyya et al. [41] described this method using flexible bronchoscopy in 67 patients with a 6-month follow-up. The success rate of long-term follow-up was 79 %. There were procedure failures in 22 %, the cause being false localization (46 %), proximal or inappropriate placement of the glue (31 %), and difficult cannulation (23 %).

Laser Bronchoscopy

Bronchoscopic CO_2 laser was originally used in 1970s by Strong and his colleagues [42]. Utilization of neodymium–yttrium–aluminum–garnet (Nd–YAG) laser for bronchoscopic coagulation was first reported by Dumon et al. in 1985 [43]. Wavelength of Nd–YAG laser (1,064 nm) imparts tissue–laser interactions making it optimal for bronchoscopic use. The Nd:YAG laser has a lower absorptive coefficient than scatter coefficient allowing for deeper penetration and a wide coagulation zone and it is an effective treatment option for hemoptysis when the source of bleeding is bronchoscopically visible. It allows photocoagulation of the bleeding mucosa with resulting hemostasis, and can help achieve photoresection and vaporization of the underlying lesion, thus providing a definitive approach to hemoptysis management. Laser probe is inserted through working channel of the flexible bronchoscope or the rigid bronchoscope and the tip of probe is kept beyond the distal end of the scope and approximately 5 mm proximal to the lesion. FiO_2 is reduced below 40 % and initially low wattage of laser (20 W) is used in a pulsed fashion. Strength of laser could be increased slowly depending upon the tissue response. After complete coagulation, tissue can be debulked and removed using forceps. Various studies have shown that laser photocoagulation is an effective method for control of bleed from tumor vessels and for debulking the lesions. Han et al. reported improvement in hemoptysis in 94 % of cancer patients who underwent endobronchial Nd–YAG laser treatment, with complete cessation of bleeding in 74 % [44]. In another study Hetzel and smith noticed arrest of bleed from inoperable tumors for a month after laser treatment [45].

Table 14.3 Comparison between Nd–YAG laser and argon plasma coagulation

Nd–YAG laser	Argon plasma coagulation
Noncontact laser	Noncontact coagulation
Uses thermal energy	Electrical energy
Deeper tissue penetration	Superficial and lateral spread
High temperature	Access to remote location and lateral lesions
	Homogenous tissue desiccation

In recent years Nd:YAP (yttrium–aluminum–perovskite) laser has been introduced to the armamentarium of the Interventional Pulmonologists. Its wavelength of 1,340 nm is 20 times more absorbed by water than standard 1,064 nm YAG lasers providing a better effectiveness-to-power ratio. Theoretically it should be highly effective in producing photocoagulation of the endobronchial lesion. More experience is being gathered with the use of this novel laser device.

Argon Plasma Coagulation

Argon plasma coagulation (APC) has several advantages over conventional electrocautery and Nd–YAG laser (Table 14.3). It is a noncontact electrocoagulation tool, uses high-frequency electrical current rather than thermal energy, is more accessible to laterally located tissue or around anatomic corners, and tissue desiccation is homogenous than that achieved with lasers. Blood is a good conductor of electrical energy and once the bleeding bronchus becomes desiccated it becomes less conductive of electrical energy and deeper tissue penetration is prevented [46, 47].

Several studies have demonstrated that APC is an effective tool in definitive management of endobronchial lesions causing hemoptysis, helpful in obtaining hemostasis as well as debulking the tumor lesion. Morice and his colleagues have documented an immediate arrest of bleed from an endoluminal source in 31/31 patients with the help of APC with no recurrence of bleeding observed after a mean follow-up period of 97 days [47]. Keller et al. reported a case of endobronchial polypoidal lesion in a patient of heart transplantation who was successfully treated with APC and there was no recurrence of hemoptysis until 10-month follow-up [46].

Electrocautery

Electrocautery can be used through the flexible bronchoscope. Homasson has reported a case series of 56 patients of advanced tracheobronchial malignancies and benign tumors having hemoptysis in which electrocautery helped control hemoptysis in 75 % of patients [48].

Other Modalities

Freezing has been shown to produce vasoconstriction and microthrombi formation in capillaries and venules, thus achieving hemostasis [49, 50]. Accordingly, bronchoscopic cyrotherapy may control chronic hemoptysis in some patients with endobronchial tumors. Similarly, brachytherapy, although effective as a palliation treatment for hemoptysis in advanced lung cancer, is not a treatment option for massive hemoptysis [51]. Photodynamic therapy (PDT) has been suggested in the management of hemoptysis. Due to the need for the protoporphyrin injected 48 h prior to the nonthermal laser application, it has no role in the management of massive hemoptysis. However, it can be used for control of low-grade chronic hemoptysis in suitable candidates with endobronchial tumors.

Non-bronchoscopic Interventions

Even though with advanced technology bronchoscopic interventions have proven to be promising in achieving control of hemoptysis in all types of patients, in a subgroup of patients who have a refractory bleed or a recurrent hemoptysis, endovascular interventions such as bronchial artery embolization (BAE) might be necessary to arrest the bleeding. As described earlier, bronchial arteries are commonly the source of bleeding. Angiographically these vessels are dilated and ectatic and often have extensive collateral formation. Rupture of these friable vessels may result in massive hemoptysis. Angiographic placement of gelfoam, absorbable gelatin sponges, cyanoacrylates, steel coils, polyvinyl alcohol, and other sclerosing agents have been used to occlude vessels in areas of localized bleeding. This method is useful in hemoptysis with bronchoscopically non-visible bleeding site and in those with bronchiectasis, tuberculosis, aspergilloma, and situations where endobronchial methods are less satisfactory [52, 53].

Summary and Conclusion

Hemoptysis is a common and alarming symptom. There are no accepted volume-based definitions of non-massive or massive hemoptysis. For practical purpose, it is better to define massive hemoptysis on the basis of magnitude of effect rather than the amount of expectorated blood. Acute bronchitis is the most common cause of non-massive hemoptysis. The common causes of massive hemoptysis include bronchiectasis, tuberculosis, lung cancer, and mycetoma. Bronchoscopy plays a central role in diagnostic evaluation and management of hemoptysis. Direct inspection allows localization of the bleeding site and isolation of bleeding segment to prevent flooding of non-bleeding lung and asphyxiation. Rigid bronchoscope is preferred over flexible bronchoscope for management of massive hemoptysis but its utility is limited by nonavailability of trained personnel in majority of medical centers. In the absence of facilities for rigid bronchoscopy, it is prudent to secure airway with a large endotracheal tube, perform early flexible bronchoscopy, and initiate aggressive resuscitative measures. Several bronchoscopic techniques such as balloon tamponade, topical application of cold saline, vasoconstrictors, and procoagulant substances may be applied for temporary control of bleeding. Interventional techniques such as laser photoresection and APC may be helpful in selected cases. Temporary control of bleeding may facilitate institution of definitive therapies such as bronchial artery embolization and surgery in selected patients.

References

1. Stoller JK. Diagnosis and management of massive hemoptysis: a review. Respir Care. 1992;32:564–81.
2. Conlan AA, Hurwitz SS, Krige L, et al. Massive hemoptysis. Review of 123 cases. J Thorac Cardiovasc Surg. 1983;85:120–4.
3. Yeoh CB, Hubaytar RT, Ford JM, et al. Treatment of massive hemorrhage in pulmonary tuberculosis. J Thorac Cardiovasc Surg. 1967;54:503–10.
4. Holsclaw DS, Grand RJ, Shwachman H. Massive hemoptysis in cysticfibrosis. J Pediatr. 1970;76: 829–38.
5. Marshall TJ, Jackson JE. Vascular intervention in the thorax: bronchial artery embolization for hemoptysis. Eur Radiol. 1997;7:1221–7.
6. Sakr L, Dutau H. Massive hemoptysis: an update on the role of bronchoscopy in diagnosis and management. Respiration. 2010;80:38–58.
7. Crocco JA, Rooney JJ, Fankushen DS, DiBenedetto JR, Lyons HA. Massive hemoptysis. Arch Intern Med. 1968;121:495–8.
8. Corder R. Hemoptysis. Emerg Med Clin North Am. 2003;21:421–35.
9. Levitzky MG. Pulmonary physiology. Blood flow to the lung. McGraw-Hill 1995;4:87–114.
10. Cauldwell EW, Sickert RG, Lininger RE, et al. The bronchial arteries: an anatomic study of 150 human cadavers. Surg Gynecol Obstet. 1948;86:395–412.
11. Hirshberg B, Biran I, Glazer M, et al. Hemoptysis: etiology, evaluation, and outcome in a tertiary referral hospital. Chest. 1997;112:440–4.
12. Rumbak M, Kohler G, Eastrige C, et al. Topical treatment of life threatening hemoptysis from aspergillomas. Thorax. 1996;51:253–5.
13. Ong TH, Eng P. Massive hemoptysis requiring intensive care. Intensive Care Med. 2003;29:317–20.
14. Savale L, Parrot A, Khalil A, et al. Cryptogenic hemoptysis: from a benign to a life threatening pathologic vascular condition. Am J Respir Crit Care Med. 2007;175:1181–5.
15. Marshall TJ, Flower CD, Jackson JE. The role of radiology in the investigation and management of patients with hemoptysis. Clin Radiol. 1996;51:391–400.
16. Haponik EF, Britt EJ, Smith PL, Bleecker ER. Computed chest tomography in the evaluation of hemoptysis: impact on diagnosis and treatment. Chest. 1987;91:80–5.
17. Revel MP, Fournier LS, Hennebicque AS, Cuenod CA, Meyer G, Reynaud P, et al. Can CT replace bronchoscopy in the detection of the site and cause of bleeding in patients with large or massive hemoptysis? Am J Roentgenol. 2002;179:1217–24.
18. Khalil A, Soussan M, Mangiapan G, Fartoukh M, Parrot A, Carette MF. Utility of high-resolution chest CT scan in the emergency management of hemoptysis in the intensive care unit: severity, localization and etiology. Br J Radiol. 2007;80:21–5.
19. RemyJardin M, Bouaziz N, Dumont P, Brillet PY, Bruzzi J, Remy J. Bronchial and non-bronchial systemic arteries at multi-detector row CT angiography: comparison with conventional angiography. Radiology. 2004;233:741–9.
20. Khalil A, Parrot A, Nedelcu C, Fartoukh M, Marsault C, Carette MF. Severe hemoptysis of pulmonary arterial origin: signs and role of multidetector row CT. Chest. 2008;133:212–9.
21. Hsiao EI, Kirsch CM, Kagawa FT, Wehner JH, Jensen WA, Baxter RB. Utility of fiberoptic bronchoscopy before bronchial artery embolization for massive hemoptysis. Am J Roentgenol. 2001;177:861–7.
22. Naidich DP, Funt S, Ettenger NA, Arranda C. Hemoptysis: CT-bronchoscopic correlations in 58 cases. Radiology. 1990;177:357–62.
23. Gong Jr H, Salvatierra C. Clinical efficacy of early and delayed fiberoptic bronchoscopy in patients with hemoptysis. Am Rev Respir Dis. 1981;124:221–5.
24. Dweik R, Stoller JK. Role of bronchoscopy in massive hemoptysis. Clin Chest Med. 1999;20:89–105.
25. Conlan AA, Hurwitz SS. Management of massive hemoptysis with the rigid bronchoscope and cold saline lavage. Thorax. 1980;35:901–4.
26. Zavala DC. Pulmonary hemorrhage in fibreoptic transbronchial biopsy. Chest. 1976;70:584–8.
27. Mazkereth R, Paret G, Ezra D, et al. Epinephrine blood concentrations after peripheral bronchial versus endotracheal administration of epinephrine in dogs. Crit Care Med. 1992;20:1582–7.
28. Kalyanaraman M, Carpenter RL, McGlew MJ, Guertin SR. Cardiopulmonary compromise after use of topical and submucosal α agonists: possible added complication by the use of β-blocker therapy. Otolaryngol Head Neck Surg. 1997;117:56–61.
29. Breuer HW, Charchut S, Worth H, Trampisch HJ, Glänzer K. Endobronchial versus intravenous application of the vasopressin derivative glypressin during diagnostic bronchoscopy. Eur Respir J. 1989;2:225–8.
30. Sharkey AJ, Brennen MD, O'Neill MP, et al. A comparative study of the haemostatic properties and cardiovascular effects of adrenaline and ornipressin in children using enflurane anaesthesia. Acta Anaesthesiol Scand. 1982;26:368–70.
31. Tuller C, Tuller D, Tamm M, Brutsche MH. Hemodynamic effects of endobronchial application of ornipressin versus terlipressin. Respiration. 2004;71: 397–401.
32. Wong LT, Lillquist YP, Culham G, DeJong BP, Davidson AG. Treatment of recurrent hemoptysis in a child with cystic fibrosis by repeated bronchial artery embolizations and long-term tranexamic acid. Pediatr Pulmonol. 1996;22:275–9.
33. Chang AB, Ditchfield M, Robinson PJ, Robertson CF. Major hemoptysis in a child with cystic fibrosis from

multiple aberrant bronchial arteries treated with tranexamic acid. Pediatr Pulmonol. 1996;22:416–20.
34. Graff GR. Treatment of recurrent severe hemoptysis in cystic fibrosis with tranexamic acid. Respiration. 2001;68:91–4.
35. Solomonov A, Fruchter O, Zuckerman T, Brenner B, Yigla M. Pulmonary hemorrhage: a novel mode of therapy. Respir Med. 2009;103:1196–200.
36. Tsukamoto T, Sasaki H, Nakamura H. Treatment of hemoptysis patients by thrombin and fibrinogen-thrombin infusion therapy using a fiberoptic bronchoscope. Chest. 1989;96:473–6.
37. Bense L. Intrabronchial selective coagulative treatment of hemoptysis. Chest. 1990;97:990–6.
38. Freitag L, Tekolf E, Stamatis G, Montag M, Greschuchna D. Three years experience with a new balloon catheter for the management of hemoptysis. Eur Respir J. 1994;7:2033–7.
39. Dutau H, Palot A, Haas A, Decamps I, Durieux O. Endobronchial embolization with a silicone spigot as a temporary treatment for massive hemoptysis. Respiration. 2006;73:830–2.
40. Valipour A, Kreuzer A, Koller H, Koessler W, Burghuber OC. Bronchoscopy-guided topical hemostatic tamponade therapy for the management of life-threatening hemoptysis. Chest. 2005;127:2113–8.
41. Sarkar BP, Ghosh D, Nag S, Chowdhury S, et al. Evaluation of the technical details of bronchoscopic endobronchial sealing: review of 67 patients. Indian J Chest Dis Allied Sci. 2007;49:137–42.
42. Strong MS, Jako GJ. Laser surgery in the larynx. Early clinical experience with CO_2 laser. Ann Otol Rhinol Laryngol. 1972;86:791–8.
43. Dumon JF, Meric B, Surpas P, Ragni J. Endoscopic resection in bronchology using the YAG laser. Evaluation of a five year experience. Schweiz Med Wochenschr. 1985;115:1336–44.
44. Han CC, Prasetyo D, Wright GM. Endobronchial palliation using Nd-YAG laser is associated with improved survival when combined with multimodal adjuvant treatments. J Thorac Oncol. 2007;2: 59–64.
45. Hetzel MR, Smith SGT. Endoscopic palliation of tracheobronchial malignancies. Thorax. 1991;46: 325–33.
46. Keller CA, Hinerman R, Singh A, Alvarez F. The use of endoscopic argon plasma coagulation in airway complications after solid organ transplantation. Chest. 2001;119:1968–75.
47. Morice RC, Ece T, Ece F, Keus L. Endobronchial argon plasma coagulation for treatment of hemoptysis and neoplastic airway obstruction. Chest. 2001;119: 781–7.
48. Homasson JP. Endobronchial electrocautery. Semin Respir Crit Care Med. 1997;18:535–43.
49. Mathur PN, Wolf KM, Busk MF, Briete WM, Datzman M. Fiberoptic bronchoscopic cryotherapy in the management of tracheobronchial obstruction. Chest. 1996;110:718–23.
50. Maiwand MO, Asimakopoulos G. Cryosurgery for lung cancer: clinical results and technical aspects. Technol Cancer Res Treat. 2004;3:143–50.
51. Cardona AF, Reveiz L, Ospina EG, Ospina V, Yepes A. Palliative endobronchial brachytherapy for non-small cell lung cancer. Cochrane Database Syst Rev. 2008; 16:CD004284.
52. Cremaschi P, Nascimbene C, Vitulo P, et al. Therapeutic embolization of bronchial artery: a successful treatment in 209 cases of relapse hemoptysis. Angiology. 1993;44:295–9.
53. Yu-Tang Goh P, Lin M, Teo N, En SWD. Embolization for hemoptysis: a six year review. Cardiovasc Intervent Radiol. 2002;25:17–25.

Index

A.C. Mehta and P. Jain (eds.), *Interventional Bronchoscopy: A Clinical Guide*, Respiratory Medicine 10, DOI 10.1007/978-1-62703-395-4, © Springer Science+Business Media New York 2013

Printed by Publishers' Graphics LLC